Genetic Counseling for Adult Neurogenetic Disease

Jill S. Goldman
Editor

Genetic Counseling for Adult Neurogenetic Disease

A Casebook for Clinicians

Springer

Editor
Jill S. Goldman
Taub Institute
Columbia University Medical Center
New York, NY
USA

Videos to this book can be accessed at http://www.springerimages.com/videos/978-1-4899-7481-5

ISBN 978-1-4899-7481-5 ISBN 978-1-4899-7482-2 (eBook)
DOI 10.1007/978-1-4899-7482-2
Springer New York Heidelberg Dordrecht London

Library of Congress Control Number: 2014952454

Printed on acid-free paper

Springer is part of Springer Science+Business Media (www.springer.com)

This book would never have been conceived or written without the encouragement of my husband, Lee Goldman. Not only is he a role model for me, but the impetus and support for my professional growth. I, therefore, dedicate this book to Lee and to our children—Jeff, Daniel, and Robyn and their spouses, Abbey and Tobin, who also provided unending and unconditional support while listening to me complain.

Accompanying Video

The video clips that accompany this book feature aspects of genetic counseling for several of the neurogenetic conditions discussed in the book. Please refer to these video clips as appropriate. Dr. Sampson's full neurological examination may be of particular interest for genetic counselors who have not been exposed to neurology.

The video clips include both segments of actual genetic counseling sessions and counseling simulations. The clips intend to show some of the unique aspects of counseling for these diseases. We cover diagnostic genetic testing, presymptomatic testing, return of results, impact of testing on family members, genetic research studies, reproductive counseling, and treatment and management. Additionally, a video clip demonstrates the neurological examination. Because of limited access to patients, we could not film every disease discussed in this book.

Participants in the video:
Jill S. Goldman, M.S., M.Phil., C.G.C.
Jacinda B. Sampson, M.D., Ph.D.
Ashley L. Wilson, M.S., C.G.C.
Megan Truitt Cho, Sc.M., C.G.C.
Sarah E. Teed
Kara Ansett
Gracious patients

Contents

List of Contributors

Amanda Bergner Department of Neurology and the McKusick-Nathans Institute of Genetic Medicine, Johns Hopkins University School of Medicine, Baltimore, MD, USA

Matthew Bower Department of Genetics and Metabolism, University of Minnesota Medical Center, Fairview, Minneapolis, MN, USA

Elise Caccappolo Department of Neurology, Columbia University Medical Center, New York, NY, USA

Joline Dalton Paul and Sheila Wellstone Muscular Dystrophy Center, University of Minnesota, Minneapolis, MN, USA

Jamie C. Fong Department of Neurology, Memory and Aging Center, University of California, San Francisco, San Francisco, CA, USA

Jill S. Goldman Taub Institute, Columbia University Medical Center, New York, NY, USA

Alison LaPean Kirschner Department of Neurology, Center for Patient Care and Outcomes Research (PCOR), Medical College of Wisconsin, Milwaukee, WI, USA

Trisha J Multhaupt-Buell Department of Neurology, Breakefield Group, Massachusetts General Hospital, Charlestown, MA, USA

Jacinda B. Sampson Department of Neurology, Columbia University Medical Center, New York, NY, USA

Alice B. Schindler Neurogenetics Branch, NINDS, NIH, Bethesda, MD, USA

Carly E. Siskind Stanford Hospital and Clinics Neuroscience Center, Stanford University, Stanford, CA, USA

Paul Tuite Department of Neurology, University of Minnesota Medical Center, Fairview, Minneapolis, MN, USA

Jeff Waugh Department of Child Neurology, Boston Children's Hospital, Boston, MA, USA

Elisabeth McCarty Wood Center for Neurodegenerative Disease Research, University of Pennsylvania, Philadelphia, PA, USA

Heather Workman Department of Medical Genetics, Dayton Children's Hospital, Dayton, OH, USA

Additional Video Contributors

Ashley Wilson
Megan Truit
Sarah Teed

Part I
The Movement Disorders

Chapter 1
Overview of Movement Disorders

Matt Bower and Paul Tuite

Movement disorders are defined as conditions in which there is either a paucity or excess of voluntary or involuntary movements unrelated to corticospinal tract injuries (that occur in stroke, cerebral palsy, or motor neuron disease) or weakness (from peripheral nerve or muscle conditions) [1]. Classification systems have been developed based upon clinical findings, anatomy, pathology, etiology, and genetics. Unfortunately, these systems are not comprehensive or flawless in any sense. For example, a clinical feature such as rhythmical shaking (defined as tremor) may arise from dysfunction in deep brain nuclei (basal ganglia) or the cerebellum. As another example, the pathological finding of alpha-synuclein deposits in the brain can be present in an assortment of clinically distinct conditions such as Parkinson disease or multiple system atrophy. Thirdly, a variety of genetic mutations have been described that may present with a similar clinical phenotype. Conversely, some single genetic mutations may present with clinically distinct phenotypes. Thus, putting together clinical features with pathology and genetics remains a work in progress.

M. Bower (✉)
Department of Genetics and Metabolism, University of Minnesota Medical Center, Fairview, 420 Delaware St SE (MMC 485), Minneapolis, MN 55455, USA
e-mail: MBOWER1@Fairview.org

P. Tuite
Department of Neurology, University of Minnesota Medical Center, Fairview, 420 Delaware St SE (MMC 206), Minneapolis, MN 55455, USA
e-mail: tuite002@umn.edu

J.S. Goldman (ed.), *Genetic Counseling for Adult Neurogenetic Disease*,
DOI 10.1007/978-1-4899-7482-2_1

1.1 Classification of Movement Disorders

1.1.1 Clinical Classification

Movement disorders are typically grouped into two broad categories based on the speed of movements: slow (hypokinetic) and fast (hyperkinetic) movement disorders. The classic hypokinetic condition characterized by a paucity of movement is Parkinson disease (PD) in which there is loss of facial movement, reduced blinking, shuffling gait, and small handwriting (micrographia). This paucity of movement results from a failure of brain structures to initiate movements, sustain movements, or create movement of sufficient amplitude to achieve a desired purpose (speech, walking). There are numerous hypokinetic conditions that fall under the broad category of "parkinsonism." Hyperkinetic movement disorders are characterized by excessive or unwanted movements. This broad category encompasses numerous clinically distinct types of movements including chorea, dystonia, myoclonus, tics, and dyskinesias.

1.1.2 Anatomic Classification

Movement disorders can also be classified by the anatomical structures that are affected. Movement disorders related to basal ganglia dysfunction are characterized as "extra-pyramidal" as opposed to "pyramidal" conditions caused by disease of the corticospinal tracts. The extrapyramidal system consists of the thalamus and the basal ganglia consisting of the striatum (caudate nucleus and putamen), globus pallidus, subthalamic nucleus, substantia nigra, and nucleus accumbens. While the cerebellum is not generally included among the extrapyramidal structures, it does have an important function in the coordination of movements. Lesions in specific brain structures, regardless of the underlying cause, tend to result in characteristic clinical presentations. Cerebellar disease results in ataxia (incoordination of movement), lesions in the substantia nigra result in parkinsonism (slowness of movement), pallidal lesions are often associated with abnormal postures and dystonia, and disease of the caudate nucleus may result in brief flitting movements (chorea). While this may be a helpful way to correlate clinical findings with anatomy, it is important to remember that all of these structures are interconnected and communicate with structures outside the extra-pyramidal system. Thus, complete correlation between specific brain structures and specific clinical syndromes may not exist.

1.1.3 Pathological Classification

Accumulation of misfolded proteins in affected neurons has emerged as a common theme in neurodegenerative diseases. Considerable debate still exists about whether such inclusions are the cause of neurodegeneration or whether they are simply a compensatory (even a protective) mechanism to the underlying disease processes. Nevertheless, the presence of pathological findings is another means of classifying seemingly unrelated diseases. Polyglutamine diseases, caused by expansions of CAG repeat sequences in specific genes, are a diverse group of movement disorders including Huntington disease, dentatorubral pallidoluysian atrophy (DRPLA), and spinocerebellar ataxia (SCA) types 1, 2, 3, 6, 7, and 17. Pathologic accumulation of alpha synuclein may be seen in Parkinson disease, Lewy body dementia, and multiple system atrophy. Deposition of microtubule associated protein *tau* can be found in progressive supranuclear palsy, frontotemporal degeneration, and corticobasal degeneration.

While pathology may identify common mechanisms in clinically distinct movement disorders, it may also demonstrate that seemingly related conditions have very different underlying disease processes. For example, the brains of patients with autosomal recessive juvenile onset Parkinson disease caused by *PARK2* mutations lack the diagnostic finding of Lewy bodies [2].

1.1.4 Classification by Symptomology

Movement disorders may be classified by the underlying symptom. For example, chorea can have a heritable cause (Huntington disease), be secondary to an autoimmune process (Sydenham chorea), or have an unknown etiology (idiopathic). Such classification schemes may be useful in identifying movement disorders that may be amenable to therapeutic interventions.

Functional movement disorders (also known as "conversion disorders" or "psychogenic movement disorders") are conditions for which no causative lesion can be identified. Individuals may present with any type of movement ranging from chorea to parkinsonism. The precise cause of such movement disorders is widely debated, but they may be maladaptive responses to emotional stress, abuse, or significant life events. Patients often resent this diagnosis because they perceive that they are being told that they are "faking it" or "it's all in your head." Genetic counselors should be aware that individuals with functional movement disorders may be clinically indistinguishable from individuals with neurologic disease. Thus, all patients should be evaluated by an experienced movement disorder neurologist.

1.1.5 Genetic Classification

The discovery of causative and risk-altering genes provides another means for classification of movement disorders. In some cases, classification by underlying genetic etiology will group together individuals with varying clinical presentations. Such is the case with individuals having mutations in the *SPG7* gene. Mutations in this gene have been associated with both spastic paraparesis and ataxia [3]. In contrast, classification by symptomology may also result in grouping conditions caused by different underlying genetic etiologies, e.g., hereditary spastic paraplegias (HSP). Genetic analysis of HSP has demonstrated that the same clinical phenotype can result from mutations affecting axonal transport, mitochondrial function, and vesicle formation.

1.2 Genetic Counseling Issues in Movement Disorders

One complicated aspect of genetic counseling for movement disorders is that many conditions, such as Parkinson disease, have both Mendelian and multifactorial causes that result in the same clinical syndrome. The pattern of inheritance may be difficult to discern when there is no family history. Another challenge is the late age of onset for many movement disorders. A family history may appear to be negative due to the early death of a family member or due to unrecognized symptoms that never prompted formal neurologic evaluation. A recollection bias towards or against a diagnosis of PD may also influence accurate ascertainment of a family history.

Perhaps one of the most challenging aspects of genetic counseling for movement disorders is the presence of exceptions to nearly every rule of Mendelian inheritance. Mendelian movement disorders are often characterized by dramatically reduced penetrance and/or variable expression. *DYT1* dystonia is a classic example in which the penetrance of the generalized dystonia phenotype is less than 40 % [4]. Individuals with the same *DYT1* mutation may present with a disabling generalized dystonia or a focal dystonia that only affects handwriting. Another example of genetic complexity relates to *GBA* mutations that can cause a recessive disease (Gaucher disease) or act as autosomal dominant *risk factor*s for idiopathic PD [5]. Yet another example is the association of intermediate CAG repeat numbers in the *ATXN2* gene with non-ataxia phenotypes. While larger expansions in this gene are classically associated with autosomal dominant spinocerebellar ataxia type 2, more modest expansions have recently been identified as a risk factor for motor neuron disease [6]. Genes associated with movement disorders may demonstrate parent-of-origin specific imprinting effects, as is the case with *SGCE* mutations causing myoclonus dystonia [7]. Gender-specific penetrance has been described in *GCH1* related dopa-responsive dystonia [8]. Finally, mutations in some genes have been described as having both autosomal dominant and recessive patterns of inheritance depending on the type of mutation identified. Examples of this phenomenon include mutations in the *AFG3L2*, *SETX*, and *SPTBN2* genes [9–11].

Finally, considerable overlap exists in the clinical presentations of many movement disorders. Indeed, many movement disorders defy classification into even the most basic of neurological clinical schemes. As an example, Mendelian ataxia may coexist in a family with parkinsonism, neuropathy, and/or motor neuron disease. Thus, determining what genes to test can be difficult.

1.3 Family History Questions Specific to Movement Disorders

Most people's knowledge of movement disorders is limited, thus specific questions such as "Did any other family members have dystonia or ataxia?" may not elicit the desired response. Rather than focusing on specific clinical findings and medical terminology, it is often useful to begin by asking broad questions such as:

- Have any family members ever seen a neurologist?
- Have any family members needed to use a walker, cane, or wheelchair?
- Do you remember any family members with tremors?

Additionally, rather than focusing on a diagnosis reported by a patient such as "Parkinson's," it is important to focus on symptoms:

- Did they walk in an unusual way?
- Did they have a tremor?
- Was the disease static or progressive?

Individuals may be biased by their perception of a particular disease. For example, eliciting a family history of parkinsonism may be challenging due to the common perception that tremor is the most common feature of Parkinson disease. A focus on family members with visible tremors may ignore individuals whose primary issues are rigidity and bradykinesia. Additional clinical findings that may suggest parkinsonism include a shuffling gait, soft voice, small handwriting, "masked" facial appearance, loss of sense of smell, and unusual sleep behaviors. Family members may also be biased by the presentation of symptoms in a proband. A patient with severe generalized dystonia may neglect to mention milder symptoms such as writer's cramp or "stiff neck" in other family members. To the patient, these milder symptoms seem unrelated to their severe disease. Family members also may have attributed neurologic findings to other causes. A common example is a family member with tremor, dysarthria, or ataxic gait being labeled as an alcoholic. The genetic counselor should include all attributed symptoms on the pedigree.

Finally, eliciting ethnic background may provide important clues in some cases. As an example, a North-African individual with an apparently idiopathic case of

Parkinson disease has a high likelihood of harboring a mutation in the *LRRK2* gene [12].

The following chapters will introduce the reader to the most common Movement Disorders and the genetic counseling issues that are associated with these conditions. We begin with Huntington disease (HD) because it is the prototype for genetic counseling for neurogenetic disease and the best studied of these diseases. Additionally, HD symptoms include both movement disorders and dementia, thus intersecting the first two chapters of the book.

References

1. Fahn, S. (2011). Classification of movement disorders. *Movement Disorders, 26*(6), 947–957.
2. Mori, H., Kondo, T., Yokochi, M., Matsumine, H., Nakagawa-Hattori, Y., Miyake, T., et al. (1998). Pathologic and biochemical studies of juvenile Parkinsonism linked to chromosome 6q. *Neurology, 51*(3), 890–892.
3. Roxburgh, R. H., Marquis-Nicholson, R., Ashton, F., George, A. M., Lea, R. A., Eccles, D., et al. (2012). The p.Ala510Val mutation in the SPG7 (paraplegin) gene is the most common mutation causing adult onset neurogenetic disease in patients of British ancestry. *Journal of Neurology, 260*, 1286–1294. epublished Dec 27 2012.
4. Risch, N. J., Bressman, S. B., de Leon, D., Brin, M. F., Burke, R. E., Greene, P. E., et al. (1990). Segregation analysis of idiopathic torsion dystonia in Ashkenazi Jews suggests autosomal dominant inheritance. *American Journal of Human Genetics, 46*, 533–538.
5. Sidransky, E., et al. (2009). Multicenter analysis of glucocerebrosidase mutations in Parkinson disease. *The New England Journal of Medicine, 361*(17), 1651–1661.
6. Elden, A. C., Kim, H. J., Hart, M. P., Chen-Plotkin, A. S., Johnson, B. S., Fang, X., et al. (2010). Ataxin-2 intermediate-length polyglutamine expansions are associated with increased risk for ALS. *Nature, 466*(7310), 1069–1075.
7. Grabowski, M., Zimprich, A., Lorenz-Depiereux, B., Kalscheuer, V., Asmus, F., Gasser, T., et al. (2003). The epsilon-sarcoglycan gene (SGCE), mutated in myoclonus-dystonia syndrome, is maternally imprinted. *European Journal of Human Genetics, 11*(2), 138–144.
8. Furukawa, Y., Lang, A. E., Trugman, J. M., Bird, T. D., Hunter, A., Sadeh, M., et al. (1998). Gender-related penetrance and de novo GTP-cyclohydrolase I gene mutations in dopa-responsive dystonia. *Neurology, 50*, 1015–1020.
9. Chen, Y. Z., Hashemi, S. H., Anderson, S. K., Huang, Y., Moreira, M. C., Lynch, D. R., et al. (2006). Senataxin, the yeast Sen1p orthologue: characterization of a unique protein in which recessive mutations cause ataxia and dominant mutations cause motor neuron disease. *Neurobiology of Disease, 23*(1), 97–108.
10. Pierson, T. M., Adams, D., Bonn, F., Martinelli, P., Cherukuri, P. F., Teer, J. K., et al. (2011). Whole-exome sequencing identifies homozygous *AFG3L2* mutations in a spastic ataxia-neuropathy syndrome linked to mitochondrial m-AAA proteases. *PLoS Genetics, 7*(10), e1002325. doi:10.1371/journal.pgen.1002325. Epub 2011 Oct 13.
11. Lise, S., Clarkson, Y., Perkins, E., Kwasniewska, A., Sadighi Akha, E., et al. (2012). Recessive mutations in *SPTBN2* implicate β-III spectrin in both cognitive and motor development. *PLoS Genetics, 8*(12), e1003074. doi:10.1371/journal.pgen.1003074. Epub 2012 Dec 6.
12. Lesage, S., Leutenegger, A. L., Ibanez, P., Janin, S., Lohmann, E., Dürr, A., et al. (2005). *LRRK2* haplotype analyses in European and North African families with Parkinson disease: A common founder for the G2019S mutation dating from the 13th century. *The American Journal of Human Genetics, 77*(2), 330–332.

Chapter 2
Huntington Disease

Matt Bower and Paul Tuite

The discovery of a CAG repeat expansion in the *HTT* (*IT15*) gene in 1993 marked the end of a decades-long scientific quest to identify the Huntington disease (HD) gene and the beginning of the era of predictive genetic medicine. In recognition of the complex medical and psychosocial issues surrounding predictive genetic testing for HD, guidelines for offering the predictive test were published and most major centers established "protocols" that included visits with physicians, genetic counselors, and mental health providers prior to the disclosure of results [1].

In some ways, HD represents a relatively "simple" neurogenetic disease when compared with multifactorial conditions like Parkinson disease or Alzheimer disease. It is a highly penetrant, monogenic condition caused by the same mutation in all affected individuals. Despite this "simple" etiology, 20 years have passed since the discovery of the HD gene, and fundamental questions about Huntington disease remain unanswered: "What is/are the function(s) of the normal *HTT* gene?" and "How do expanded CAG repeats cause neurodegeneration?" As with other neurodegenerative diseases, an effective strategy to prevent or slow the course of neurodegeneration remains an unachieved goal.

The prevalence of HD varies widely throughout the world with the highest incidences noted in individuals with Western European ancestry (3–7:100,000)

Electronic supplementary material is available in the online version of this chapter at 10.1007/978-1-4899-7482-2_2. Videos can also be accessed at http://www.springerimages.com/videos/978-1-4899-7481-5.

M. Bower (✉)
Department of Genetics and Metabolism, University of Minnesota Medical Center, Fairview, 420 Delaware St SE (MMC 485), Minneapolis, MN 55455, USA
e-mail: MBOWER1@Fairview.org

P. Tuite
Department of Neurology, University of Minnesota Medical Center, Fairview, 420 Delaware St SE (MMC 206), Minneapolis, MN 55455, USA
e-mail: tuite002@umn.edu

J.S. Goldman (ed.), *Genetic Counseling for Adult Neurogenetic Disease*,
DOI 10.1007/978-1-4899-7482-2_2

and in the Lake Maracaibo region of Venezuela. The higher incidence of HD in these populations can be attributed to specific predisposing haplotypes more common in Western Europe and to specific founder effects seen in the Lake Maracaibo population, respectively [2, 3].

2.1 Clinical Presentation

(HD Video clip Part 1)

Huntington disease is an autosomal dominant neurodegenerative disease characterized by abnormal movements, psychiatric symptoms, and cognitive changes.

Motor findings: In an 1872 publication, Dr. George Huntington first described the choreiform movements in the disease that bears his name [4]. Chorea, from the Greek word to dance, refers to involuntary random flitting movements that may affect any part of the body. While chorea is often the most obvious outward manifestation of HD, it is not universally present, and it is often not the first motor feature of the disease to manifest. Abnormalities of eye movements (e.g., slowed rapid eye movements or saccades) often precede the onset of chorea [5]. In addition to chorea, other abnormal involuntary movements, such as dystonia (abnormal postures), rigidity (stiffness), and bradykinesia (slowness), may be observed. Dysphagia (difficulty swallowing) is a common finding, which usually develops later in the disease and may lead to aspiration pneumonia.

Psychiatric findings: In his initial description of Huntington disease, Dr. Huntington also noted depression in addition to chorea. More recent studies have documented that the incidence of major depression in HD is twice that of the general population, while the risk for suicide is 4–6 times that of the general population [6, 7]. It is not known to what extent this depression is caused by Huntington disease or is a response to the diagnosis. Additional psychiatric findings in HD patients may include psychosis, bipolar disorder, apathy, irritability, and perseveration [8].

Cognitive findings: Early cognitive changes in Huntington disease typically include difficulties with attention and executive functions, such as planning, executing sequential tasks, and judgment [9]. Individuals with HD often lack insight into their own disease, which can cause significant adaptive issues for both themselves and friends/family [10]. The cognitive difficulties are progressive, and patients are eventually unable to speak or care for themselves.

Huntington disease most often presents in the fourth or fifth decade of life. Age of onset is typically defined as the onset of neurologic disease, though subtle cognitive and motor findings may predate neurologic onset by many years [11]. Age of onset is inversely correlated with CAG repeat size, with larger repeat numbers associated with younger age of onset [12]. However, CAG repeat number only accounts for about 70 % of the variability in age of onset [13]. Approximately 25 % of individuals present with symptoms after age 50 and typically have a milder course, while 5–10 % of individuals present with juvenile onset HD and a more rapid clinical course. Anticipation, or the occurrence of earlier ages of onset in subsequent generations, is a phenomenon seen in HD, especially when the disease is transmitted through the father. Anticipation is due to the instability of the CAG expansion.

Classic descriptions of HD note a typical clinical course of 10–15 years. However, good care including nutrition and physical therapy may extend this time frame. It is increasingly clear that there is an identifiable prodromal "stage" that is present prior to the frank onset of HD symptoms. This period of time may predate the formal diagnosis of HD by many years and is characterized by subtle changes in cognitive and motor performance and psychiatric disturbances [14]. The early clinical stages of Huntington disease are typically marked by mild motor findings (e.g., slowing of eye movements) and more pronounced behavioral/mood changes (e.g., depression, agitation, apathy, anxiety). The middle stage is characterized by increasing choreiform movements, difficulties with speech and swallowing, and weight loss. In the final stages of HD, individuals typically have more issues with rigidity and bradykinesia than chorea. At this stage, patients are unable to speak, ambulate, or care for themselves; weight loss, swallowing, and choking continue to be significant concerns.

2.2 Diagnosis

Since the discovery of the pathogenic CAG repeat expansion in 1993, the gold standard for HD diagnosis is the presence of an expanded *HTT* allele containing 36 or more CAG repeats. In the absence of genetic testing, a diagnosis of HD may be strongly suspected in the presence of characteristic cognitive/psychiatric changes, motor findings, and positive family history.

Diagnosis without genetic testing is more difficult in individuals who do not have a clear family history of Huntington disease. The lack of family history may be due to adoption, non-paternity, loss of contact with family members, unrecognized symptoms, or *de novo* expansions. In individuals with characteristic clinical findings and a negative family history, other causes of chorea, such as stroke, infection, and autoimmune processes, must be excluded. A lack of family history should not preclude gene testing as a substantial proportion of patients may report negative or uncertain family histories [15].

The clinical examination can support a diagnosis of Huntington disease, but in most cases, it is not sufficient to clearly establish the diagnosis. In addition to the presence of chorea, key findings on clinical exam include slowing of eye movements, motor impersistence (e.g., cannot hold tongue out for 10 seconds), and difficulties with specific motor tasks (e.g., the Luria task in which the patient mimics a series of hand gestures demonstrated by the physician). MRI imaging may demonstrate caudate atrophy, but this is typically not the primary means of diagnosis for Huntington disease [16].

In addition, larger intermediate alleles are closer to the disease threshold and even a relatively modest expansion of 1–3 repeats may be sufficient to expand into the disease range. In contrast, an allele with 27 repeats would need to expand by 9 repeats to be in the disease-causing range.

(b) *Gender of the transmitting parent*: Segregation analysis has consistently demonstrated that CAG repeat instability, and particularly the propensity for CAG repeat expansion, is greater with male transmission [27]. To date, all documented expansions from intermediate to disease alleles have occurred with male transmissions [28]. The fact that substantial expansions of maternally transmitted alleles with as few as 36 repeats have occurred provides evidence that expansions of large maternal intermediate alleles into the disease range are theoretically possible [29].

(c) *Age of the transmitting parent*: Some studies have suggested a specific effect of paternal age on the risk for intermediate allele expansion, with increasing paternal age associated with higher instability of the CAG repeat number [27].

(d) *Predisposing haplotypes-*: Intermediate alleles that are ascertained *because they had already undergone an expansion* are more likely to demonstrate instability than alleles that are incidentally ascertained from the general population [28] Further work has delineated specific haplotypes that are prone to expansion [2]. *Cis*-acting factors present with some HD alleles may be important in determining the propensity for expansion upon transmission.

Several large studies have reached differing overall conclusions about the propensity of intermediate alleles to expand to disease-causing mutations [30, 31].

Since the last publishing of HD guidelines, numerous case reports have been published documenting the presence of HD symptoms in individuals with intermediate CAG repeat numbers [32–37]. The authors have presented clinical, imaging, and pathologic evidence of Huntington disease in the presence of *HTT* alleles with less than 36 repeats. The authors report exclusion of varying HD phenocopies to support the notion that HD can be diagnosed in some cases with intermediate repeat numbers.

Other authors have cautioned that some of these cases may represent the coincidental finding of HD-like symptoms in individuals with intermediate repeat numbers and that the evidence must be carefully reviewed before attributing HD symptoms to intermediate repeat numbers [28]. Whether these cases represent coincidental discovery of neurologic disease in individuals with intermediate repeats, or whether these cases suggest that alleles with less than 36 repeats can be disease-causing in some circumstances remains to be determined.

3. *Reduced penetrance alleles* (*36–39 repeats*):

As the name implies, reduced penetrance alleles may or may not cause Huntington disease within a normal lifespan. Estimates of penetrance depend to some extent on how the onset of Huntington disease is defined. Penetrance data for the onset of neurologic (rather than psychiatric) disease suggests that, while the majority of individuals with 39 repeats will manifest HD by age 75–80, the majority of individuals with 36-repeat disease alleles will remain free of neurologic disease at this age [38].

4. *Full penetrance alleles* (*40 or more repeats*):

   The presence of a single full penetrance allele is sufficient to cause Huntington disease in all individuals within a typical lifespan. The age of onset correlates with the size of the CAG repeat expansion such that larger CAG repeats are associated with younger ages of onset. Age-specific penetrance data has been published, though the authors urge caution in applying this model-derived data in specific clinical cases [38]. While there has been some discussion in the past as to whether the CAG repeat number on the "normal" allele influences age of onset, recent data suggests that the length of the longer HD allele determines age of onset in a dominant manner [12].

2.5 Genetic Counseling Issues

Establishing the correct diagnosis in a family: In most cases where a *clinical* diagnosis of Huntington disease is established, molecular testing of the *HTT* gene provides confirmation for a diagnosis of Huntington disease. In cases where the characteristic *HTT* CAG repeat expansion is absent, consideration should be given to documented HD phenocopies, including dentatorubral pallidoluysian atrophy (DRPLA), spinocerebellar ataxia type 17 (SCA17), neuroferritinopathy, Huntington disease-like 1 (due to expansions of an octapeptide domain in the *PRNP* gene), and Huntington disease-like 2 (due to CAG repeat expansions in the *JPH3* gene) [39]. All of these conditions mimic the clinical features of HD and the autosomal dominant pattern of inheritance. Other phenocopies have been described, but can typically be distinguished from HD by their patterns of inheritance, clinical presentations, or laboratory findings. When counseling patients for predictive testing, it is important to make the best effort to obtain records confirming the molecular diagnosis of HD in affected family members. If such records cannot be obtained, patients should be counseled about the small possibility that a normal *HTT* gene test may not exclude the neurologic disease that is in the family.

Predictive testing: Perhaps the most surprising finding following the identification of the Huntington disease gene in 1993 was the *lack* of individuals who came forward for predictive testing. Prior to identification of the *HTT* gene, a majority of at-risk individuals indicated that they would want molecular testing for Huntington disease when the gene was discovered [40]. Subsequent analyses demonstrated that the uptake of molecular genetic predictive testing was much lower than expected. A review of the Canadian experience demonstrated that approximately 1–2 % of at-risk individuals will present for testing in a given year, and that only 20 % of at-risk individuals have chosen to have molecular genetic predictive testing [41]. Studies evaluating the characteristics of individuals who seek a predictive

counselor and the family will discuss the reasons why genetic testing is being considered, explore the reasons for and expectations of testing, and try to anticipate how the family will react to the test results when they become available. After visiting the genetic counselor, John will meet with a neurologist who will take his medical history and perform a neurological examination. Finally, he will meet with a psychologist to assess his coping skills and psychiatric state. Following these evaluations, if all parties agree that it is reasonable to proceed, John can choose to have blood drawn for genetic testing. He would then return with his wife for post-test counseling and results.

The genetic counselor asks how the diagnosis of Huntington disease first came to light in the family. John indicates that his mother was a first-generation immigrant to the USA and he has only limited contact with her family in Europe. His mother was healthy until her early 60s when the family began noticing erratic behaviors and clumsiness. Several neurologists evaluated her, but no formal diagnosis was ever made. Her symptoms progressed over the next 10 years, and she died unexpectedly from a heart attack at age 70.

Five years ago, a maternal cousin contacted John with unexpected news: the cousin had been diagnosed with Huntington disease at age 50. He had developed symptoms in his late 40s and had just recently had a genetic test confirming the diagnosis. This cousin's father (John's mother's brother) had been estranged from the family and his medical information was not available. As John and his wife read more about Huntington disease, the pieces of his mother's story began to fall into place. The erratic behaviors, the restless fidgety movements, and forgetfulness that marked her later years all fit with a diagnosis of Huntington disease.

John is aware that his family history places him at a 50 % risk for Huntington disease, but after reading that the average age of onset is 35-55 years of age, he is hopeful that he has outlived his risk. John and his wife have three adult children (ages 22, 24, and 27) and they have struggled with what information they should share with their children. The children are all aware that their grandmother had a neurologic disease at the time of her death, but it had always been assumed to be a "sporadic" illness. John and his wife considered telling their children on several occasions, but eventually 5 years passed and the children were still not aware of the diagnosis of Huntington disease in the family. In the meantime, their oldest child (a son) has started a family and has two healthy children. Their middle child (a daughter) has recently become engaged, while their youngest child just entered medical school.

At age 61, John feels relatively confident that he has outlived his risk for Huntington disease. He indicates that his primary motivation for testing is to rule out the diagnosis so that when he shares the information about his cousin's diagnosis with his children, he can immediately reassure them that they are not at risk. When asked about any possible neurologic symptoms, John indicates that he has not noticed anything other than "the usual forgetfulness that comes with age."

In reviewing his social history, John discusses his career as an engineer. He worked up until a year ago, when he accepted an early retirement package. Towards the end of his employment, he was having increasing difficulties with his work duties, which he attributed to difficulty in keeping up with newer and newer computer systems. Since his retirement, he spends significant time "puttering" in his workshop.

John and his wife have been married for 35 years. His wife indicates that recently they have had increasing difficulties with communication and her husband has been more agitated and withdrawn. She had asked him to come with her to couple's therapy to improve their communication, but he refused. Besides his wife and children, John reports few close friends.

During the neurologist's exam, John is "fidgety," and at one point spills a bottle of water that he had brought with him to the appointment. He is unaware of the movements and, when asked about them, he attributes them to "nerves." Additional examination findings include: (1) slowed saccades: slight slowing of eye movements when he was asked to quickly fix his eyes between two targets, (2) impairment of sequential movements, i.e., a motor sequencing task called the Luria, and (3) motor impersistence (e.g., inability to keep his tongue protruded for 10 seconds). The neurologist discusses the findings with John and his wife and indicates that they are subtle and suggestive of HD, but are not diagnostic, and that genetic testing would be able to provide a more definitive means to confirm or exclude a diagnosis of Huntington disease.

At one point during the examination, the neurologist takes John to the hallway to evaluate his gait. John's wife confides to the genetic counselor that she has grown concerned about her husband's health. He is spending increasing time alone in his workshop, even during a recent family Thanksgiving dinner. Additionally, he becomes agitated when they discuss financial matters. During his retirement dinner, several colleagues commented that John appeared to be "drunk," slurring his speech, stumbling, and behaving in an odd manner. She has tried to discuss her concerns with John, but he consistently rebuffs her attempts.

The genetic counselor next meets with John, his wife, and a clinical psychologist. When asked how he would respond to a potential abnormal HD test, John dismisses the possibility. His wife, however, begins to cry. She says that she feels that they have "betrayed" their children by not sharing information about John's mother's probable HD. She feels selfish that she and her husband never shared the news because they were afraid that their children would be unnecessarily worried. She feels the "betrayal" is amplified by the fact that her children have made major life decisions about children and careers in the past 5 years. Like her husband, she hoped that he had already outlived the risk, but secretly, she has grown increasingly concerned about a possible HD diagnosis given his change in personality.

Questions:

- How should this couple relay information about HD to their children? Should this issue be discussed before testing or after testing?
- If the team is not certain that John is in an ideal situation to receive results of HD testing, do they have the right to withhold or delay testing for a legally competent adult? Is it fair to John and his family to withhold testing or is this a paternalistic approach?

- If the team believes that John's testing is likely to be abnormal, what is their obligation to communicate this to John versus allow him to believe that he is "just fine?"
- What support mechanisms should be put in place before delivering results?

The team agrees that, regardless of his HD status, John would benefit from treatment with an antidepressant medication. In addition, couples therapy is recommended to help John and Jane better communicate about a potential HD diagnosis and discuss strategies for sharing this information with their children. John returns alone one month later to have his blood drawn for HD testing. He and his wife met with a couple's therapist. He indicates that he feels less "agitated" now that he is taking an antidepressant. After reviewing the informed consent for testing, the genetic counselor discusses the fact that results will only be disclosed in person and that John needs to come to the results visit with his wife or another support person.

Two weeks later, John and his wife return to clinic to review results of genetic testing. Unfortunately, the testing reveals that John has 16 CAG repeats in one *HTT* allele and 40 CAG repeats in other *HTT* allele, confirming that John has inherited the HD gene. In the context of the subtle findings noted on exam, the neurologist indicates that John has "symptomatic HD." Additionally, his test results mean that each of his children has a 50 % risk of having inherited Huntington disease. John is shocked, stating that he truly believed he had outlived his risk, and had never considered that he might have to discuss this with his children. Jane is visibly upset by the results. She expresses her concern that it will be very difficult to help her husband if he continues to act as though nothing is wrong. In addition, she feels that the burden of sharing this news with their children will fall on her shoulders. The couple turns to the team and asks, "Where do we go from here?"

Discussion questions:

- What are the most important "first steps" for this couple? How can the team facilitate these steps?
- Should the team have done more to prepare John for the fact that his result was likely to be abnormal?
- What strategies would you suggest for communicating the information about Huntington disease to John's children? What are the potential risks of these strategies?

The genetic counselor suggests that John and his wife tell their children the diagnosis, but then schedule a genetic counseling family meeting with her to help them discuss both the diagnosis and the implications for the children.

The family returns the following week with John, Jane, their children (David, Sarah, and Lucy), their daughter-in-law, and their future son-in-law. The tension is immediately apparent. The genetic counselor welcomes everyone and reviews the purpose of the meeting. She then asks what David, Sarah, and Lucy understand about their father's diagnosis, and whether they have particular questions they want addressed. Since being told, Lucy has done a lot of research. She is quite concerned not only about her father's disease, but about the possibility of anticipation. At this point in the discussion, David's wife starts crying. She blurts out that she has not slept since Lucy told them about the possibility that David and his siblings could get the disease at an earlier age and that their children could get it even earlier. The genetic counselor says that she is correct, but suggests that they start at the beginning and go over the genetics and the possible next steps. She also states that she is sure that the diagnosis had evoked many feelings-fear, sadness, guilt, and even anger. David gives his father a seething look, as if to say, "Why couldn't you have told us before the kids?"

The counselor then reviews both the symptoms and genetics of HD, carefully explaining the possibility of anticipation. She discusses the reasons why some people choose to have presymptomatic testing, and suggests that David might wish to pursue testing both to plan for the future and know whether the children are at risk. She validates David's concern for his children by sharing that such feelings are common when a new diagnosis is made in a family, and then reviews some of the reasons why predictive genetic testing is typically not done on young asymptomatic children. She also discusses the very personal nature of presymptomatic testing and how it is not the right choice for many people. Prior to having predictive testing, it is important to consider the potential impact that either a positive or negative result could have on mental health, relationships, employment, and financial matters (e.g., life insurance). She also discusses the need to obtain long-term care and/or life insurance before being tested if they ever wanted it. Lastly she turns to Sarah and Lucy and talks about reproductive options including PGD. Once again, David looks at his father. This time the genetic counselor addresses the obvious reaction saying, "It's incredibly hard to find out that there is a genetic disease in the family—it's hard for the person with the disease and hard for those who are at risk. John and Jane, I know you feel terrible for trying to protect your children from worry by not telling them about your cousin. David, Sarah, and Lucy, you must feel conflicted—sad for your father but resentful that you did not know he was at risk. Let's talk about it." At that point, David explodes yelling, "Dad how could you not tell us! You knew Sue and I wanted children!" John tries to explain that he really didn't think he could get the disease and wanted to protect his kids. Lucy interrupts saying that this was now over and they need to come together as a family and support each other. She says that at the present time, she would not want presymptomatic testing, but thought that she would if in a relationship. Sarah adds that she wants to think about it and discuss it with her fiancé. David says he isn't sure. The counselor offers to be available by phone for any questions, and would be glad to have future meetings with anyone in the family.

Discussion questions:

- In what ways should a genetic counselor address the emotions raised during a session?
- How does the possibility of anticipation affect genetic counseling for HD?

David and his wife return for counseling about 2 months later. They have come to terms with David's risk and also with their anger at John. They have decided that it is better for David to know his status and prepare for the future than for them to worry about David and their children. The couple feels that they could cope with a positive result, although they would be even more worried for the children. However if he were to test positive, they intend to become part of an HD study so that they can be connected to experts in the field. The couple decides not to share a positive result with John and Jane for fear that this would cause great depression. David goes through the HD protocol, is tested, and discovers that he has not inherited the expanded HD gene.

2.7 Patient Resources

1. Huntington Disease Society of America (HDSA)
   www.hdsa.org
   - Web site for patients, families, friends, and caregivers. Information about support groups and links to educational materials for download or purchase.
2. Huntington Disease Youth Organization (HDYO)
   www.hdyo.org
   - Web site specifically targeted for younger persons. Forums, message boards, and information specifically targeted to youth.
3. Understanding Behavior in Huntington Disease
   http://www.hdsa.org/images/content/1/1/11704.pdf
   - Free booklet authored by Jane Paulsen, PhD discussing difficult behaviors in HD and strategies for intervention.
4. Mapping Fate: A Memoir of Family, Risk, and Genetic Research
   - Written by Alice Wexler, who herself was at 50 % risk for Huntington disease, about growing up with HD and then participating in the quest to find the HD disease gene. A powerful tale for at-risk young people who ask the question "what can I do?"

References

1. International Huntington Association and World Federation of Neurology. (1994). International Huntington Association and the World Federation of Neurology Research Group on Huntington's Chorea. Guidelines for the molecular genetics predictive test in Huntington's disease. *Journal of Medical Genetics, 31*(7), 555–559.

2. Warby, S. C., Montpetit, A., Hayden, A. R., Carroll, J. B., Butland, S. L., Visscher, H., et al. (2009). CAG expansion in the Huntington disease gene is associated with a specific and targetable predisposing haplogroup. *The American Journal of Human Genetics, 84*(3), 351–366.
3. Wexler, N. S., Lorimer, J., Porter, J., Gomez, F., Moskowitz, C., Shackell, E., et al. (2004). Venezuelan kindreds reveal that genetic and environmental factors modulate Huntington's disease age of onset. *Proceedings of the National Academy of Sciences of the United States of America, 101*(10), 3498–3503.
4. Huntington, G. (1872). On chorea. *Medical and Surgical Reporter (Philadelphia), 26*(15), 317–321.
5. Blekher, T., Johnson, S. A., Marshall, J., White, K., Hui, S., Weaver, M., et al. (2006). Saccades in presymptomatic and early stages of Huntington disease. *Neurology, 67*(3), 394–399.
6. Paulsen, J. S., Nehl, C., Hoth, K. F., Kanz, J. E., Benjamin, M., Conybeare, R., et al. (2005). Depression and stages of Huntington's disease. *The Journal of Neuropsychiatry and Clinical Neurosciences, 17*(4), 496–502.
7. Schoenfeld, M., Myers, R. H., Cupples, L. A., Berkman, B., Sax, D. S., & Clark, E. (1984). Increased rate of suicide among patients with Huntington's disease. *Journal of Neurology, Neurosurgery and Psychiatry, 47*(12), 1283–1287.
8. Rosenblatt, A. (2007). Neuropsychiatry of Huntington's disease. *Dialogues in Clinical NeuroSciences, 9*(2), 191–197.
9. Peinemann, A., Schuller, S., Pohl, C., Jahn, T., Weindl, A., & Kassubek, J. (2005). Executive dysfunction in early stages of Huntington's disease is associated with striatal and insular atrophy: A neuropsychological and voxel-based morphometric study. *Journal of the Neurological Sciences, 239*(1), 11–19.
10. Ho, A. K., Robbins, A. O., & Barker, R. A. (2006). Huntington's disease patients have selective problems with insight. *Movement Disorders, 21*(3), 385–389.
11. Stout, J. C., Paulsen, J. S., Queller, S., Solomon, A. C., Whitlock, K. B., Campbell, J. C., et al. (2011). Neurocognitive signs in prodromal Huntington disease. *Neuropsychology, 25*(1), 1–14.
12. Lee, J. M., Ramos, E. M., Lee, J. H., Gillis, T., Mysore, J. S., Hayden, M. R., et al. (2012). CAG repeat expansion in Huntington disease determines age at onset in a fully dominant fashion. *Neurology, 78*(10), 690–695.
13. Rosenblatt, A., Kumar, B. V., Mo, A., Welsh, C. S., Margolis, R. L., & Ross, C. A. (2012). Age, CAG repeat length, and clinical progression in Huntington's disease. *Movement Disorders, 27*(2), 272–276.
14. Paulsen, J. S. (2010). Early detection of Huntington's disease. *Future Neurology, 5*(1), 85–104.
15. Siesling, S., Vegter-van de Vlis, M., Losekoot, M., Belfroid, R. D., Maat-Kievit, J. A., Kremer, H. P., et al. (2000). Family history and DNA analysis in patients with suspected Huntington's disease. *Journal of Neurology, Neurosurgery and Psychiatry, 69*(1), 54–59.
16. Almqvist, E. W., Bloch, M., Brinkman, R., Craufurd, D., & Hayden, M. R. (1999). A worldwide assessment of the frequency of suicide, suicide attempts, or psychiatric hospitalization after predictive testing for Huntington disease. *The American Journal of Human Genetics, 64*(5), 1293–1304.
17. Phillips, W., Shannon, K. M., & Barker, R. A. (2008). The current clinical management of Huntington's disease. *Movement Disorders, 23*(11), 1491–1504.
18. Huntington Study Group. (2006). Tetrabenazine as antichorea therapy in Huntington disease: A randomized controlled trial. *Neurology, 66*(3), 366–372.
19. Bonelli, R. M., & Hofmann, P. (2007). A systematic review of the treatment studies in Huntington's disease since 1990. *Expert Opinion on Pharmacotherapy, 8*(2), 141–153.
20. DiFiglia, M., Sena-Esteves, M., Chase, K., Sapp, E., Pfister, E., Sass, M., et al. (2007). Therapeutic silencing of mutant huntingtin with siRNA attenuates striatal and cortical

neuropathology and behavioral deficits. *Proceedings of the National Academy of Sciences of the United States of America, 104*(43), 17204–17209.

21. Andrew, S. E., Goldberg, Y. P., Theilmann, J., Zeisler, J., & Hayden, M. R. (1994). A CCG repeat polymorphism adjacent to the CAG repeat in the Huntington disease gene: Implications for diagnostic accuracy and predictive testing. *Human Molecular Genetics, 3*(1), 65–67.
22. Nance, M. A., Seltzer, W., Ashizawa, T., Bennett, R., McIntosh, N., Myers, R. H., et al. (1998). ACMG/ASHG statement. Laboratory guidelines for Huntington disease genetic testing. *The American Journal of Human Genetics, 62*(5), 1243–1247.
23. Potter, N. T., Spector, E. B., & Prior, T. W. (2004). Technical standards and guidelines for Huntington disease testing. *Genetics in Medicine, 6*(1), 61–65.
24. Kremer, B., Goldberg, P., Andrew, S. E., Theilmann, J., Telenius, H., Zeisler, J., et al. (1994). A worldwide study of the Huntington's disease mutation. The sensitivity and specificity of measuring CAG repeats. *The New England Journal of Medicine, 330*(20), 1401–1406.
25. Kelly, T. E., Allinson, P., McGlennen, R. C., Baker, J., & Bao, Y. (1999). Expansion of a 27 CAG repeat allele into a symptomatic Huntington disease-producing allele. *American Journal of Medical Genetics, 87*(1), 91–92.
26. Chong, S. S., Almqvist, E., Telenius, H., LaTray, L., Nichol, K., Bourdelat-Parks, B., et al. (1997). Contribution of DNA sequence and CAG size to mutation frequencies of intermediate alleles for Huntington disease: Evidence from single sperm analyses. *Human Molecular Genetics, 6*(2), 301–309.
27. Goldberg, Y. P., Kremer, B., Andrew, S. E., Theilmann, J., Graham, R. K., Squitieri, F., et al. (1993). Molecular analysis of new mutations for Huntington's disease: Intermediate alleles and sex of origin effects. *Nature Genetics, 5*(2), 174–179.
28. Semaka, A., Creighton, S., Warby, S., & Hayden, M. R. (2006). Predictive testing for Huntington disease: Interpretation and significance of intermediate alleles. *Clinical Genetics, 70*(4), 283–294.
29. Laccone, F., & Christian, W. (2000). A recurrent expansion of a maternal allele with 36 CAG repeats causes Huntington disease in two sisters. *The American Journal of Human Genetics, 66*(3), 1145–1148.
30. Semaka, A., Warby, S., Leavitt, B. R., & Hayden, M. R. (2008). Re: Autopsy-proven Huntington's disease with 29 trinucleotide repeats. *Movement Disorders, 23*(12), 1794–1795.
31. Brocklebank, D., Gayán, J., Andresen, J. M., Roberts, S. A., Young, A. B., Snodgrass, S. R., et al. (2009). Repeat instability in the 27-39 CAG range of the HD gene in the Venezuelan kindreds: Counseling implications. *American Journal of Medical Genetics Part B: Neuropsychiatric Genetics, 150B*(3), 425–429.
32. Andrich, J., Arning, L., Wieczorek, S., Kraus, P. H., Gold, R., & Saft, C. (2008). Huntington's disease as caused by 34 CAG repeats. *Movement Disorders, 23*(6), 879–881.
33. Groen, J. L., de Bie, R. M., Foncke, E. M., Roos, R. A., Leenders, K. L., & Tijssen, M. A. (2010). Late-onset Huntington disease with intermediate CAG repeats: True or false? *Journal of Neurology, Neurosurgery and Psychiatry, 81*(2), 228–230.
34. Herishanu, Y. O., Parvari, R., Pollack, Y., Shelef, I., Marom, B., Martino, T., et al. (2009). Huntington disease in subjects from an Israeli Karaite community carrying alleles of intermediate and expanded CAG repeats in the HTT gene: Huntington disease or phenocopy? *Journal of the Neurological Sciences, 277*(1–2), 143–146.
35. Kenney, C., Powell, S., & Jankovic, J. (2007). Autopsy-proven Huntington's disease with 29 trinucleotide repeats. *Movement Disorders, 22*(1), 127–130.
36. Ha, A. D., & Jankovic, J. (2011). Exploring the correlates of intermediate CAG repeats in Huntington disease. *Postgraduate Medicine, 123*(5), 116–121.
37. Squitieri, F., Esmaeilzadeh, M., Ciarmiello, A., & Jankovic, J. (2011). Caudate glucose hypometabolism in a subject carrying an unstable allele of intermediate CAG33 repeat length in the Huntington's disease gene. *Movement Disorders, 26*(5), 925–927.
38. Langbehn, D. R., Brinkman, R. R., Falush, D., Paulsen, J. S., Hayden, M. R., & International Huntington's Disease Collaborative Group. (2004). A new model for prediction of the age of

onset and penetrance for Huntington's disease based on CAG length. *Clinical Genetics, 65*(4), 267–277.

39. Schneider, S. A., Walker, R. H., & Bhatia, K. P. (2007). The Huntington's disease-like syndromes: What to consider in patients with a negative Huntington's disease gene test. *Nature Clinical Practice Neurology, 3*(9), 517–525.
40. Babul, R., Adam, S., Kremer, B., Dufrasne, S., Wiggins, S., Huggins, M., et al. (1993). Attitudes toward direct predictive testing for the Huntington disease gene. Relevance for other adult-onset disorders. *JAMA, 270*(19), 2321–2325.
41. Creighton, S., Almqvist, E. W., MacGregor, D., Fernandz, B., Hogg, H., Beis, J., et al. (2003). Predictive, pre-natal and diagnostic genetic testing for Huntington's disease: The experience in Canada from 1987 to 2000. *Clinical Genetics, 63*(6), 462–475.
42. Quaid, K. A., & Morris, M. (1993). Reluctance to undergo predictive testing: The case of Huntington disease. *American Journal of Medical Genetics, 45*, 41–45.
43. Klitzman, R., Thorne, D., Williamson, J., Chung, W., & Marder, K. (2007). Decision-making about reproductive choices among individuals at-risk for Huntington's disease. *Journal of Genetic Counseling, 16*(3), 347–362.
44. Decruyenaere, M., Evers-Kiebooms, G., Boogaerts, A., Philippe, K., Demyttenaere, K., Dom, R., et al. (2007). The complexity of reproductive decision making in asymptomatic carriers of the Huntington mutation. *European Journal of Human Genetics, 15*(4), 453–462.
45. Broadstock, M., Michie, S., & Marteau, T. (2000). Psychological consequences of predictive genetic testing: A systematic review. *European Journal of Human Genetics, 8*(10), 731–738.
46. Duncan, R. E., & Delatycki, M. B. (2006). Predictive genetic testing in young people for adult-onset conditions: Where is the empirical evidence? *Clinical Genetics, 69*(1), 8–16.
47. Mand, C., Gillam, L., Duncan, R. E., & Delatycki, M. B. (2013). "It was the missing piece": Adolescent experiences of predictive genetic testing for adult-onset conditions. *Genetics in Medicine, 15*(8), 643–649.
48. Nance, M. A., & Myers, R. H. (2001). Juvenile onset Huntington's disease: Clinical and research perspectives. *Mental Retardation and Developmental Disabilities Research Reviews, 7*(3), 153–157.
49. Lehman, K., & Nance, M. (2013). Family history and juvenile Huntington disease: Do the signs point to "yes" or "very doubtful?". *Neurology, 80*(11), 976–977.

Chapter 3
Parkinson Disease

Matt Bower and Paul Tuite

Although some earlier historic references exist, it was Dr. James Parkinson, in his 1817 manuscript, "An Essay on the Shaking Palsy," who provided the first detailed clinical description of the disease that now bears his name. In this work, he described the tremor, slow movements, stooped posture, and characteristic gait associated with what is now known as "Parkinson disease." Parkinson disease (PD) is the second most common neurodegenerative disease after Alzheimer disease, affecting approximately 1 % of individuals over 60 years of age [1, 2].

3.1 Clinical Presentation

(PD video clip Part 1)

PD falls under the broader diagnostic category of "parkinsonian" conditions, all of which share some of the features of PD, but each has additional features that distinguish it from PD. Thus parkinsonian individuals, i.e., those with parkinsonism, have some combination of the triad of clinical findings including tremor,

---

Electronic supplementary material Supplementary material is available in the online version of this chapter at 10.1007/978-1-4899-7482-2_3. Videos can also be accessed at http://www.springerimages.com/videos/978-1-4899-7481-5.

M. Bower (✉)
Department of Genetics and Metabolism, University of Minnesota Medical Center, Fairview, 420 Delaware St SE (MMC 485), Minneapolis, MN 55455, USA
e-mail: MBOWER1@Fairview.org

P. Tuite
Department of Neurology, University of Minnesota Medical Center, Fairview, 420 Delaware St SE (MMC 206), Minneapolis, MN 55455, USA
e-mail: tuite002@umn.edu

J.S. Goldman (ed.), *Genetic Counseling for Adult Neurogenetic Disease*,
DOI 10.1007/978-1-4899-7482-2_3

bradykinesia (slow movements), and muscle rigidity. The distinct clinical parkinsonian entities include:

Parkinson disease: PD is the most common form of parkinsonism. The diagnosis is based upon the presence of a resting tremor (although 25 % of patients lack tremor), bradykinesia, and muscle rigidity [3]. Additional clinical findings that increase the accuracy of diagnosis include a good response to dopaminergic medication, asymmetric onset of limb symptoms, and absence of findings suggestive of atypical parkinsonism (see below) [4]. The gold standard for diagnosis is postmortem neuropathology demonstrating gliosis in the substantia nigra, loss of dopamine-producing neurons in the substantia nigra, and the presence of Lewy bodies in surviving neurons [5].

Atypical parkinsonism or "Parkinson plus" syndromes: Several distinct clinical and pathological entities have been described in which the core features of parkinsonism are accompanied by additional neurologic findings:

Progressive Supranuclear Palsy (PSP): PSP is distinguished from Parkinson disease by the presence of vertical gaze palsy (inability to look up or down), a tendency early in the course of the disease toward backward falls, and a lack of response to typical PD medications [6]. Pathologically, PSP is characterized by tau inclusions, rather than the Lewy body pathology seen in Parkinson disease. While PSP is typically a sporadic disease, familial cases have been described and mutations in the *MAPT* gene have been identified in a limited number of families [7, 8].

Corticobasal syndrome (CBS): CBS is the name given to the combination of clinical symptoms that accompany the pathologic entity corticobasal degeneration (CBD). CBS may or may not have CBD pathology. Key findings that distinguish CBS from PD include the "alien limb" phenomenon, in which a patient feels that an arm or leg is foreign or has a "mind of its own," apraxia (loss of ability to perform a previously acquired motor task, such as imitating hand or foot movements), and cortical sensory deficits (e.g., inability for a patient with closed eyes to identify an object in their palm or a number drawn on their hand; the patient can feel the tracing or object, but cannot identify specifically what is happening or what is in their hand.) Patients may also have primary progressive aphasia, a progressive language disorder [9, 10]. While most cases of CBS are sporadic, rare mutations have been identified in the *MAPT*, *GRN*, and *C9orf72* genes in autosomal dominant families [11–13].

Multiple system atrophy (MSA): MSA has a cerebellar (MSA-C), autonomic (MSA-A), and parkinsonian (MSA-P) presentation. MSA is typically distinguished from PD by the presence of parkinsonism with early autonomic impairment (bladder/sexual dysfunction and/or blood pressure dysregulation), ataxia, brisk reflexes, and a lack of response to dopaminergic therapy [14]. Pathologically, MSA is characterized by alpha-synuclein inclusions in glial cells. MSA is typically a sporadic condition.

Lewy body dementia: Lewy body dementia (LBD) is the second most common form of dementia and is usually accompanied by features of parkinsonism. LBD is pathologically characterized by the presence of Lewy bodies in the brainstem and the cerebral cortex. Individuals with LBD usually have onset of motor features (parkinsonian features) and cognitive changes within a year or two of one another, and typically have fluctuating cognition and vivid visual hallucinations [15]. Mutations in the *GBA* gene have been identified as risk factors for Lewy body dementia [16].

Parkinsonism as a feature of a complex syndrome: Parkinsonism may be a component of numerous Mendelian conditions including mitochondrial conditions, recessive conditions (e.g., neurodegeneration with brain iron accumulation), autosomal dominant conditions (e.g., spinocerebellar ataxia type 3), and X-linked conditions (e.g., fragile X tremor ataxia syndrome).

3.2 Diagnosis

The early features of PD are often subtle so establishing a firm diagnosis may require following a patient over several months or years, depending on how early the patient presents and how quickly the disease progresses. Initial complaints that may prompt clinical evaluation include fatigue, stiffness, loss of dexterity, and dragging of the foot [17]. Friends, coworkers, and family members may note changes in facial expressions, smaller handwriting, softening in the tone or volume of speech, and flexed arm posture with reduced arm swing when walking.

In retrospect, many patients and families can recall "prodromal" features of PD that may have seemed irrelevant at the time, such as a loss of the sense of smell or unusual REM sleep behaviors. These prodromal findings reflect the fact that PD pathology is often present in other parts of the nervous system before the subcortical motor systems, i.e., the basal ganglia.

On the clinical examination, physicians look for slowed movements or "bradykinesia." While bradykinesia may be apparent to the experienced clinician simply from observing the patient in the examination room, a formal assessment of bradykinesia includes asking patients to tap their finger and thumb together quickly, or tap their foot on the ground. Patients with PD have slower than expected movements with a reduction in amplitude after repetition of the task. These findings are typically more obvious on one side of the body.

Resting tremor, which is often the most recognizable sign of PD to lay observers, is not universally present. The PD tremor is primarily a "pill-rolling" movement of the hand when the arm is at rest, but action tremor may also be seen in the arm, leg, or jaw. In some cases, physicians need to employ strategies to elicit a resting tremor, such as asking a patient to perform a motor task with the opposite limb. Rigidity, or muscle stiffness, is another cardinal feature of PD, and can be assessed through physical examination.

Diagnostic imaging, e.g., MRI or CT scanning, is used to exclude potentially treatable causes of parkinsonism (e.g., stroke, infection, tumors). However, traditional imaging techniques do not provide confirmation of PD. Through changes in binding of a radioactive tracer, the new scanning technique, DaTSCAN™, can now demonstrate a loss of dopamine in the basal ganglia. This test can provide supportive evidence of a degenerative parkinsonian condition, but cannot distinguish PD from MSA or any other atypical parkinsonian disorders [18].

3.3 Treatment and Management

There is currently no cure for PD and no intervention known to delay the progression of the disease. While the disease itself cannot be cured, many of the troubling motor symptoms respond to treatment.

Medications: Many patients decide to forgo any active treatment until motor symptoms reach a point of significantly interfering with daily living. At that point, treatment addresses dopamine depletion with dopamine-enhancing medications. While most patients have some benefit, these medicines (levodopa, dopamine agonists, etc.) can result in side effects that some patients may not tolerate, including dyskinesia and personality changes. Numerous pharmacologic options can aid in the management of motor findings [18, 19].

Physical/Occupational therapy: Clinical trials have shown efficacy of specific interventions such as the LSVT BIG and LSVT LOUD programs [20, 21]. These programs focus on retraining the motor components of limb movements and voice. Because people with PD have slow, low-amplitude movements, these therapies train patients to make exaggerated movements (or use exaggerated speech) in order to "retrain the brain" to produce larger movements and to retrain the sensory system to recognize such movements as normal [22].

Deep brain stimulation (DBS) surgery: Neurosurgical treatment of Parkinson disease was first attempted in the 1950s with some success. Initial efforts caused a physical lesion in specific brain regions to eliminate abnormal basal ganglia motor signals. More recently, deep brain stimulation (DBS) has emerged as a treatment option for patients whose motor symptoms cannot be effectively managed with clinical therapies. DBS surgery involves the implantation of electrodes in basal ganglia structures. This surgery is not without risks, and patients are typically carefully screened to ensure that all attempts to manage their symptoms medically have been considered. Not all aspects of PD respond to DBS surgery, and it is critical that patients have realistic expectations of the potential risks and benefits of this surgery [23].

3.4 Genetics

(PD video clip Part 2)

Historically, PD has been viewed as a "non-genetic" disease because, with the exception of rare Mendelian families, most affected individuals do not report an affected family member amongst their close relatives. However, early epidemiological studies suggested a role for genetics in the etiology of idiopathic PD [24, 25]. Subsequent studies have confirmed the importance of genetic factors in early-onset cases, while the role of genetics in later-onset cases appears to be minimal [26, 27]. Despite many large genome wide association studies, the genetic basis of idiopathic later-onset PD remains largely unknown [28].

3.4.1 Autosomal Dominant Mendelian PD

The first Mendelian form of Parkinson disease was described in 1997 in four Italian and Greek families [29]. These families demonstrated an autosomal dominant pattern of inheritance with typical Lewy body pathology. A heterozygous p. Ala53Thr mutation in the a-synuclein gene (*SNCA*) was identified in affected family members from all four families. Subsequent haplotype analysis suggested a common founder. Since that time, additional Swiss and Korean families with the p.Ala53Thr mutation have been identified, suggesting that this mutation arose independently in other populations.

Since the initial reports, a limited number of additional *SNCA* point mutations and pathogenic copy number variations (both duplications and triplications) have been identified [29, 30]. Overall, *SNCA* mutations appear to be a rare cause of PD. Nevertheless, the discovery of *SNCA*-related PD led to the understanding that the pathologic hallmark of PD, Lewy bodies, is composed of alpha-synuclein protein [31].

A heterozygous p.Ile93Met mutation in the *UCHL1* gene has been reported in a single family with apparently autosomal dominant PD [32]. As no other PD-causing mutations have ever been reported in this gene, some have cast doubt on the pathogenicity of the original mutation [33]. Several other rare autosomal dominant PD genes have been described [39], and mutations in genes such as *GRN* and *MAPT* may result in autosomal dominant frontotemporal dementia with parkinsonism or in dominant forms of atypical parkinsonism [34].

3.4.2 Autosomal Dominant "Risk Factors"

Perhaps the most significant advance in PD genetics came with the discovery of two genes that confer autosomal dominant susceptibility to PD: *LRRK2* and *GBA*. These findings were most notable for how common they were, and despite their frequency, how long they remained undetected by clinicians and scientists [35, 36]. The *LRRK2* gene is a large gene with 51 coding exons throughout which numerous missense variants have been identified. To date, there is convincing evidence of pathogenicity for a limited number of *LRRK2* variants and most laboratories limit their analysis to these variants. Comprehensive studies of additional *LRRK2* variants have been published, but the evidence for pathogenicity of other variants is limited enough that full sequencing of the *LRRK2* gene is not recommended in most cases [37].

Several studies have sought to quantify both the frequency of *LRRK2* mutations in sporadic and familial PD and the penetrance of PD in mutation carriers. Most studies have focused on common variants, such as the p.Gly2019Ser mutation. This particular mutation is seen in approximately 1 % of individuals with sporadic PD and 4 % of individuals with familial PD [38]. The frequency of particular mutations varies widely by ethnicity with the highest mutation frequency for the p. Gly2019Ser mutation noted in those with North African or Ashkenazi Jewish ancestry (37 % and 18 % of familial PD, respectively) [38, 39]. Due to founder effects, other mutations may be seen with higher frequency in other ethnicities, such as the p.Arg1441Gly mutation in individuals with Basque ancestry [35]. The most comprehensive penetrance data has been published for individuals with the p. Gly2019Ser mutation. While studies have reached differing numerical conclusions regarding penetrance, penetrance is age-dependent, but incomplete [38]. Published lifetime penetrance figures range from 30 to 74 %. Despite this incomplete penetrance, much of the literature considers *LRRK2* an autosomal dominant gene [40].

While it was surprising that a common genetic risk factor such as *LRRK2* remained undetected until 2004, it was even more surprising that the link between *GBA* mutations and Parkinson disease was not firmly established until 2009 [41]. Homozygous and compound heterozygous *GBA* mutations had long been known to cause the lysosomal storage disease Gaucher disease. The possibility that glucocerebrosidase deficiency could contribute to parkinsonism was raised based on clinical observations of parkinsonism in some individuals with Gaucher disease [42]. It became clear that PD was much more common in the relatives of people with Gaucher disease and, therefore, that a heterozygote *GBA* mutation conferred risk of PD. Since Ashkenazi Jews have a much higher carrier frequency than other populations (with the N370S mutation being the most common founder mutation in this population), the prevalence of a *GBA* mutation in Ashkenazi Jews with PD is 10.7–31.3 % depending on study methodology. Prevalence of a mutation in other populations is 2.3–9.4 %. PD caused by *GBA* mutation tends to have an earlier age of onset and more frequent occurrence of dementia than idiopathic PD [43]. The actual risk of a *GBA* carrier to develop PD is unknown, but appears to be low. Thus, genetic testing of asymptomatic individuals is generally not advised.

3.4.3 Autosomal Recessive Mendelian PD

Mutations in the *PARK2* (Parkin) gene were first identified in autosomal recessive juvenile onset (<20 years) Parkinson disease and later in individuals with "young onset" Parkinson disease (<45 years). While *PARK2* mutations are said to cause juvenile onset "Parkinson disease," important clinical and pathological differences exist between Parkin-related PD and idiopathic PD disease. First, patients with Parkin-related disease usually lack the characteristic neuropathologic finding of Lewy bodies that define PD [44]. Second, in spite of a relatively young age of onset, patients with Parkin-related PD often have a prolonged and more benign course than individuals with typical PD. This is in contrast to many other neurodegenerative diseases where younger age of onset is often correlated with a more rapid clinical course. Finally, patients with Parkin-related disease differ clinically from patients with typical PD in that they typically do not lose their sense of smell (anosmia), often present with dystonia and brisk reflexes early in the course of the disease, and typically respond very well to sustained treatment with oral levodopa [45, 46].

Mutations in two other genes have now been convincingly associated with autosomal recessive early-onset PD. Mutations in the *PARK7* (*DJ-1*) gene were initially described in consanguineous families from Italy and the Netherlands [47]. Subsequently, mutations in the *PINK1* (*PARK6*) gene were identified in several consanguineous families with early onset parkinsonism [48]. Interestingly, the *PARK7* and *PINK1* genes reside physically close to one another on chromosome 1p36. With over 30 mutations of every variety, from point mutations to copy number variants, *PINK1* is the second most common autosomal recessive cause of PD [49].

Some controversy exists as to whether or not carrier status for a single recessive early-onset PD mutation is a risk factor for later onset "idiopathic" PD. This observation was initially based on findings of single mutations in individuals with PD, as well as an increased risk for PD in carrier relatives of probands with autosomal recessive PD. However, findings based on different methodologies are still inconclusive [50] (Table 3.1).

Table 3.1 Genetic risk factors for PD

Rare Mendelian parkinsonism			
Dominant typical PD	*Dominant atypical PD*	*Recessive typical PD*	*Recessive atypical PD*
SNCA mutations	*ATXN2* (SCA2)	*PARK2* (PARKIN)	*PLA2G6*
SNCA duplication/triplication	*ATXN3* (SCA3)	PARK6 *(PINK1)*	*ATP13A2*
LRRK2		*PARK7* (DJ1)	

Dominant risk factors
Common variants with moderate effects
GBA carrier status

Possible risk genes		
Carrier status for recessive PD	*Dominant genes with limited evidence*	*Common SNPS with small effect*
PARK2	*UCHL1*	*MAPT*
PINK1	*VPS35*	*SNCA* (common variants)
PARK7	*FBX07*	Others

3.5 Genetic Counseling Issues

Since PD is a common disorder, family history can be complicated by the co-occurrence of both the genetic and sporadic forms of the disease in the same pedigree. Reduced penetrance and late disease onset may mask the presence of hereditary forms of parkinsonism. Finally, exclusion of the familial genetic risk factor does not preclude development of the idiopathic form of the disease.

When reviewing a family history for Parkinson disease, genetic counselors should be aware that some individuals with parkinsonism might not have actually received a formal diagnosis. Thus, in addition to asking about other family members with Parkinson disease, genetic counselors should ask about the presence of specific symptoms such as stooped posture, shuffling gait, "masked" facial appearance, and tremor. Genetic counselors should be aware that contrary to common perceptions, a significant proportion of patients with PD do not manifest tremor. The presence of other neurologic diseases in the family (e.g., dementia, motor neuron disease, ataxia) that might point to a specific Mendelian cause should also be explored. Ethnic background may provide important clues, as is the case of common *LRRK2* variants in the Basque, Ashkenazi Jewish, or North African populations.

Several distinctive aspects of genetic counseling for PD include:

- The variety of inheritance patterns documented in familial parkinsonism including autosomal dominant, autosomal recessive, and autosomal dominant with reduced penetrance.

- The possibility that Mendelian forms of PD may not behave as traditional dominant or recessive conditions (e.g., carriers of *PARK2* mutations may have a risk for later-onset PD).
- The fact that some of the most common genetic PD risk factors, *GBA* mutations, are often evaluated as part of prenatal or pre-conception genetic testing. Thus, carrier status for these risk factors may be identified in the unrelated context of reproductive decision-making. It is not clear to what extent couples are counseled about the risk for PD when having this testing.
- The extremely common nature (and reduced penetrance) of some genetic risk factors for PD, including *LRRK2* mutations and *GBA* mutations.
- The availability of direct-to-consumer testing for some of the PD genes including *LRRK2*.

3.6 Case History (Fig. 3.1)

Sandy is a 58-year-old woman who presents for a movement disorders evaluation. In the past year, she noticed difficulty buttoning blouses, her right leg drags "causing her to trip" when walking, and difficulty getting out of bed in the morning because of stiffness. She has a slight right-handed rest tremor, especially when she is meeting with clients at work. She is aware that her colleagues have noticed the tremor and this has been embarrassing for her. Although she does not write very often, her handwriting has become smaller and her typing is slower.

Sandy's husband and two adult children, Ben and Lucille, accompany her to clinic. Sandy is concerned about the possibility of Parkinson disease (PD) because both her father and her brother were diagnosed with PD. Due to the significant family history, the neurologist asks the genetic counselor to join the conversation.

Sandy reports that, other than the symptoms mentioned above, she is in good health. Upon further questioning, she reveals that her sense of smell has diminished over the past few years. Her husband adds that Sandy has been "acting out her dreams" at night. At one point, she struck her husband during a particularly vivid dream. Since that time, they have slept in separate beds.

Neurologic examination reveals subtle findings suggestive of PD. Sandy's finger tapping is slower on her right side and her right arm swing is reduced when she walks. Sandy has a right-sided rest tremor. The neurologist explains that, given her family history, the features on examination suggest PD. He discusses additional evaluations that might provide insight. Much to the family's frustration, he explains that sometimes it takes several visits to confidently establish or exclude a diagnosis of PD.

By this point in the visit, Sandy is quite distraught. She saw this same process play out in her father and brother, and says, "I know how this story ends." The neurologist and genetic counselor suggest that it might be helpful to schedule

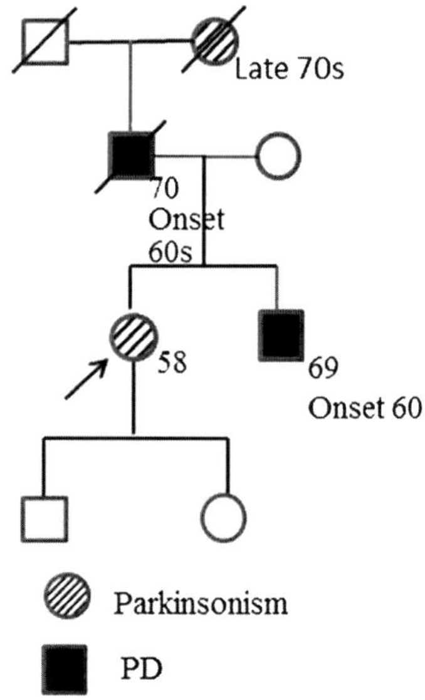

Fig. 3.1 PD case history pedigree

another visit in 2–4 weeks to further discuss the family history and potential genetic implications. The family agrees and schedules a return appointment.

At the return visit, Sandy indicates that her father was the first person in the family to be diagnosed with PD. He had a hand tremor beginning in his 60s. Subsequently, he developed a shuffling gait and a "masked" facial expression. His symptoms improved somewhat with medication, but they eventually progressed and he passed away in his mid-70s from respiratory complications. During his last years, the family noticed growing cognitive difficulties. Many years later, Sandy's brother was evaluated for PD at age 60. After seeking several "second" opinions, he was formally diagnosed with PD at age 62. At age 68, he had deep brain stimulation surgery to improve his tremor. The surgery provided with him with significant benefit.

In asking about extended family history, Sandy notes that her paternal grandmother was "stiff and slow" near the end of her life. Otherwise, no other neurologic disease was reported in the family. Sandy indicates that her father's family was Ashkenazi Jewish and that her mother's family was Norwegian (Fig. 3.1).

The discussion then turns to the genetics of PD. Sandy and her family had been reassured in the past that PD was "not a genetic disease." However, the recent diagnosis of her brother has created significant concern. The genetic counselor begins by stating that, in most cases, PD is a multifactorial condition caused by the interaction of numerous genetic and environmental factors. However, genetic forms of PD do occur. Because of the family history and late age of onset, an autosomal dominant form of the disease is possible in Sandy's family.

The counselor discusses the recent discovery of autosomal dominant risk factors for PD, including the *LRRK2* and *GBA* genes. These genes are of particular concern given the Ashkenazi Jewish ancestry in the family. The counselor explains that variants in these genes confer an increased *risk* for PD, but they are not fully penetrant risk factors.

At this point, the genetic counselor notes that Sandy's son has become withdrawn and looks quite upset. When the counselor asks Ben about his reaction, he states that he and his wife are planning a family. As part of the planning, he had carrier testing for the more common Ashkenazi Jewish diseases. His testing revealed that he is a carrier of Gaucher disease, with a single copy of the *GBA* N370S mutation. While this news had initially been surprising to him, his wife had tested negative for *GBA* mutations so they had been reassured that Ben's carrier status for Gaucher disease was unlikely to be of any consequence to his future children. The relationship between *GBA* mutations and Parkinson disease risk had not been discussed. At this point, Sandy's husband interrupts Ben saying, "This isn't about you!" Ben quietly withdraws, while his younger sister begins to cry.

Discussion questions:

- What are the most effective strategies to confront the different issues facing each of the family members?
- What responsibilities do genetic counselors in reproductive and/or pediatric settings have to discuss risks for adult onset neurologic disease when testing patients for potential reproductive risks (e.g., GBA mutations and PD or FMR1 premutations and fragile X tremor ataxia syndrome)?
- What value is there in identifying genetic susceptibility to adult onset neurologic disease when there is not a clear intervention that will prevent or delay the onset of the disease?
- What approaches might be effective to introduce the idea of genetic susceptibility when families believe a disease to be "non-genetic"?

The genetic counselor acknowledges the significance of this unanticipated potential connection between Ben's Gaucher carrier status and his mother's parkinsonism. What had been an abstract concept of genetic risk for PD has become a very concrete reality with a specific name: *GBA*. The counselor acknowledges that Ben's *GBA* mutation could explain, in part, the PD in the family. Without formally testing Sandy, however, this is only an assumption. The counselor also acknowledges that this information has a direct impact on everyone present. Sandy and her husband indicate to the counselor that they would like to take some time to think about this information and they are not yet ready to have genetic testing. Ben and Lucille agree that it would be best to have time to absorb this information. The counselor tells the family that she will check in with them when they come for follow-up care with the neurologist.

Eventually, Sandy decides that she wants testing for the *GBA* N270S mutation and also for *LRRK2* mutations. As expected, her testing demonstrates that she is heterozygous for the *GBA* N270S mutation, but negative for *LRRK2*. She indicates that, while she was initially upset, her son has become involved in a research project for individuals with genetic risk for PD. Sandy's daughter, on the other hand, has decided that she would rather not know her status for the time being. She understands that even if she carries the gene mutation, she might never develop PD.

3.7 Patient Resources

1. Parkinson's Disease Foundation: www.pdf.org
2. Michael J. Fox Foundation for Parkinson's research: http://www.michaeljfox.org
3. We Move: Worldwide Education and Awareness for Movement Disorders: http://www.wemove.org
4. National Parkinson Foundation: http://www.parkinson.org

References

1. De Lau, L. M., & Breteler, M. M. (2006). Epidemiology of Parkinson's disease. *Lancet Neurology, 5*(6), 525–535.
2. Van Den Eeden, S. K., Tanner, C. M., Bernstein, A. L., Fross, R. D., Leimpeter, A., Bloch, D. A., et al. (2003). Incidence of Parkinson's disease: variation by age, gender, and race/ethnicity. *American Journal of Epidemiology, 157*(11), 1015–1022.
3. Hughes, A. J., Daniel, S. E., Ben-Shlomo, Y., & Lees, A. J. (2002). The accuracy of diagnosis of parkinsonian syndromes in a specialist movement disorder service. *Brain, 125*(Pt. 4), 861–870.
4. Hughes, A. J., Ben-Shlomo, Y., Daniel, S. E., & Lees, A. J. (2001). What features improve the accuracy of clinical diagnosis in Parkinson's disease: A clinicopathologic study. 1992. *Neurology, 57*(10 Suppl 3), S34–S38.
5. Braak, H., & Braak, E. (2000). Pathoanatomy of Parkinson's disease. *Journal of Neurology, 247*(Suppl 2), II3–II10.
6. Burn, D. J., & Lees, A. J. (2002). Progressive supranuclear palsy: Where are we now? *Lancet Neurology, 1*(6), 359–369.
7. Tuite, P. J., Clark, H. B., Bergeron, C., Bower, M., St George-Hyslop, P., Mateva, V., et al. (2005). Clinical and pathologic evidence of corticobasal degeneration and progressive supranuclear palsy in familial tauopathy. *Archives of Neurology, 62*(9), 1453–1457.
8. Poorkaj, P., Muma, N. A., Zhukareva, V., Cochran, E. J., Shannon, K. M., Hurtig, H., et al. (2002). An R5L tau mutation in a subject with a progressive supranuclear palsy phenotype. *Annals of Neurology, 52*(4), 511–516.
9. Armstrong, M. J., Litvan, I., Lang, A. E., et al. (2013). Criteria for the diagnosis of corticobasal degeneration. *Neurology, 80*(5), 496–503.
10. Mahapatra, R. K., Edwards, M. J., Schott, J. M., & Bhatia, K. P. (2004). Corticobasal degeneration. *Lancet Neurology, 3*(12), 736–743.
11. Lesage, S., Le Ber, I., Condroyer, C., Broussolle, E., Gabelle, A., Thobois, S., et al. (2013). C9orf72 repeat expansions are a rare genetic cause of parkinsonism. *Brain, 136*(Pt 2), 385–391.
12. Lindquist, S., Duno, M., Batbayli, M., Puschmann, A., Braendgaard, H., Mardosiene, S., et al. (2013). Corticobasal and ataxia syndromes widen the spectrum of C9ORF72 hexanucleotide expansion disease. *Clinical Genetics, 83*(3), 279–283.
13. Bugiani, O., Murrell, J. R., Giaccone, G., Hasegawa, M., Ghigo, G., Tabaton, M., et al. (1999). Frontotemporal dementia and corticobasal degeneration in a family with a P301S mutation in tau. *Journal of Neuropathology and Experimental Neurology, 58*(6), 667–677.

14. Stefanova, N., Bücke, P., Duerr, S., & Wenning, G. K. (2009). Multiple system atrophy: An update. *Lancet Neurology, 8*(12), 1172–1178.
15. McKeith, I., Mintzer, J., Aarsland, D., Burn, D., Chiu, H., Cohen-Mansfield, J., et al. (2004). Dementia with Lewy bodies. *Lancet Neurology, 3*(1), 19–28.
16. Tsuang, D., Leverenz, J. B., Lopez, O. L., Hamilton, R. L., Bennett, D. A., Schneider, J. A., et al. (2012). GBA mutations increase risk for Lewy body disease with and without Alzheimer disease pathology. *Neurology, 79*(19), 1944–1950.
17. Lees, A. J., Hardy, J., & Revesz, T. (2009). Parkinson's disease. *Lancet, 373*(9680), 2055–2066.
18. Benamer, T. S., Patterson, J., Grosset, D. G., Booij, J., de Bruin, K., van Royen, E., et al. (2000). Accurate differentiation of parkinsonism and essential tremor using visual assessment of [123I]-FP-CIT SPECT imaging: the [123I]-FP-CIT study group. *Movement Disorders, 15*(3), 503–510.
19. Jankovic, J., & Poewe, W. (2012). Therapies in Parkinson's disease. *Current Opinion in Neurology, 25*(4), 433–447.
20. Ramig, L. O., Sapir, S., Countryman, S., Pawlas, A. A., O'Brien, C., Hoehn, M., et al. (2001). Intensive voice treatment (LSVT®) for individuals with Parkinson's disease: A two year follow-up. *Journal of Neurology, Neurosurgery & Psychiatry, 71*(4), 493–498.
21. Farley, B. G., & Koshley, G. F. (2005). Training BIG to move faster: The application of the speed-amplitude relation as a rehabilitation strategy for people with Parkinson's disease. *Experimental Brain Research, 167*(3), 462–467.
22. Fox, C., Ebersbach, G., Ramig, L., & Sapir, S. (2012). LSVT LOUD and LSVT BIG: Behavioral treatment programs for speech and body movement in parkinson disease. *Parkinson's Disease, 2012*, 391946.
23. Miocinovic, S., Somayajula, S., Chitnis, S., & Vitek, J. L. (2013). History, applications, and mechanisms of deep brain stimulation. *JAMA Neurology, 70*(2), 163–171.
24. Marder, K., Tang, M.-X., Mejia, H., Alfaro, B., Côté, L., Louis, E., et al. (1996). Risk of Parkinson's disease among first-degree relatives: A community-based study. *Neurology, 47*(1), 155–160.
25. Payami, H., Larsen, K., Bernard, S., & Nutt, J. (1994). Increased risk of Parkinson's disease in parents and siblings of patients. *Annals of Neurology, 36*(4), 659–661.
26. Rocca, W. A., McDonnell, S. K., Strain, K. J., Bower, J. H., Ahlskog, J. E., Elbaz, A., et al. (2004). Familial aggregation of Parkinson's disease: The Mayo Clinic Family Study. *Annals of Neurology, 56*(4), 495–502.
27. Tanner, C. M., Ottman, R., Goldman, S. M., Ellenberg, J., Chan, P., Mayeux, R., et al. (1999). Parkinson disease in twins. An etiologic study. *The Journal of the American Medical Association, 281*(4), 341–346.
28. Maraganore, D. M., de Andrade, M., Lesnick, T. G., Strain, K. J., Farrer, M. J., Rocca, W. A., et al. (2005). High-resolution whole-genome association study of Parkinson disease. *The American Journal of Human Genetics, 77*, 685–693.
29. Polymeropoulos, M. H., Lavedan, C., Leroy, E., Ide, S. E., Dehejia, A., Dutra, A., et al. (1997). Mutation in the alpha-synuclein gene identified in families with Parkinson's disease. *Science, 276*(5321), 2045–2047.
30. Singleton, A. B., Farrer, M., Johnson, J., Singleton, A., Hague, S., Kachergus, J., et al. (2003). alpha-Synuclein locus triplication causes Parkinson's disease. *Science, 302*(5646), 841.
31. Giasson, B. I., Duda, J. E., Murray, I. V. J., Chen, Q., Souza, J. M., Hurtig, H. I., et al. (2000). Oxidative damage linked to neurodegeneration by selective alpha-synuclein nitration in synucleinopathy lesions. *Science, 290*(5493), 985–989.
32. Leroy, E., Boyer, R., Auburger, G., Ulm, G., Mezey, E., Harta, G., et al. (1998). The ubiquitin pathway in Parkinson's disease. *Nature, 395*(6701), 451–452.
33. Healy, D. G., Abou-Sleiman, P. M., & Wood, N. W. (2004). Genetic causes of Parkinson's disease: UCHL-1. *Cell and Tissue Research, 318*(1), 189–194.

34. Rademakers, R., Cruts, M., & van Broeckhoven, C. (2004). The role of tau (MAPT) in frontotemporal dementia and related tauopathies. *Human Mutation, 24*(4), 277–295.
35. Paisan-Ruiz, C., Jain, S., Evans, E. W., Gilks, W. P., Simón, J., van der Brug, M., et al. (2004). Cloning of the gene containing mutations that cause PARK8-linked Parkinson's disease. *Neuron, 44*(4), 595–600.
36. Zimprich, A., Biskup, S., Leitner, P., Lichtner, P., Farrer, M., Lincoln, S., et al. (2004). Mutations in LRRK2 cause autosomal-dominant parkinsonism with pleomorphic pathology. *Neuron, 44*(4), 601–607.
37. Ross, O. A., Soto-Ortolaza, A. I., Heckman, M. G., Aasly, J. O., Abahuni, N., Annesi, G., et al. (2011). Association of LRRK2 exonic variants with susceptibility to Parkinson's disease: A case–control study. *Lancet Neurology, 10*(10), 898–908.
38. Healy, D. G., Falchi, M., O'Sullivan, S. S., Bonifati, V., Durr, A., Bressman, S., et al. (2008). Phenotype, genotype, and worldwide genetic penetrance of LRRK2-associated Parkinson's disease: A case–control study. *Lancet Neurology, 7*(7), 583–590.
39. Puschmann, A. (2013). Monogenic Parkinson's disease and parkinsonism: Clinical phenotypes and frequencies of known utations. *Parkinsonism & Related Disorders, 19*(4), 401–415.
40. Houlden, H., & Singleton, A. B. (2012). The genetics and neuropathology of Parkinson's disease. *Acta Neuropathologica, 124*(3), 325–338.
41. Sidransky, E., Nalls, M. A., Aasly, J. O., Aharon-Peretz, J., Annesi, G., Barbosa, E. R., et al. (2009). Multicenter analysis of glucocerebrosidase mutations in Parkinson's disease. *The New England Journal of Medicine, 361*(17), 1651–1661.
42. Tayebi, N., Walker, J., Stubblefield, B., Orvisky, E., LaMarca, M. E., Wong, K., et al. (2003). Gaucher disease with parkinsonian manifestations: Does glucocerebrosidase deficiency contribute to a vulnerability to parkinsonism? *Molecular Genetics and Metabolism, 79*(2), 104–109.
43. Sidransky, E., & Lopez, G. (2012). The link between the GBA gene and parkinsonism. *Lancet Neurology, 11*(11), 986–998.
44. Poulopoulos, M., Levy, O. A., & Alcalay, R. N. (2012). The neuropathology of genetic Parkinson's disease. *Movement Disorders, 27*(7), 831–842.
45. Alcalay, R. N., Siderowf, A., Ottman, R., Caccappolo, E., Mejia-Santana, H., Tang, M. X., et al. (2011). Olfaction in Parkin heterozygotes and compound heterozygotes: the CORE-PD study. *Neurology, 76*(4), 319–326.
46. De Rosa, A., Volpe, G., Marcantonio, L., Santoro, L., Brice, A., Filla, A., et al. (2006). Neurophysiological evidence of corticospinal tract abnormality in patients with Parkin mutations. *Journal of Neurology, 253*(3), 275–279.
47. Bonifati, V., Rizzu, P., van Baren, M. J., Schaap, O., Breedveld, G. J., Krieger, E., et al. (2003). Mutations in the DJ-1 gene associated with autosomal recessive early-onset parkinsonism. *Science, 299*(5604), 256–259.
48. Valente, E. M., Abou-Sleiman, P. M., Caputo, V., Muqit, M. M., Harvey, K., Gispert, S., et al. (2004). Hereditary early-onset Parkinson's disease caused by mutations in PINK1. *Science, 304*(5674), 1158–1160.
49. Crosiers, D., Theuns, J., Cras, P., & Van Broeckhoven, C. (2011). Parkinson disease: Insights in clinical, genetic and pathological features of monogenic disease subtypes. *Journal of Chemical Neuroanatomy, 42*(2), 131–141.
50. Klein, C., Lohmann-Hedrich, K., Rogaeva, E., Schlossmacher, M. G., & Lang, A. E. (2007). Deciphering the role of heterozygous mutations in genes associated with parkinsonism. *Lancet Neurology, 6*(7), 652–662.

Chapter 4
Dystonia

Jeff L. Waugh and Trisha Multhapt-Buell

Dystonia is a movement disorder recognized by abnormal fixed positions and twisting movements. It is often elicited by specific actions—for example, attempts at writing may cause the hand to flex or twist into painful and non-functional positions, while other movements with the same hand are performed normally. Simultaneous contraction of agonist–antagonist muscle pairs is common, as is overflow of movement from the desired muscles to others in close proximity. Dystonia can affect any muscle, but favors those involved in finely controlled or coordinated movements, such as the hand, vocal cords, or foot and ankle. Dystonia is the third-most common movement disorder, following Parkinson disease and essential tremor.

The typical site of onset for dystonia varies by age: in adults, the most common sites are the neck, face and/or eyelids, and hand; in children, onset in the leg or foot is most common, followed in frequency by the hand. Adult dystonia tends to remain focal, with little spread beyond contiguous body parts. Childhood-onset dystonia, loosely defined as having onset before the mid-20s, typically generalizes to both sides of the body and/or large segments of the body. Although most inherited dystonias can present with a wide range of body locations and age at onset, they generally have "textbook" presentations.

Electronic supplementary material Supplementary material is available in the online version of this chapter at 10.1007/978-1-4899-7482-2_4. Videos can also be accessed at http://www.springerimages.com/videos/978-1-4899-7481-5.

J.L. Waugh (✉)
Department of Child Neurology, Boston Children's Hospital, 300 Longwood Ave., Boston, MA 02155, USA
e-mail: Jeff.Waugh@childrens.harvard.edu

T. Multhapt-Buell
Department of Neurology, Breakefield Group, Massachusetts General Hospital, 110 6th Street, Rm 213C, Charlestown, MA 02129-4522, USA
e-mail: tmulthaupt@partners.org

J.S. Goldman (ed.), *Genetic Counseling for Adult Neurogenetic Disease*,
DOI 10.1007/978-1-4899-7482-2_4

When dystonia is the only neurologic symptom it is termed *primary dystonia*. This definition allows for tremor in the affected body part, though such a tremor should generally be less problematic than the dystonia. Conditions that include other movement disorders with dystonia are referred to as *dystonia plus syndromes*. *Secondary dystonias* occur when the movement disorder follows an identified or suspected injury, such as stroke, trauma, or premature birth. Additionally, secondary dystonias can result from an occult injury (or ongoing, progressive injury, such as an expanding tumor), making brain MRI an important but not obligatory part of an evaluation. Though secondary dystonias will not be discussed further in this chapter, these nonheritable causes of dystonia should be excluded before any genetic testing. When the diagnostic workup recognizes a more widespread neurologic disorder resulting in abnormal development or progressive loss of function, the term *heredodegenerative dystonia* is applied.

By characterizing a patient on these few axes—age at onset, location at onset, rate of progression, and presence of other neurologic symptoms—one can often narrow down the possible causal genes or loci. In this chapter, we will review the most commonly encountered genetic dystonias, as well as a few treatable syndromes that should never be overlooked (Fig. 4.1).

4.1 General Genetic Counseling Issues for All Dystonia

The majority of people with primary dystonia will not qualify for genetic testing. Dystonia genes are still being identified, and clinical genetic testing may not be readily available for some dystonia genes. Most adults with dystonia have symptom onset after age 30 and have no relatives with a childhood-onset dystonia, and thus, do not qualify for genetic testing. Children with symptoms of primary dystonia or another non-secondary dystonia qualify for testing with or without a family history of dystonia, given the reduced penetrance of many dystonia genes.

For dystonia, genetic testing can confirm a clinical diagnosis and provide individuals and families information about recurrence risk. However, in most cases, the genetic test result will not change treatment recommendations. Therefore, insurance may not pay for testing. Additionally, it is important to remind patients of the possibility of false negative results due to testing methodology or unidentified dystonia-related genes.

For relatives interested in predictive testing, in all but a few exceptional cases, mutations must be identified first in an affected family member before testing an unaffected individual. This recommendation is due to the following: (1) Most dystonias do not have associated gene mutations (the associated gene has not been identified). (2) Finding variants of unknown significance is becoming more common in these genes, and will become even more common when testing is performed using whole genome or exome sequencing.

When presymptomatic testing is an option, patients must understand the reduced penetrance and variable expressivity associated with dystonia gene mutations and

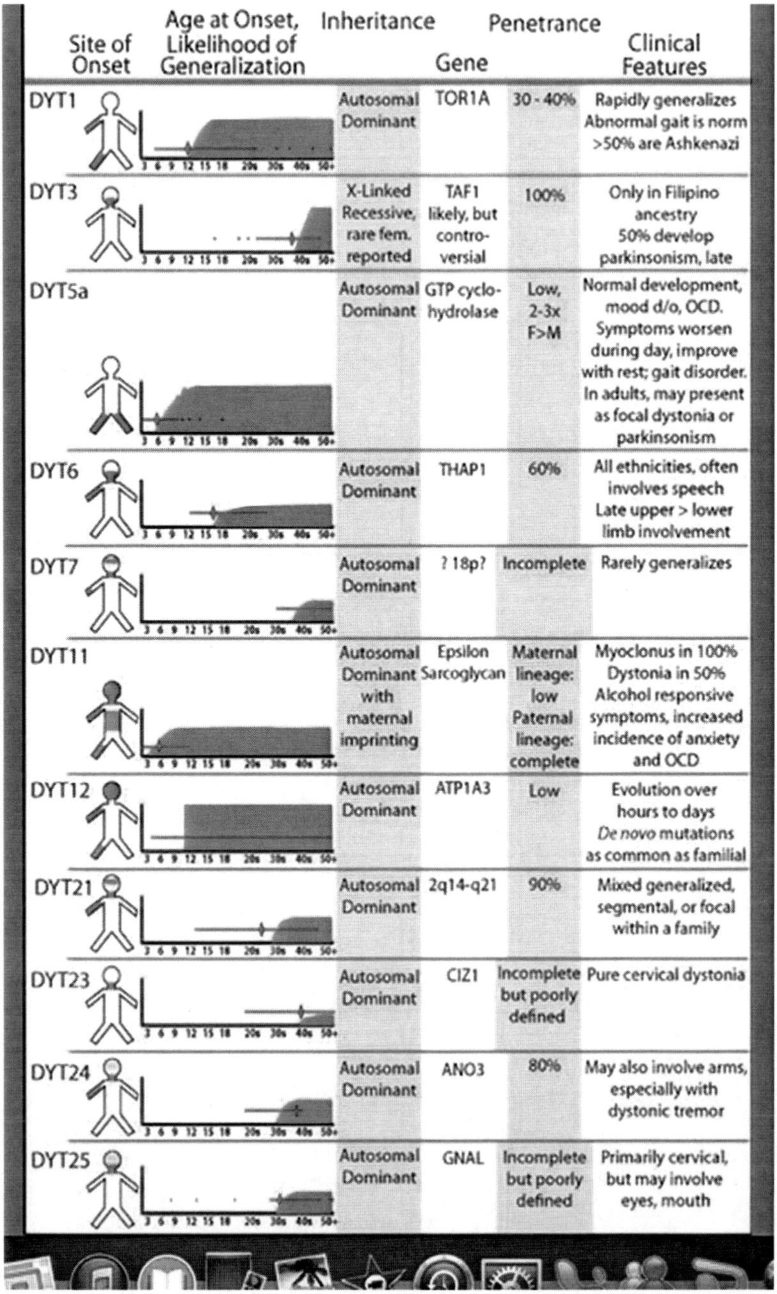

Fig. 4.1 Syndromes with Dystonia as the Presenting or a Predominant Feature—Primary dystonias or dystonia-plus syndromes that commonly begin with dystonia and can onset in adulthood are listed. The most common sites of dystonia-onset are indicated on the homunculus in *red*, with less-common sites of onset in *green*. The distribution in age of onset is indicated by a *blue bar*, with mean age

the possibility of phenocopies. To accomplish this, clinicians should first require a pretest genetic counseling session and then clinical evaluation by a movement disorder specialist. It should be explained that symptoms of dystonia can be subtle such that assumed presymptomatic testing may become symptomatic testing after the neurological evaluation. Whenever possible, a face-to-face result counseling session should be utilized.

Most patients are compliant with this protocol, and many choose not to go forward with testing after genetic counseling. Those who choose not to test often feel that identification of a mutation would only increase their worry without means to ameliorate their anxiety or reduce their risk. Parents of affected children may choose to forego genetic testing to avoid the burden of guilt. Those patients who proceed with testing usually cope well with their results. Common reasons for testing include discomfort with uncertainty and clarification of recurrence risk for their children.

4.1.1 Family History Questions Pertinent to Dystonia

Pertinent family history questions should document any neurological or psychiatric condition with age of onset and age of death. When taking the pedigree, the patient and informant should be asked the following questions:

- Did anybody have dystonia, tremor, or Parkinson disease?
- Did anybody have any movement problems?
- Did anyone have difficulty with handwriting, walking, or eating?
- Did anyone have difficulty with speech or speech quality?
- Did anybody have a mental illness, especially chronic depression, anxiety, or obsessive-compulsive disorder?
- Was anyone in a nursing home or mental institution? If so, why?
- Was anyone alcoholic?

4.2 The Primary Dystonias

Dystonia unaccompanied by other neurological symptoms is called a primary dystonia. Primary dystonia's prevalence is estimated to be 152–330 per million [1]. Primary dystonia can be subdivided depending on symptom distribution, such

---

Fig. 4.1 (continued) indicated by a *blue diamond*, and rare but reported outliers indicated by extralinear *blue dashes*. Typical rates of progression and likelihood of generalization are indicated by *red plots*. Note that homunculi and plots represent the most common clinical presentations, but variations on these axes are not uncommon

as generalized, hemi-dystonia, segmental, multifocal, and focal dystonia. We will focus on those types for which genes have been identified; however, there will be many patients who have primary dystonia and no genetic diagnosis. For example, adult-onset focal dystonia is the most common type of dystonia, and most of these dystonias are primary without known genetic associations (Tables 4.1 and 4.2).

4.2.1 Clinical Presentation

Primary dystonia, also known as idiopathic or primary torsion dystonia (PTD), has a broad clinical expression. Symptoms can begin in any voluntary muscle and can remain locally restricted or can spread. The progression of symptoms is typically gradual over the course of months or years. Onset can occur at any age, but age of onset is commonly categorized as early-onset dystonia occurring before age 26 and late-onset dystonia occurring after age 26.

In children and adolescents, PTD usually begins in an arm or a leg and spreads to other body regions. Early-onset PTD represents a small percentage of all dystonia cases, but a large portion of these can be attributed to the genes, *TOR1A* and *THAP1*. Recently, a causal gene for late-onset PTD was identified, *GNAL* [2].

DYT1 (TOR1A)-associated dystonia:

DYT1 dystonia is the most common cause of early-onset generalized dystonia. Approximately 50 % of individuals with early-onset generalized dystonia beginning in a limb have a heterozygous *TOR1A* mutation. For people who are of Ashkenazi Jewish descent and have early-onset generalized dystonia, as many as 80 % have a *TOR1A* mutation [1].

Only 30–40 % percent of individuals with DYT1 develop PTD; thus, reduced penetrance is a significant issue. In 90 % of individuals with DYT1 dystonia, symptoms begin in a limb before age 21 (mean 13 years), and in about 65 %, symptoms progress to generalized or multifocal involvement [1].

DYT6 (THAP1)-associated dystonia

Another type of early-onset PTD, *THAP1*-associated dystonia, accounts for about 1 % of all primary dystonias and up to 25 % of multiplex families with early-onset and non-focal dystonia [1]. The penetrance of DYT6 mutations is estimated to be 60 %.

Symptoms of DYT6 usually begin in the arm (50 %) or cranial or neck muscles (25 % each) at an average age of 16 (range: 5–62 years) [2]. Symptom onset in the leg is rare, but speech involvement is common. Symptoms progress to other body regions in over 50 % of cases.

GNAL-associated dystonia

Identified in 2012, mutations in *GNAL* cause late-onset PTD (mean 31 years, range 7–54).

Cervical muscles are the most common site of onset (82 %), with cranial onset including face, jaw/tongue and larynx being the second most common site (18 %).

Table 4.1 Primary dystonia

Designation	Dystonia type	Inheritance	Penetrance	Gene locus	Gene/product
DYT1	Early-onset generalized primary torsion dystonia	AD	Reduced (30 %)	9q	*TOR1A*/torsinA
DYT2	Early-onset primary torsion dystonia	AR	n/a	Unknown	Unknown
DYT4	"Non-DYT1" primary torsion dystonia: whispering dysphonia, extrusional tongue dystonia and "hobby horse gait"	AD	Complete (100 %)	19p13.12–13	*TUBB4*/β-tubulin 4a
DYT6	Adolescent-onset torsion dystonia of mixed type	AD	Reduced (60 %)	8p21–q22	*THAP1*/THAP1
DYT7	Adult-onset focal torsion dystonia: prominent cervical involvement	AD	n/a	18p	Unknown
DYT13	Adolescent onset multifocal/segmental dystonia: prominent craniocervical involvement	AD	Reduced	1p36.32–p36.13	Unknown
DYT17	Adolescent onset segmental dystonia: prominent cervical-laryngeal involvement	AR	n/a	20p11.22–q13.12	Unknown
DYT21	Later-onset primary torsion dystonia: prominent cranial/cervical or hand involvement	AD	Slightly Reduced	2q14.3–q21.3	Unknown
DYT23	Late-onset primary torsion dystonia: prominent cervical involvement	AD		9q34.11	*CIZ1*/ CDKN1A-interacting zinc finger protein 1
DYT24	Late-onset primary torsion dystonia: prominent craniocervical involvement	AD		11p	*ANO3*
DYT25	Late-onset primary torsion dystonia: prominent cervical-cranial involvement	AD	Slightly reduced	18p11.21	*GNAL*/$G\alpha_{olf}$

Table 4.2 Dystonia plus syndromes

Designation	Dystonia type	Inheritance	Penetrance	Gene locus	Gene/ product
Dystonia plus–parkinsonism					
DYT3	X-linked dystonia parkinsonism	X-recessive	Complete (age-related)	Xq13.1	*TAF1 or DYT3*/
DYT5/14	Dopa-responsive dystonia, Segawa syndrome	AD	Reduced	14q22.2	*GCH1*/ GTPCH
DYT12	Rapid-onset dystonia parkinsonism	AD (*de novo* mutations occur)	Reduced	19q13.2	*ATP1A3*/
DYT16	Early-onset generalized dystonia with parkinsonism	AR	n/a	2q31.2	*PRKRA*/
Dystonia plus—myoclonus					
DYT11	Myoclonus-dystonia	AD	Reduced: maternal imprinting	7q21.3	*SGCE*/
DYT15	Myoclonus-dystonia	AD	n/a	18p11	Unknown

Symptom onset in the arm has not been observed and symptom spread to the arm is infrequent (32 %), which distinguishes *GNAL* from *THAP1* [2].

4.2.2 *Diagnosis*

A neurologist or movement disorder specialist typically makes a diagnosis of dystonia. As there is no definitive diagnostic test, diagnosis is based on a clinical physical examination and review of medical history. Brain imaging, such as an MRI or CT scan, and blood work may be ordered to rule out other conditions.

When ordering genetic testing for early-onset PTD, decisions about which gene (s) to test should be made based on the patient's age and region of symptom onset. Age of onset before 26 years in clinically ascertained patients provides 100 % sensitivity and specificity of 63 % in Ashkenazi Jews and 43 % in non-Jews for DYT1 [3].

4.2.3 *Treatment and Management*

Primary dystonia has no cure or remission. However, treatments can reduce the symptoms of dystonia and improve quality of life. Anticholinergic medications, such as trihexyphenidyl (Artane) and benztropine (Cogentin), and muscle relaxants, such as baclofen or clonazepam (Klonopin), are commonly used to treat dystonia.

Most oral medications have limited benefit and are dose-limited by cognitive side effects. Most individuals require a combination of daily oral medications to achieve the best result.

People with focal or segmental dystonia can receive intramuscular injections of botulinum toxin to weaken the overactive muscle. Botulinum toxin injections must be repeated every 3-4 months, but save the patient the side effects of a systemic medication.

Surgical intervention for primary dystonia is becoming more common, especially for individuals who do not respond to other forms of treatment. Deep brain stimulation (DBS) works by blocking brain signals that cause the abnormal movements or postures with mild electrical stimulation. A neurosurgeon implants a thin wire with four electrodes into the globus pallidus. The wire runs under the skin to a battery-operated electric stimulator (similar to a pacemaker) implanted near the collarbone. After surgery, the stimulator is programmed to control symptoms. Benefits from DBS slowly accumulate over the first 6–12 months of use. DBS is being recommended more frequently as a treatment for genetically defined PTD, with some groups arguing that early implantation prevents disease progression and limits motor disability [4]. For idiopathic, secondary, or adult-onset focal dystonias, DBS appears to provide less benefit than in the primary genetic dystonias. Benefits appear to be stable for at least a decade, but the technique is still too new to know whether children with DBS will continue to benefit throughout their life [5].

Pallidotomy and thalamotomy work by selectively lesioning the pallidum or thalamus using heat. This treatment is very rarely recommended today, but patients with an early-onset dystonia who are now age 50 or older may have had one of these irreversible surgeries.

Adjuvant treatments, such as physical therapy and stress reduction techniques, may provide limited benefit to some.

4.2.4 Genetics

DYT1 is due to a GAG deletion in *TOR1A*. Inheritance is autosomal dominant with penetrance of approximately 30 %. The individuals with a DYT1 mutation typically develop early-onset generalized dystonia, but in rare cases can develop adult-onset focal dystonia or dopamine-responsive dystonia. The D216H polymorphism within the *TOR1A* gene has been shown to reduce penetrance when it is in trans with the GAG deletion [6].

DYT6 is caused by mutations in *THAP1*. Inheritance is autosomal dominant with approximately 60 % penetrance. Many different sizes and types of pathogenic mutations have been identified within *THAP1*.

DYT25 is caused by mutations in *GNAL* and is autosomal dominant. Pathogenic nonsense, frameshift, missense and in-frame deletion mutations have been identified in *GNAL*. In the first series of families with *GNAL* mutations reported, imprinting does not appear to play a role in expression [2].

4.2.5 *Genetic Counseling Issues*

Most adults with PTD will not qualify for genetic testing, so genetic counselors must be prepared to respond to patient and doctors' question, "Why aren't we testing?" Similarly, genetic counselors need to be prepared to explain to patients and families why genetic testing results may be negative, but the diagnosis of dystonia is unchanged.

Determining dystonia etiology allows for accurate recurrence risk assessment and may avoid other diagnostic testing; however, there is no specific treatment for any of the genetic subtypes of PTD. Genetic testing has limited potential to alter treatment recommendations. DYT1 dystonia responds well to DBS (in ~80 % of patients), but other dystonias respond less well. Therefore, the decision of whether to use DBS is made easier by a confirmed DYT1 mutation, but genetic testing is less informative for all other primary dystonias.

People with symptoms of PTD who qualify for genetic testing must be counseled about the impact of the information on their current and future family. Minors are often tested for PTD genes. For families who are struggling to understand their child's symptoms, confronting a genetic etiology can be demoralizing. Prior to testing, parents need to be aware that etiological determination could reveal their own likelihood to develop dystonia, as well as the risk to their extended family. Because DYT1 and DYT6 dystonias typically have an early onset, a positive result usually does not cause anxiety about parental risk, but does cause guilt for passing on a faulty gene and concern for their other children. When feelings of blame prevent parents from undergoing carrier testing, estimating recurrence risk for extended family becomes difficult. If parental resistance to carrier testing is absolute, offering counseling and education to extended family about dystonia signs and symptoms can help ameliorate uncertainty. The parents and minor also need to recognize that a positive test result will impact the child's future family planning. Whenever possible and appropriate, the child should be included in this discussion. Patients or parents should be counseled about informing extended family members of positive genetic test results. Counselors can offer to facilitate that process.

A positive genetic test result for a PTD can lead to presymptomatic testing of unaffected adults. Due to reduced penetrance and the inability to prevent disease, presymptomatic genetic testing of minors is not recommended. Presymptomatic testing of adults may occur in situations where an aunt/uncle of an affected child wants to determine risk to their own children. These patients should be advised of the Genetic Information Nondiscrimination Act (GINA) and the option to self-pay in order to keep this information confidential. Though under GINA, employment and healthcare insurance can no longer be influenced by presymptomatic genetic diagnosis, this is not true for disability, long term care, and life insurance.

4.2.6 Case History 1 (Fig. 4.2)

Lindsay is a 35-year-old woman who comes with her parents to a dystonia research center. Her brother, now age 31, developed dystonia at age 11. Her brother's mobility and speech have been significantly affected, and these disabilities impact his daily life. He has tried many different treatment options, including DBS. Since her brother first developed symptoms, her parents have been dystonia research advocates and raised money to promote research efforts. Due to family estrangement, family history of movement abnormalities is vague. The cause of her brother's dystonia has remained unknown until recently when he was found to have a mutation in the *THAP1* gene. Lindsay has never had a neurological evaluation and genetic counseling related to DYT6-associated dystonia.

Discussion Questions:

- What do you estimate Lindsay's risk of carrying a mutation to be?
- What do you anticipate are going to be the most salient issues to Lindsay?
- What issues do you want to be sure to communicate to Lindsay?
- Are the family dynamics and involvement in the dystonia research community important? If so, why?
- What do you anticipate Lindsay's reaction/response will be if the testing is negative? If positive?

Lindsay describes how her parents were very grateful to learn the cause of their son's dystonia. Given their children's "natural" differences, they believe that Lindsay does not carry the DYT6 mutation. Five years ago, she was in a serious motor vehicle accident in which she shattered multiple bones in her leg and face, but recovered and has only minor long-standing sequelae. She feels that such a major physical trauma would have 'triggered' dystonia if she were a carrier. A neurologist evaluates Lindsay and reports that she has no signs of dystonia or other neurological issues. Lindsay agrees to provide a blood sample for a research study and her parents ask to self-pay for clinical genetic testing. Lindsay agrees to receive clinical results and you make a plan to call her when the results are available.

Discussion Questions:

- What do you say to Lindsay about her beliefs about physical trauma and dystonia?
- Why would Lindsay's parents want to self-pay for Lindsay's clinical testing? Do you agree with their decision?
- How do you ensure that clinical testing and research participation are what Lindsay wants to do and not what her family expects?

You receive Lindsay's test results and they are positive; she has the same DYT6 mutation as her brother.

Discussion Questions:

- How do you prepare for the phone call to provide Lindsay with her results? What issues do you want to be sure to communicate to Lindsay?
- Will you ask Lindsay to come in for in-person follow-up? She lives 3 hours away.
- Lindsay's brother is routinely seen in clinic and his parents always accompany him. Do you address Lindsay's results with the rest of the family?

4.3 The Dystonia-Plus Syndromes

Dystonia that occurs with other neurological symptoms is designated as a dystonia-plus syndrome. We will review the dystonia-plus syndromes that occur with parkinsonism or myoclonus.

4.3.1 Clinical Presentation

DYT3 (TAF1-associated dystonia; X-linked dystonia parkinsonism, XDP; Lubag dystonia):

DYT3 dystonia affects males with maternal Filipino ancestry; very rarely, Filipino females with Turner syndrome or paternal unipaternal disomy have exhibited symptoms that are later in onset and less severe. XDP presents with severe focal dystonia, often in the jaw or neck, with average age of onset in the mid-30s (range, 12–52 years). Over a course of about 4 years, the dystonia progresses and becomes multifocal or generalized dystonia. Within 10 years, symptoms of parkinsonism develop in approximately 50 % of people with XDP [7].

The first sign of XDP is almost always an abnormality of rapid alternating limb movements [8]. Some individuals with XDP only exhibit parkinsonism or may only develop dystonia late in their disease course. Those who develop the classic symptoms of XDP, profound orolingual and cervical dystonia with parkinsonism within the first year or two of symptom onset, have the worst prognosis. Symptom

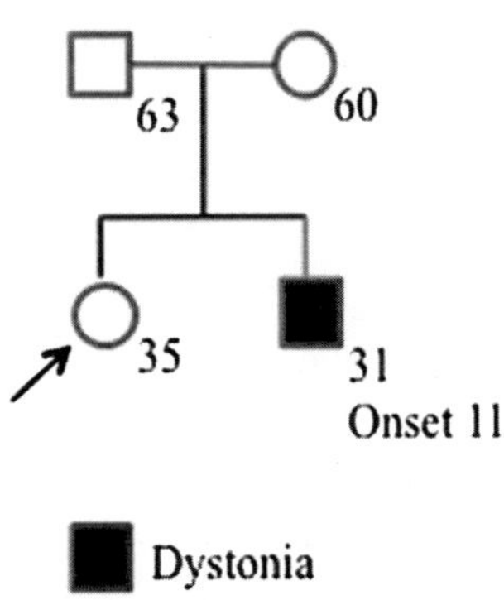

Fig. 4.2 Dystonia case history 1 pedigree

response to treatment with medication is limited, and lifespan is reduced with death often occurring from aspiration or immobility-related illness. XDP is the only DYT locus in which postmortem neurodegeneration (atrophy of the caudate and putamen) has been found.

DYT5 (GCH1-associated dystonia; DOPA-responsive dystonia, DRD)

Dopa-responsive dystonia (DRD), also known as Segawa disease, is characterized by childhood onset generalized dystonia that may exhibit diurnal fluctuation of symptoms [1]. DRD must be distinguished from DYT1 and DYT6 dystonia. This is done clinically by administration of oral levodopa to which there is significant sustained symptom reduction. Features of parkinsonism may be present at onset or develop if DRD is not treated.

DYT12 (ATP1A3-associated dystonia; rapid-onset dystonia parkinsonism, RDP):

Rapid-onset dystonia parkinsonism (RDP) is suspected in individuals who experience some event, such as exertion, childbirth or emotional stress, and then present with dystonia and/or parkinsonism that develops quickly over a few hours to a day. The symptoms progress rapidly beginning in the face, then spreading to the arm and leg. Symptoms stabilize, often in a hemi-dystonic distribution that includes dysarthria and dysphagia. Most people (85 %) with *ATP1A3* mutations experience symptom onset prior to age 30 [9]. Treatment benefits tend to be very limited.

DYT11 (SGCE-associated dystonia; myoclonus-dystonia):

(Myoclonus-dystonia video clip Part 1 and 2)

People with myoclonus-dystonia experience childhood-onset myoclonic jerks, typically in the face, neck, and upper greater than lower extremities. Girls may develop symptoms earlier than boys (age 5 versus age 8) and may be more likely to experience onset in a lower extremity [10]. Fifty percent of people with M-D will also experience dystonia, usually in a focal or segmental pattern. Myoclonus, and to a lesser extend dystonia, is responsive to alcohol. Individuals with DYT11 are at increased risk for alcoholism, though whether this is due to the reduction in abnormal movements or as a consequence of the increase in mood and anxiety disorders is unclear. Myoclonus-dystonia without epsilon sarcoglycan mutations is known as DYT15 and has been mapped to a locus on chromosome 18p.

DYT16 (PRKRA-associated dystonia):

PRKRA mutations were originally reported in three Brazilian families who had one of two early-onset phenotypes, generalized dystonia or dystonia-parkinsonism [11]. In two of the three cases of dystonia-parkinsonism, symptoms of dystonia appeared first. In all cases, dystonia began in a limb and generalized. The parkinsonian symptoms do not respond to levodopa treatment.

4.3.2 Diagnosis

A neurologist or movement disorder specialist typically makes a dystonia-plus diagnosis. Clinical presentation and an immediate positive response to dopamine replacement (i.e., Sinemet or levodopa) can definitely diagnose dopa-responsive dystonia. However, not all DRD is caused by *GCH1* mutations, and juvenile-onset Parkinson disease must be ruled out after positive response to levodopa.

If there is a plausible suspicion of a *DYT5*, *11*, or *12* gene mutation, genetic testing can be used to confirm etiology. Presently, clinical *DYT3* and *DYT16* testing are only available through German labs, so CLIA certification or insurance coverage may be lacking. However, if testing is negative or unavailable, the clinical diagnosis stands.

Genetic testing for *ATP1A3* mutations is recommended for individuals who experience abrupt onset of dystonia with parkinsonism in a rostro-caudal pattern with significant bulbar features [9].

4.3.3 Treatment and Management

Daily treatment with carbidopa/levodopa can ameliorate all or almost all symptoms of dopa-responsive dystonia. Treatment of the other types of dystonia-plus syndromes can be challenging.

As with primary dystonias a combination of oral medications and botulinum toxin injections are first line treatments. Neither XDP nor RDP nor M-D responds particularly well to medication or injection. Deep brain stimulation can be considered for patients with dystonia-plus syndromes, but it can only be used to ameliorate either parkinsonian OR dystonic symptoms. At this time, DBS lead placement and programming does not allow for good control of both types of symptoms. Only a handful of individuals with dystonia-plus syndromes have had DBS surgery, so that it is too early to determine expected surgical outcomes.

4.3.4 Genetics

DYT3 (*TAF1*):

Inheritance of DYT3 is X-linked recessive due to a founder mutation among the Filipino population on the island of Panay [7]. The exact molecular abnormality causing XDP is still being debated. There are five disease specific changes (DSC) in the XDP critical region of the X chromosome associated with XDP [12]. However, DSC3 is the only one located within an exon. The 38 exon *TAF1* gene is found within the XDP critical region, and a SVA retrotransposon in intron 32 reduces TAF1 expression [13].

Currently, genetic testing of *TAF1* for DYT3 dystonia is available in Germany. Depending on insurance and hospital regulations, it may be difficult to order an out-of-country genetic test in a non-CLIA certified laboratory. Some patients may be required to self-pay for testing.

DYT5 (*GCH1*):

GTP cyclohydrolase (GCH1) mutations are the most common cause of dopa-responsive dystonia, having been identified in about 60 % of people with DRD. GCH1 mutations are autosomal dominant with reduced sex-related penetrance such that about 90 % of girls and 40 % of boys with a GCH1 mutation develop DRD. Sequencing and del/dup analysis is required because of the variety of mutations found in *GCH1* [14].

The GTP cyclohydrolase 1 protein plays an important role in the synthesis of dopamine. It is also a cofactor for phenylalanine and tryptophan hydroxylase.

DYT12 *(ATP1A3)*

Six missense mutations in the *ATP1A3* gene that encodes the Na+/K+-ATPase alpha3 subunit have been described. *ATP1A3* mutations are autosomal dominant, but *de novo* mutations do occur.

DYT11 *(SGCE)*

SGCE encodes epsilon-sarcoglycan. *SGCE* mutations are autosomal dominant with reduced penetrance due to maternal imprinting [15]. Males and females are affected equally, but almost 100 % of people develop M-D if the mutation is inherited from their father. If the mutation is inherited from the mother, there is only about a 5 % chance of symptom expression, though in at least one pedigree, it appears that maternal inheritance is less protective [16, 17]. While *SGCE* mutations account for about 40 % of familial myoclonus-dystonia, a much smaller fraction of idiopathic, nonfamilial myoclonus is due to *SGCE* mutations [18, 19].

DYT16 (*PRKRA*)

In the original families, PRKRA mutations are autosomal recessive [11].

4.3.5 Genetic Counseling Issues

Dystonia-plus syndromes are very rare among people with dystonia, parkinsonism, or myoclonus. To ensure that testing is appropriate, classic presentation or family history of related disease must be noted during the patient work-up. Patients who express a desire for genetic testing of "all dystonia genes" require an explanation of test indication and the poor yield of blind testing. Patients with the classic presentation of symptoms of primary dystonia often have normal genetic test results. Testing is ordered much less frequently in dystonia-plus syndromes, but positive genetic test results are more likely.

As with PTD, confirmation of diagnosis and accurate recurrence risk assessment are reasons to perform genetic testing in dystonia-plus syndromes. However, with the exception of DRD, no gene-specific treatment is recommended. Individuals must understand that etiologic confirmation of diagnosis will identify other family members at risk without a method for disease prevention. Additionally because of limited beneficial treatment options, the prognosis of dystonia-plus syndromes is worse than primary dystonias. Most families with dystonia-plus syndromes have family members with adult-onset disease, making it likely that the next generation of affected individuals has already been born. Issues of guilt, blame, and family communication must be addressed during pretest counseling.

Given that XDP is only found among people of Filipino ancestry, genetic counselors with knowledge of common Filipino cultural themes and practices will better negotiate these sessions.

Individuals and families with any type of dystonia must manage the emotional stress associated with a visible physical disorder, and genetic counselors can normalize this stress. In individuals and families with *SGCE* mutations, there can be concomitant psychiatric disease (such as anxiety or obsessive-compulsive disorder), in addition to situational mental health issues. Due to the symptom-ameliorating effects of alcohol, alcoholism is common in *SGCE* pedigrees. Given the possible psychosocial repercussions of familial alcoholism, special effort may be required to document medical and family history. Patient-reported medical history may be incomplete or inconsistent, and family relationships should be verified. Non-paternity and maternal imprinting need to be carefully considered.

4.3.6 Case History 2 (Fig. 4.3)

An out-of-state physician calls a genetic counselor to refer a 65-year-old patient for genetic testing of the DTY3 gene. Her patient is Filipino, and he developed parkinsonism at age 45. The genetic counselor (GC) calls the patient to schedule the appointment and collect some medical history information.

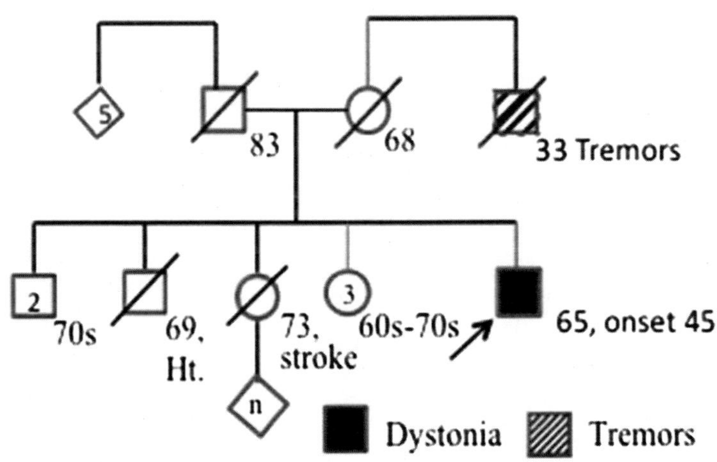

Fig. 4.3 Dystonia case history 2 pedigree

Discussion Questions:

- What does the genetic counselor want to know before seeing this patient? Why?
- What should the patient know before the appointment?

The GC calls the patient's home and speaks with his wife. During the conversation, she learns that in the past 1–2 years, the patient has developed cervical dystonia and blepharospasm. Botulinum toxin injections for cervical dystonia improve pain, but not posture. With oral medications, the patient's tremor is well controlled, but he experiences freezing while walking. The couple has no children. The patient has three brothers: two are in their 70s and one died of a heart attack at age 69. He has three sisters in their 60–70s and one sister who is deceased of complications after a stroke. None of his siblings had dystonia, parkinsonism, or another related movement issue. Only one of his sisters has biological children and none of them have neurological issues.

Discussion Questions:

- Should the genetic counselor discuss these issues with the patient's wife?
- At this point, would you recommend DYT3 testing? Reasons for? Against?

Finally GC turns the conversation to the patient's maternal relatives. His mother died at age 68 of pancreatic cancer. The patient's wife says her husband's mother had no siblings. Immediately, GC hears garbled speech in the background and is aware that the patient is speaking to his wife. The wife says, "I didn't know that she had a brother," and she returns her attention to the phone conversation. She explains that it is difficult to translate, but that her husband had a maternal uncle who died at age 33 of "natural causes" because he was "hungry." This uncle had tremors, and he was very shy, so shy that he wouldn't eat outside of his own house.

Discussion Questions:

- What do you need to know about DYT3 dystonia, parkinsonism, and/or Filipino culture to know whether or not this is relevant?
- Is it plausible that someone with a significant hand tremor related to Parkinson disease would not want to eat in public?
- Is it plausible that someone with Parkinson disease would die of hunger? Someone with DYT3 dystonia?
- The patient has seven siblings, his father had five siblings. The Philippines is a predominantly Catholic country. Is it plausible that the patient's mother would have been an only child? (which the wife believed until you called)
- At this point, would you recommend DYT3 testing? Reasons for? Against?

4.3.7 *Case History 3 (Fig. 4.4)*

Phillipe is a 9-year-old boy who presents to a movement disorders clinic with his mother for difficulty walking. They meet with a genetic counselor and neurologist. He developed this symptom 1 year ago, and has slowly but progressively lost the ability to walk without assistance. He describes an inward rotation of his right foot and leg that worsens as he walks. At the worst moments his right leg will also extend backward and hook behind his left leg. A lesser problem for him, but a visibly striking one, is a marked backward pulling of his shoulders while walking, which leads him to sway backward in a "C" position. He is able to maintain an upright posture while seated.

On examination, the physician comments on quick, jerking movements of the boy's arms and neck. His mother interjects that these movements started when Phillipe was a toddler, but that they were separate from the gait problem and not worrisome—her husband had the same childhood movements, and that "it's a French-Canadian thing." She is of mixed Irish-Norwegian ancestry and knows little of this history. She phones her husband for more information; he confirms that he is of Quebecois origin, that these excessive movements started in primary school, and that his Montreal pediatrician had diagnosed him with hyperekplexia, an excessive startle syndrome. He has never had the problems walking or twisting movements like those seen in Phillipe.

The genetic counselor feels that this information is essential for Phillipe's diagnosis, and requests that the family makes another appointment when his father can attend. She suggests that they all meet with the neurologist at the same time so that he can explain the symptoms he is observing.

Discussion Questions:

- Is this likely one genetic syndrome or two?
- What is the best clinical descriptor for Phillipe's symptoms?

The family returns for their meeting with the neurologist and genetic counselor. The genetic counselor starts by taking a more extensive family history. Phillipe's father repeats that he has a little muscle twitching, as does one of his sisters and father. Additionally, an aunt had both the jerking and twisted when she walked. He jokes that all it takes to have his twitching stop is a beer or two. The neurologist explains that the jerking that he observed in his family was probably myoclonus, not hyperekplexia. He tells them that hyperekplexia is a syndrome of excessive startle that begins in the newborn period or early infancy, not in childhood as with this family. Some varieties are more common in Quebecois. He asks Phillipe's father if he has been to a neurologist since he was young, and he says he has not. The neurologist suggests that he might want a full evaluation. He then informs the family that Phillipe's gait disorder, and probably that of Phillipe's great aunt, is a common manifestation of childhood-onset dystonia. Since both myoclonus and dystonia are found in the family, the most likely diagnosis is myoclonus-dystonia.

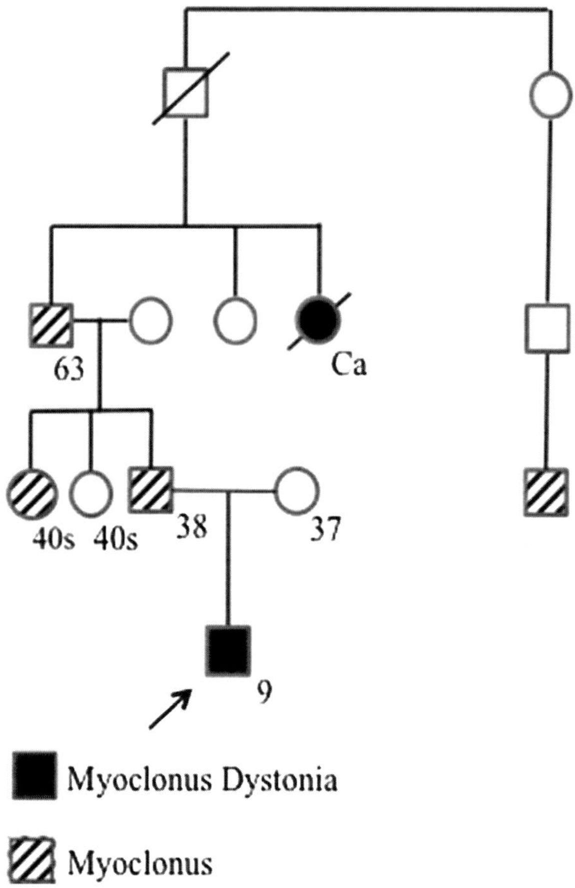

Fig. 4.4 Myoclonus-dystonia case history pedigree

The genetic counselor then discusses how myoclonus-dystonia is a dominantly inherited condition with variable penetrance. Protective maternal imprinting leads to infrequent or absent symptoms in the children of a carrier female. Phillipe's father's and aunt's mild symptoms were due to variable expressivity of the gene. Phillipe's mother becomes visibly upset and describes her desire to have a large family. She is now terrified of having another child with myoclonus-dystonia. Examining the pedigree, she notes the larger number of symptomatic males. She asks whether embryo selection to assure a female fetus would be possible.

Discussion Questions:

- How would you advise this couple?
- What is the likelihood that Phillipe's parents will bear another child with dystonia?

The genetic counselor explains that there are several reproductive options, but that sex selection would not be beneficial. The probability of inheriting the dominant gene for myoclonus-dystonia is 50 % whether the child is male or female. The probability of manifesting dystonia if the child carries the myoclonus-dystonia gene is about 50 %. Therefore, the product of these probabilities predicts a 25 % likelihood that any one of their children will have dystonia. She also explained the variability of symptoms and points to the likelihood that Phillipe's father, grandfather, and aunt all carried the gene, but were more mildly affected. She then explains reproductive options including PGD, prenatal testing, sperm donation, and adoption. She also says that they will have to identify the gene in the family before PGD or prenatal testing would be possible.

The family agrees to have Phillipe tested. They return for results and are told that a mutation was found in the *SGCE* gene. The counselor says that Phillipe's father can also test if he wishes but that in all likelihood, he carries the gene. She reviews the family history and maternal imprinting. She also talks about other symptoms that could be part of the disorder including psychiatric issues and alcoholism. She discusses how symptoms respond to alcohol and how easy it is to self-medicate. Phillipe's mother says she will watch her husband carefully. He said, "No worries!" The couple is referred for reproductive counseling.

Discussion Questions:

- To what extent should a genetic counselor go into the psychiatric aspects of a movement disorder?
- To what extent should the GC explore family issues of alcoholism and psychiatric disease?

4.4 The Heredodegenerative Dystonias

Many hereditary degenerative syndromes can produce dystonia, and dystonia may be a key feature in their diagnosis. However, it is unusual for dystonia to be the only manifestation present at the time of assessment. Frequently cognitive, emotional, and other motor symptoms will co-occur with dystonia. Advising families about expectations with these disorders is difficult, as relatives often vary significantly in the pace of decline and order of symptom presentation. The most relevant of these disorders is arranged in Table 4.3 by typical age at onset, but presentation at other ages is not unusual. All nomenclature conforms to OMIM conventions (Adapted from [20–22]).

Onset in Adulthood

Many of the conditions noted in Table 4.3 can present in adulthood, though this is very unusual. Other conditions, such as rapid-onset dystonia-parkinsonism (DYT12) can present at any age. Similarly, many mitochondrial disorders can present in adulthood, with rare instances manifesting as dystonia. Dentatorubral-pallidoluysian atrophy (DRPLA) is a dominantly inherited degenerative condition caused by mutations in *ATN1*. DRPLA typically produces myoclonus, chorea, and ataxia, but may have dystonia as a lesser feature. In 10–20 %, idiopathic Parkinson

Table 4.3 Heredodegenerative dystonias

Disorder (including parallel nomenclatures)	Relationship of dystonia to other features	Gene	Inheritance pattern
Onset before 2 years of life			
Aromatic L-amino acid decarboxylase (AADC) deficiency	Variably present, follows other symptoms: hypotonia, developmental delay, occulogyric crises	*DDC*	Recessive
Glutaric academia type I	Dystonia usually progressive, often after acute encephalopathic crisis	*GCDH*	Recessive
Idiopathic basal ganglia calcification, familial Fahr disease	Coexists with severe developmental delay, epilepsy, hypotonia	Unknown	Recessive
NBIA2A and -B, PLAN, infantile neuroaxonal dystrophy (INAD)	Wide array of phenotypes: psychomotor regression, ataxia with abnormal eye movement and optic atrophy (INAD); early global developmental delay and hypotonia, progressing to myoclonic epilepsy, ataxia, chorea, and dystonia (PLAN); adult-onset dystonia-parkinsonism	*PLA2G6*	Recessive
Methylmalonic aciduria	Dystonia common and may be transient with metabolic crises, persistent after basal ganglia infarction	*MUT*, several others	Recessive
Lesch–Nyhan Disease	Psychomotor retardation typically precedes dystonia/chorea	*HPRT*	X-linked
Hypomyelinative leukodystrophy (HLD1), Pelizaeus–Merzbacher disease	Choreoathetoid movements are more common, dystonia is rare	*PLP1*	X-linked, rare symptomatic carrier females
Rett syndrome	Dystonia occurs late and most likely affects the legs	*MECP2*	X-linked dominant
Subacute necrotizing encephalomyelopathy			
Leigh syndrome	Dystonia, chorea, ataxia , unlikely to be found in isolation	Many	Mitochondrial or recessive
Onset between 2 and 10 years of age			
Wilson disease	Uncommon finding, late onset of neurological symptoms	*ATP7B*	Recessive
Friedreich ataxia	Multiple movement disorders following onset of ataxia: postural tremor—	*FXN*	Recessive

(continued)

Table 4.3 (continued)

Disorder (including parallel nomenclatures)	Relationship of dystonia to other features	Gene	Inheritance pattern
	most common, dystonia—common, chorea—unusual		
Ataxia telangiectasia	Dystonia and/or chorea develop in ~90 %, well after ataxia is evident	*ATM*	Recessive
Fucosidosis	Lower extremity dystonia in a single patient	*FUCA1*	Recessive
PKAN, PANK-2 deficiency, neurodegeneration with brain iron accumulation (NBIA) type I	Gait abnormalities, psychomotor decline, chorea, and dystonia. Dystonia is a universal feature, usually generalized with prominent oromandibular dystonia	*PANK2*	Recessive
Juvenile G_{M2} gangliosidosis, Juvenile Tay-Sachs disease	Dystonia and/or chorea are rare and late findings	*HEXA*	Recessive
HDL3, Huntington disease-like 3	Dystonia presents early, often with chorea and ataxia	4p15.3	Recessive
Niemann-Pick C, types I and II	Type I: ataxia and myoclonus are common, dystonia less so Type II: chorea and facial dyskinesias common, dystonia rare	*NPC1*, *HE1*	Recessive
Woodhouse–Sakati syndrome	Cognitive impairment often present in childhood, with later development of other syndromic features. Dystonia and/or chorea are common	*C2orf37*	Recessive
Dystonia-deafness syndrome, Mohr–Tranebjaerg syndrome	Progressive deafness after 2 years of life, later dystonia	*TIMM8A*/*DDP1*	X-linked, mild symptoms in some female carriers
Marsden variant of Leber hereditary optic neuropathy	Dystonia often precedes optic atrophy. Dystonia may be isolated in an individual with familiar Leber alone or Leber plus dystonia.	*MTND1*, *MTND3*, *MTND4*, *MTND6*	Mitochondrial
Onset in adolescence			
SCA3, Machado–Joseph disease type 1	Usually follows ataxia, but dystonia may rarely be the presenting feature	*ATXN3*	Dominant with anticipation. Reduced penetrance in intermediate copy no
SCA7	Possible dystonia and/or chorea after ataxia presents, retinal degeneration and	*ATXN7*	Dominant with anticipation

(continued)

Table 4.3 (continued)

Disorder (including parallel nomenclatures)	Relationship of dystonia to other features	Gene	Inheritance pattern
	optic atrophy, bulbar palsies, and dementia. Highly variable between and within families Onset is usually in mid-life, as early as late-teens		
SCA17	Focal dystonia is the presenting symptom in rare kindreds. Typically dystonia, chorea follow ataxia, dysphagia, and/or psychiatric symptoms	*TBP*	Dominant with anticipation, reduced penetrance in intermediate copy no
Huntington disease	Dystonia is common, Younger ages are more likely to manifest as the Westphal variant of HD, with hypokinetic rigidity instead of chorea	*IT-15*	Dominant with anticipation, reduced penetrance in intermediate copy no
Neuroferrinopathy, NBIA3	Present with chorea > focal limb dystonia > parkinsonism. Typical onset 20s–30s, (some teens)	*FTL*	Dominant
PARK9, Pallidopyramidal degeneration with supranuclear upgaze paresis and dementia, Kufor-Rakeb syndrome	Parkinsonism primary, rapidly progressive, frequently develop moderate dystonia and/or myoclonus	*ATP13A2*	Recessive
PARK2	Focal dystonias, especially in feet, follow onset of parkinsonism	*PRKN*	Recessive
Choreoacanthocytosis	Chorea is near universal; dystonia, tics, and parkinsonism are less common. Onset is usually in the 20–40s	*VPS13A chorein*	Recessive, rare reports of apparent dominant inheritance

disease (PD) and inherited forms of PD may be complicated by dystonia (see Chap. 3). Mutations in parkin (*PRKN*) produce early-onset PD and are substantially more likely to produce concurrent dystonia than other forms of PD. Patients with Huntington disease will frequently have dystonia in parallel with chorea and other movement disorders (see Chap. 2). In summary, while a few hereditary degenerative conditions can produce dystonia in adults, these rare syndromes virtually never present with dystonia in isolation (Table 4.3).

4.4.1 *Diagnosis*

The assessment of heredodegenerative dystonia can be extensive. Laboratory evaluations and brain imaging are typically obtained and can include:

- CT or MRI of brain (basal ganglia calcifications or necrosis and other abnormalities)
- Muscle or peripheral nerve biopsy
- Renal and liver function tests
- Antinuclear antibodies
- Ceruloplasmin, serum copper, and 24-hour urinary copper (for Wilson disease)
- Erythrocyte sedimentation rate

4.4.2 *Treatment and Management*

Complex, idiosyncratic, and beyond the scope of this text.

4.4.3 *Genetic Counseling Issues*

Most of the neurological diseases detailed in this text have an exclusively adult-onset presentation. In contrast, there are categories of dystonia, such as heredodegenerative dystonias, where that pattern is reversed. Pediatric neurologists are often the first to diagnose cases of childhood- and adolescent-onset heredodegenerative dystonias. Genetic counselors working in neurogenetics should communicate with pediatric neurology practices or ensure that pediatric neurologists are working closely with departments of genetics (pediatric or general) for appropriate referrals related to genetic testing, return of results and management of the patients and their families.

At times, children may be referred to adult neurologists who specialize in dystonia. Genetic counselors working in adult neurology can provide patients and families the opportunity for questions, anticipatory guidance, information about recurrence risk, and genetic confirmation of diagnosis that was not available at the time of clinical diagnosis. Large academic centers may have additional specialist care available for many individuals and families with heredodegenerative dystonias. This type of referral can provide immense support to patients and families.

4.5 The Paroxysmal Dyskinesias, Which Include Dystonia

Dyskinesias are simply abnormal movements. In practice, this term refers to conditions that have a mixture of movement disorders, often in a shifting pattern. Dystonic and myoclonic (quick, jerky) movements may be combined in one episode, only to be

Table 4.4 Paroxysmal dyskinesias

Designation	Dystonia type	Inheritance	Penetrance	Gene locus	Gene/ product
DYT8	Paroxysmal nonkinesigenic dyskinesia	AD		2q35	*MR-1*
DYT9/18	Paroxysmal exercise-induced dyskinesia	AD	Slightly reduced	1p34	*SLC2A1/ GLUT1/*
DYT10	Paroxysmal kinesigenic choreoathetosis	AD		16p11.2	*PRRT2*
DYT19	Paroxysmal kinesigenic choreoathetosis	AD		16q13–q22.1	Unknown
DYT20	Paroxysmal nonkinesigenic dyskinesia	AD		2q31	Unknown

followed by a predominantly choreiform or tremulous episode (slower, flowing movements that may be dance-like). Paroxysmal dyskinesias are, therefore, episodes of mixed movement disorders, often including dystonia, that start and stop rapidly, and occur relatively briefly with periods of normal movement between. There are three subtypes, each dominantly inherited with readily available gene testing, but distinct in their manner of presentation, prognosis, and comorbidities [23].

4.5.1 Clinical Presentation

Paroxysmal kinesigenic dyskinesia (PKD, aka DYT10):

PKD is the most frequently encountered of the three paroxysmal dyskinesias. The most important distinguishing features are the triggers, frequency, and duration of attacks. Attacks are elicited by sudden movement, the plan to move, startle, flashing lights, yawning, and talking, and are exacerbated by fatigue, stress, extremes temperature, and menstruation. Patients typically give a clear report of their triggers. Episodes last only a few seconds to a few minutes, and very rarely longer than 5 minutes. In most patients, attacks occur daily, and may occur several times per hour. Attacks may be preceded by tingling, feelings of "wrongness," fatigue, or muscle tension in the affected limbs. PKD primarily affects the extremities, often asymmetrically, but can affect the face and trunk to a lesser degree. PKD is typically highly responsive to treatment, with ~90 % improving with low dose anticonvulsants. Onset may occur between infancy and the fourth decade of life, with mean onset at 8 years.

Paroxysmal non-kinesigenic dyskinesia (PNKD, aka DYT8):

The episodes of PNKD occur much less frequently (rarely more than once per day and often only 2–3 times per month), but last much longer than those in PKD (from tens of minutes to several hours, with rare cases lasting days). Unlike PKD, where attacks are likely to be unilateral or at least asymmetrical, PNKD attacks are more commonly bilateral. They may occur spontaneously, but are typically elicited by excitement, fatigue, stress or anxiety, illness, fasting, extreme temperature, and consumption of alcohol, caffeine, or chocolate. Attacks often begin with premonitory tingling, muscle cramping, sweating, diplopia, flushing, or dizziness. Typically PNKD will onset before 5 years, but cases of mid-life onset have been reported. Medications are generally ineffective, though rare improvement with benzodiazepines and levetiracetam have been reported.

Paroxysmal exertional dyskinesia (PED, aka DYT9):

PED is unusual among the paroxysmal dyskinesias in that attacks occur only after prolonged exercise (usually 5–15 minutes) and often involve only the body part that has been exercised. The legs are the most commonly affected site, but involvement of the face, arms or trunk is not rare. Symptoms are typically asymmetrical and may be unilateral, with hemidystonia a common presentation. There are no premonitory sensations. Episodes last for a few minutes, typically longer than PKD but shorter than PNKD. However, episodes lasting only a few seconds have been reported. Cessation of exercise at onset shortens attacks, which then typically resolve within 10 minutes. PED attacks occur 1–4 times per month, but increase with the individual's baseline level of exercise. In childhood, it is associated with primary generalized epilepsy or absence epilepsy, and in some cases with mild cognitive impairment. Historically PED was thought to always onset in childhood, but the growing number of cases of adult-onset dystonia associated with milder mutations suggests that the clinical spectrum extends into adulthood. Treatment with medications has only limited success (carbamazepine, levodopa, and gabapentin have been reported). Patients treated with the ketogenic diet typically have good responses for both their epilepsy and their dyskinesia.

4.5.2 Diagnosis

The paroxysmal dyskinesias are clinical diagnoses; genetic testing is useful for confirmation and for counseling regarding prognosis and heritability. PED diagnosis is typically confirmed with a lumbar puncture to compare blood and cerebrospinal fluid glucose levels. If lumbar puncture is inconclusive, radioactive glucose uptake by *in vitro* red blood cells can also be used to confirm diagnosis.

4.5.3 Treatment and Management

Low dose anticonvulsant medications are effective in PKD. Most symptoms improve in the third to fourth decade. Symptoms in PNKD are often reduced, but not eliminated, by avoiding triggers. PED symptoms may completely resolve with the ketogenic diet, but typically are only reduced. Because symptoms are paroxysmal in nature, neither botox nor surgical interventions are good alternative treatments.

4.5.4 Genetics

DYT10 (*PRRT2*)

The inheritance of PKD is autosomal dominant. The gene *PRRT2* is causative in half of cases, with penetrance of ~95 % [24]. Cases caused by *PRRT2* mutations frequently co-occur with benign infantile convulsions, benign infantile chorea, and familial hemiplegic migraine. Within affected families, individuals frequently share some but not all of these conditions, and may not recognize these diverse disorders as following a heritable pattern.

DYT8 (*MR-1*)

PNKD is caused by mutations of the *MR-1* gene (myofibrillogenesis regulator 1), which is inherited in an autosomal dominant pattern with ~90 % penetrance [25]. However, expression within and between families is variable. While *MR-1* mutations are the only recognized cause of PNKD, rare families meeting clinical diagnostic criteria have been identified who do not have mutations in *PNKD*. These families often lack the typical precipitating features seen in classic PNKD. There are no recognized co-varying neurologic conditions, unlike the other two types of paroxysmal dyskinesia.

DYT9 (*SLC2A1*)

PED is caused by mutations in *SLC2A1*, which encodes the brain-specific glucose transporter GLUT1. All symptomatic *SLC2A1* mutations are thought to reduce the amount of cerebral glucose available for neuronal function; thus, dyskinesias are thought to result from transient exhaustion of glucose stores within the striatum [26]. More disruptive mutations lead to a generalized cerebral energy deficit, and produce an intractable epilepsy in infancy and a secondary, progressive microcephaly. *SLCA2A1* mutations are inherited in a dominant pattern, though marginally disruptive mutations that are sufficient to cause PED may couple with other seemingly benign mutations in a compound heterozygous state to produce the more severe end of the phenotypic spectrum. If clinical suspicion is high and gene sequencing is negative, tertiary diagnostic assays such as red blood cell glucose transport may be helpful.

4.5.5 Genetic Counseling Issues

For people with paroxysmal dyskinesias, the diagnostic journey may include misdiagnoses such as a functional neurological (conversion) disorder or a psychological disorder. Patients can experience relief, vindication and peace if genetic testing reveals a cause for their symptoms. Alternatively, people who are clinically diagnosed with paroxysmal dyskinesias whose gene testing is normal must be reminded that the known genes for PKD explain only half of cases, and PNKD and PED cases without gene mutations have also been reported. Even so, these patients hoping to be vindicated by a genetic test might experience disappointment if the testing is negative. Normalizing these experiences can greatly improve a patient's communication and involvement in decision-making.

Paroxysmal dyskinesias can be difficult to diagnose, but because of effective treatment options and behavioral modifications, genetic confirmation of diagnosis and subsequent recurrence risk for family members have the ability to improve quality of life.

4.6 Patient Resources

General Dystonia/Movement Disorders

Dystonia Medical Research Foundation
One East Wacker Drive, Suite 2810
Chicago, IL, 60601-1905
Tel: (800) 377-3978
Fax: (312) 803-0138
E-mail: dystonia@dystonia-foundation.org
Web site: http://www.dystonia-foundation.org/
Medline Plus
Compilation Resource Site
Web site: http://www.nlm.nih.gov/medlineplus/dystonia.html
The Bachmann-Strauss Dystonia & Parkinson Foundation, Inc.
Fred French Building
551 Fifth Ave (at 45th St.), Suite 520
New York, NY 10176
Tel: (212) 682-9900
Web site: http://www.dystonia-parkinsons.org/index.cfm?fuseaction=home.viewPage&page_id=1
National Institute of Neurological Disorders and Stroke
Neurological Institute
P.O. Box 5801
Bethesda, MD 20824
Tel: (800) 352-9424
Fax: (301) 496-5751
Web site: www.ninds.nih.gov/disorders/dystonias/dystonias.htm

Blepharospasm

Benign Essential Blepharospasm Research Foundation, Inc.
PO Box 12468
Beaumont, TX 77726-2468
Tel: (409) 832-0788
Fax: (409) 832-0890
E-mail: bebrf@belpharospasm.org
Web site: http://www.blepharospasm.org/

Spasmodic Dysphonia/Laryngeal Dystonia

National Spasmodic Dysphonia Association
300 Park Boulevard, Suite 415
Itasca, IL 60143
Tel: (800) 795-6732
Fax: (630) 250-4505
E-mail: NSDA@dysphonia.org
Web site: http://www.dysphonia.org
American Speech Language and Hearing Association (ASHA)
2200 Research Boulevard
Rockville, MD 20850-3289
Tel: (800) 638-8255
Fax: (301) 296-8580
E-mail: actioncenter@asha.org
Web site: http://www.asha.org/public/speech/disorders/spasmodicdysphonia.htm
National Institute on Deafness and Other Communication Disorders (NIDCD)
31 Center Drive, MSC 2320
Bethesda, MD 20892-2320
E-mail: nidcdinfo@nidcd.nil.gov
Web site: http://www.nidcd.nih.gov/health/voice/pages/spasdysp.aspx#2

Spasmodic Torticollis/Cervical Dystonia

National Spasmodic Torticollis Association
9920 Talbert Avenue
Fountain Valley, CA 92708
Tel: 800-487-8385
E-mail: nstamail@aol.com
Web site: http://www.torticollis.org
Spasmodic Torticollis/Dystonia, Inc.
P.O. Box 28
Mukwonago, WI 53149
Tel: (888) 445-4588
E-mail: info@spasmodictorticollis.org
Web site: http://www.spasmodictorticollis.org

References

1. Fuchs, T., & Ozelius, L. J. (2011). Genetics of dystonia. *Seminars in Neurology, 31*(5), 441–448.
2. Fuchs, T., Saunders-Pullman, R., Masuho, I., Luciano, M. S., Raymond, D., Factor, S., et al. (2013). Mutations in GNAL cause primary torsion dystonia. *Nature Genetics, 45*(1), 88–92.

3. Bressman, S. B., Sabatti, C., Raymond, D., de Leon, D., Klein, C., Kramer, P. L., et al. (2000). The DYT1 phenotype and guidelines for diagnostic testing. *Neurology, 54*(9), 1746–1752.
4. Markun, L. C., Starr, P. A., Air, E. L., Marks, W. J., Jr., Volz, M. M., & Ostrem, J. L. (2012). Shorter disease duration correlates with improved long-term deep brain stimulation outcomes in young-onset DYT1 dystonia. *Neurosurgery, 71*(2), 325–330.
5. Panov, F., Gologorsky, Y., Connors, G., Tagliati, M., Miravite, J., & Alterman, R. L. (2013). Deep brain stimulation in DYT1 dystonia: A 10-year experience. *Neurosurgery, 73*(1), 86–93. discussion 93.
6. Risch, N. J., Bressman, S. B., Senthil, G., & Ozelius, L. J. (2007). Intragenic *cis* and *trans* modification of genetic susceptibility in DYT1 torsion dystonia. *The American Journal of Human Genetics, 80*(6), 1188–1193.
7. Lee, L. V., Munoz, E. L., Tan, K. T., & Reyes, M. T. (2001). Sex linked recessive dystonia parkinsonism of Panay, Philippines (XDP). *Molecular Pathology, 54*(6), 362–368.
8. Evidente, V. G., Advincula, J., Esteban, R., Pasco, P., Alfon, J. A., Natividad, F. F., et al. (2002). Phenomenology of "Lubag" or X-linked dystonia-parkinsonism. *Movement Disorders, 17*(6), 1271–1279.
9. Brashear, A., Dobyns, W. B., de Carvalho Aguiar, P., Borg, M., Frijns, C. J., Gollamudi, S., et al. (2007). The phenotypic spectrum of rapid-onset dystonia-parkinsonism (RDP) and mutations in the ATP1A3 gene. *Brain, 130*(Pt 3), 828–835.
10. Raymond, D., Saunders-Pullman, R., de Carvalho, A. P., Schule, B., Kock, N., Friedman, J., et al. (2008). Phenotypic spectrum and sex effects in eleven myoclonus-dystonia families with epsilon-sarcoglycan mutations. *Movement Disorders, 23*(4), 588–592.
11. Camargos, S., Lees, A. J., Singleton, A., & Cardoso, F. (2012). DYT16: The original cases. *Journal of Neurology, Neurosurgery & Psychiatry, 83*(10), 1012–1014.
12. Nolte, D., Niemann, S., & Muller, U. (2003). Specific sequence changes in multiple transcript system DYT3 are associated with X-linked dystonia parkinsonism. *Proceedings of the National Academy of Sciences of the United States of America, 100*(18), 10347–10352.
13. Makino, S., Kaji, R., Ando, S., Tomizawa, M., Yasuno, K., Goto, S., et al. (2007). Reduced neuron-specific expression of the TAF1 gene is associated with X-linked dystonia-parkinsonism. *The American Journal of Human Genetics, 80*(3), 393–406.
14. Furukawa, Y. (2013). GTP Cyclohydrolase 1-deficient dopa-responsive dystonia [online]. Retrieved December 6, 2013, from http://www.ncbi.nlm.nih.gov/books/NBK1508/
15. Muller, B., Hedrich, K., Kock, N., Dragasevic, N., Svetel, M., Garrels, J., et al. (2002). Evidence that paternal expression of the epsilon-sarcoglycan gene accounts for reduced penetrance in myoclonus-dystonia. *The American Journal of Human Genetics, 71*(6), 1303–1311.
16. Grabowski, M., Zimprich, A., Lorenz-Depiereux, B., Kalscheuer, V., Asmus, F., Gasser, T., et al. (2003). The epsilon-sarcoglycan gene (SGCE), mutated in myoclonus-dystonia syndrome, is maternally imprinted. *European Journal of Human Genetics, 11*(2), 138–144.
17. Foncke, E. M., Gerrits, M. C., van Ruissen, F., Baas, F., Hedrich, K., Tijssen, C. C., et al. (2006). Distal myoclonus and late onset in a large Dutch family with myoclonus-dystonia. *Neurology, 67*(9), 1677–1680.
18. Caviness, J. N., & Brown, P. (2004). Myoclonus: Current concepts and recent advances. *Lancet Neurology, 3*(10), 598–607.
19. Valente, E. M., Edwards, M. J., Mir, P., DiGiorgio, A., Salvi, S., Davis, M., et al. (2005). The epsilon-sarcoglycan gene in myoclonic syndromes. *Neurology, 64*(4), 737–739.
20. Lyon, G., Kolodny, E. H., & Pastores, G. M. (2006). *Neurology of hereditary metabolic diseases of children*. New York, NY: McGraw-Hill.
21. Schneider, S. A., & Bhatia, K. P. (2010). Rare causes of dystonia parkinsonism. *Current Neurology and Neuroscience Reports, 10*(6), 431–439.
22. Phukan, J., Albanese, A., Gasser, T., & Warner, T. (2011). Primary dystonia and dystonia-plus syndromes: Clinical characteristics, diagnosis, and pathogenesis. *Lancet Neurology, 10*(12), 1074–1085.

23. Bhatia, K. P. (2011). Paroxysmal dyskinesias. *Movement Disorders, 26*(6), 1157–1165.
24. Gardiner, A. R., Bhatia, K. P., Stamelou, M., Dale, R. C., Kurian, M. A., Schneider, S. A., et al. (2012). PRRT2 gene mutations: from paroxysmal dyskinesia to episodic ataxia and hemiplegic migraine. *Neurology, 79*(21), 2115–2121.
25. Lee, H. Y., Xu, Y., Huang, Y., Ahn, A. H., Auburger, G. W., Pandolfo, M., et al. (2004). The gene for paroxysmal non-kinesigenic dyskinesia encodes an enzyme in a stress response pathway. *Human Molecular Genetics, 13*(24), 3161–3170.
26. Suls, A., Dedeken, P., Goffin, K., Van Esch, H., Dupont, P., Cassiman, D., et al. (2007). Paroxysmal exercise-induced dyskinesia and epilepsy is due to mutations in SLC2A1, encoding the glucose transporter GLUT1. *Brain, 131*(Pt. 7), 1831–1844.

Chapter 5
Ataxia

Alison La Pean Kirschner and Jill S. Goldman

The hereditary ataxias are a complex, heterogeneous group of neurological disorders, diverse in age of onset, clinical characteristics, inheritance patterns, and pathogenic mutations. The hallmark features present in most subtypes are a slowly progressive disease course, unsteady gait with uncoordinated movements (ataxia), and dysarthria. These characteristics are usually caused by dysfunctions of the cerebellum or other parts of the central nervous system. Exact data on prevalence of the inherited ataxias does not exist, and each subtype is individually rare; however total prevalence estimates range from 4 to 9/100,000, and much higher estimates have been reported in geographically isolated areas due to founder effects [1–4]. The most common types of hereditary ataxias are the spinocerebellar ataxias (SCAs or autosomal dominant cerebellar ataxias, ADSCAs), episodic ataxias (EAs), Dentatorubral-Pallidoluysian Atrophy (DRPLA), early-onset ataxia with oculomotor apraxia and hypoalbuminemia (EAOH), Friedreich ataxia (FRDA), ataxia with vitamin E deficiency (AVED), ataxia telangiectasia (A-T), and Fragile X Tremor Ataxia Syndrome (FXTAS) [5]. Other genetic syndromes include combinations of ataxia and epilepsy, chorea, dementia, impaired metabolism, or mitochondrial disease. This chapter will focus on the SCAs, FRDA, and FXTAS.

Electronic supplementary material Supplementary material is available in the online version of this chapter at 10.1007/978-1-4899-7482-2_5. Videos can also be accessed at http://www.springerimages.com/videos/978-1-4899-7481-5.

A.L.P. Kirschner (✉)
Department of Neurology, Center for Patient Care and Outcomes Research (PCOR), Medical College of Wisconsin, 8701 Watertown Plank Rd., Rm H3155, Milwaukee, WI 53226, USA
e-mail: alapean@mcw.edu

J.S. Goldman
Taub Institute, Columbia University Medical Center, 630W. 168th St., Box 16, New York, NY 10032, USA
e-mail: jg2673@cumc.columbia.edu

J.S. Goldman (ed.), *Genetic Counseling for Adult Neurogenetic Disease*,
DOI 10.1007/978-1-4899-7482-2_5

5.1 Clinical Presentation

(Ataxia video clip Part 1)

5.1.1 *SCAs*

The hereditary SCAs are a clinically heterogeneous group of disorders, presenting with a diverse combination of symptoms (Table 5.1). However, they all share a hallmark progressive cerebellar syndrome as the fundamental phenotype. Symptoms include cerebellar gait and limb ataxia (unsteady, clumsy, wide-based gait, or dysmetria), dysarthria (impaired or slurred speech), and abnormal oculomotor control (diplopia, oscillopsia, or opthalmoplegia) caused by atrophy of the cerebellum and brainstem [5, 6]. Subtypes of SCAs may also present with a host of additional complex multisystem neurological deficits including pyramidal signs (hyper- or hyporeflexia, muscle weakness, spasticity), extrapyramidal features (involuntary movements, parkinsonism, dystonia, myoclonus, rigidity, tremor, chorea), impairment of the peripheral nervous system (most commonly peripheral sensory/sensorimotor axonal neuropathy), motor neuron disease, dysphagia, nystagmus, hearing loss, visual loss, cognitive and behavioral impairment, and seizures/epilepsy [5–7].

Although variability of age of onset from infancy to late life exists, most dominantly inherited SCAs have an age of onset between 30 and 40 years [7–10]. The most common early symptoms of SCA are gait difficulty (approximately 2/3 of patients), followed by double vision, dysarthria, impaired hand writing, and episodic vertigo [11]. In general, the SCAs are slowly progressive and lead to gradual balance and walking problems and increasing impairments in speech and swallowing. Most individuals with ataxia will require the use of walking aids, and will eventually become wheelchair bound [12]. While life span may or may not be shortened, affected individuals may experience a series of declines and plateaus in symptom progression over years or decades (typically 10–30 years) [5, 10].

5.1.2 *FRDA*

FRDA is a heterogeneous neurodegenerative disorder with clinical features of progressive ataxia, weakness, decreased sensation due to axonal neuropathy, absent reflexes in the lower extremities, dysarthria, and onset typically between 10 and 15 years of age (usually before 25 years of age) [13]. Frequently, affected individuals also experience hypertrophic cardiomyopathy (66 %), scoliosis (~66 %), pes cavus (55 %), optic atrophy (25 %), hearing loss (13 %), and glucose intolerance or diabetes mellitus (30 %) [14, 15]. FRDA may also present in an "atypical" manner

Table 5.1 Molecular genetics and clinical features of hereditary ataxias

Disease Name	Inheritance	Gene symbol or chromosomal locus	Type of mutation	Other possible symptoms in addition to cerebellar ataxia
SCA1	AD	*ATXN1*	CAG repeat	Early swallowing and respiratory signs, hyperreflexia (gait spasticity), ophthalmoparesis, chorea, ALS-like disorders; peripheral axonal neuropathy; severe disease progression
SCA2	AD	*ATXN2*	CAG repeat	Slow eye movements (slow ocular saccades); peripheral axonal neuropathy; <DTRs; verbal memory loss, executive dysfunction; severely affected pons on MRI; parkinsonism (tremor, rigidity, bradykinesia), myoclonus, chorea, dementia
SCA3	AD	*ATXN3 (*aka *MJD)*	CAG repeat	Diplopia, dystonia, nystagmus, slow eye movements; axonal neuropathy; spasticity; parkinsonism
SCA4	AD	16q22.1	–	Sensory axonal neuropathy, deafness
SCA5	AD	*SPTBN2*	Missense, in-frame deletion	Early onset, slow course, downbeat nystagmus, tremor; "pure" ataxia syndrome
SCA6	AD	*CACNA1A*	CAG repeat	Episodic ataxia, slow progression, late-onset; "pure" ataxia syndrome; downbeat nystagmus; global atrophy of the cerebellar vermis and hemispheric cerebellar atrophy on MRI
SCA7	AD	*ATXN7*	CAG repeat	Visual loss (pigmentary macular degeneration, retinopathy); dementia
SCA8	AD	*ATXN8/ ATXN8OS*	CAG·CTG (Intron)	Slowly progressive, ~brisk DTRs, <vibration sense; rare cognitive impairment; aspiration; tremor
SCA9	AD	–	–	Ophthalmoplegia, dysarthria, pyramidal tract signs, weakness, extrapyramidal signs, posterior column signs; parkinsonism
SCA10	AD	*ATXN10*	ATTCT repeat (Intron)	Seizures/epilepsy, EEG abnormalities, mood disorders, pyramidal tract signs, sensorimotor polyneuropathy
SCA11	AD	*TTBK2*	Frameshift	Milder course, remain ambulatory; "pure" ataxia syndrome

(continued)

Table 5.1 (continued)

Disease Name	Inheritance	Gene symbol or chromosomal locus	Type of mutation	Other possible symptoms in addition to cerebellar ataxia
SCA12	AD	*PPP2R2B*	CAG repeat (Intron)	Action tremor in head and hands; hyperreflexia; subtle parkinsonism; cognitive/psychiatric disorders, dementia
SCA13	AD	*KCNC3*	Missense	Mild mental retardation, delayed motor milestones, short stature, early/childhood onset
SCA14	AD	*PRKCG*	Missense	Axial myoclonus or dystonia, slow eye movements, hyperreflexia
SCA15	AD	*ITPR1*	Large deletion of the 5′ area	Allelic to SCA29; "pure" ataxia syndrome, very slow progression; head and hand tremor
SCA16	n/a	n/a	n/a	(See SCA15; original family misidentified)
SCA17	AD	*TBP*	CAA/CAG repeat mutation	Dementia (cognitive and/or behavioral impairment), spasticity, chorea, dystonia, epilepsy/seizures
SCA18	AD	7q22–q32	–	Sensory/motor neuropathy, nystagmus, <DTRs
SCA19/22	AD	*KCND3*	Missense, small deletion	Slowly progressive, rare cognitive impairment (frontal executive dysfunction), myoclonus, hyperreflexia, tremor
SCA20	AD	11q12.2–11q12.3	260-kb duplication	Early dysarthria, palatal tremor, spasmodic dysphonia, hyperreflexia, bradykinesia
SCA21	AD	–	–	Mild cognitive impairment
SCA23	AD	*PDYN*	Missense	Dysarthria, abnormal eye movements, <vibration and position sense
SCA24 (now SCAR4)	AR	1p36	–	Myoclonic jerks, fasciculations, impaired joint position sense, mild pes cavus, axonal sensorineural peripheral neuropathy
SCA25	AD	*SCA25*	–	Sensory axonal neuropathy
SCA26	AD	*EEF2*	Missense	Dysarthria, irregular visual pursuits, "pure" ataxia syndrome
SCA27	AD	*FGF14*	Missense, frameshift	Early-onset hand tremor; dyskinesia, cognitive deficits; mild axonal sensory neuropathy
SCA28	AD	*AFG3L2*	Missense	Nystagmus, ophthalmoparesis, ptosis, >tendon reflexes

(continued)

Table 5.1 (continued)

Disease Name	Inheritance	Gene symbol or chromosomal locus	Type of mutation	Other possible symptoms in addition to cerebellar ataxia
SCA29	AD	*ITPR1*	Missense	Allelic to SCA15: cognitive deficits, early age of onset
SCA30	AD	4q34.3–q35.1	–	Hyperreflexia
SCA31	AD	*BEAN1*	TGGAA repeat (Intron)	Normal sensation, pure cerebellar ataxia, hearing loss
SCA32	AD	7q32-q33	–	Variable mental impairment, azoospermia and testicular atrophy in males
SCA34	AD	6p12.3–q16.2	–	Neurocutaneous syndrome with papulosquamous erythematous ichthyosiform plaques, skin lesions disappear in early adulthood, but may reappear; classic ataxia symptoms appear later on in life
SCA35	AD	*TGM6*	Missense	Hyperreflexia, Babinski responses, cervical dystonia
SCA36	AD	*NOP56*	GGCCTG repeat (Intron)	Muscle fasiculations, tongue atrophy, hyperreflexia, motor neuron involvement
DRPLA	AD	*ATN1*	CAG repeat	Epilepsy/seizures, parkinsonism, chorea, myoclonus, dementia, other cognitive and/or behavioral impairment
FRDA	AR	*FXN/frataxin*	GAA repeat (intron); 2–4 % due to point mutations	Cardiomyopathy, hyporeflexia, Babinski responses, sensory loss; diagnosis usually in childhood before age 25
A-T	AR	*ATM*	Truncating and missense	Telangiectasia, immune deficiency, predisposition to malignancy (lymphocytic leukemia usually T-cell type, lymphoma of B-cell type, stomach mucinous adenocarcinoma), chromosomal instability, >alpha-fetoprotein; >relative risk (2.3–6.1) for malignancy in heterozygous carriers, particularly breast cancer in women
AVED	AR	*TTPA*	Frameshift, truncating, other point mutations	Similar to FRDA, head titubation, reduced plasma vitamin E concentration
FXTAS	X-linked	*FMR1*	CGG repeat	Tremor, neuropathy, parkinsonism, myoclonus, autonomic dysfunction, cognitive/psychiatric dysfunction, sleep disorder, loss of smell

(25 % of cases), either in symptomology with retained reflexes and lower incidence of cardiac involvement, or with a late age of onset from 26 years to greater than 40 years [16–19]. More rarely, affected individuals may present with spastic paraparesis, pure sensory ataxia, or chorea in the absence of cerebellar signs (though these patients may develop ataxia later in the disease course) [20–22].

Disease progression in FRDA is widely variable, but patients tend to steadily progress to wheelchair dependence in approximately 10 years after onset of symptoms [14, 23]. Patients often experience muscle weakness and atrophy, and develop cardiomyopathy as disease progresses. Life expectancy may be shortened (more often in patients with cardiomyopathy) to the mid-30s, but more recent reports document patients living into their 60s and 70s. In FRDA, age at diagnosis, which may incorporate other genetic and environmental factors, was found to be more important than GAA length in predicting development of cardiomyopathy, scoliosis, and disease progression [23].

5.1.3 FXTAS

FXTAS is due to the presence of a premutation (55–200 CGG repeats) in the *FMR1* gene. It typically presents between the ages of 60 and 65 years (range: early 50s–70s) with action tremor and ataxia. However, symptoms are variable so that tremor can be absent or mild and other symptoms (neuropathy, parkinsonism, myoclonus, autonomic problems, loss of smell, sleep issues) may be present. Additionally, psychiatric problems such as depression and irritability, and cognitive decline (especially in memory and executive function) are common. Psychiatric and cognitive problems may, in fact, precede the movement disorder by decades [24, 25]. Until recently, FXTAS was thought to occur only in male *FMR1* premutation carriers; however, female carriers are also at risk for the syndrome. Their symptoms tend to be later onset and milder than those of male premutation carriers. They are also at lower risk for cognitive impairment [25]. A childhood history of learning disabilities or ADHD may be present. The hallmark neuropathological finding is intraneuronal inclusions [24].

5.2 Diagnosis

The high phenotypic variability and overlap of clinical characteristics among hereditary ataxia subtypes, even within families, makes diagnosis based solely on clinical examination nearly impossible [7, 17, 26]. In addition to a thorough clinical neurological examination, it is important to exclude the most common nonhereditary/sporadic or acquired ataxias; therefore, skilled pedigree elicitation of at least three generations and risk assessment are essential in diagnosing ataxia patients [27]. Several other diagnostic tests, such as MRI, EMG/NCS, echocardiogram (ECG/EKG), and laboratory blood tests for vitamin deficiencies and glucose levels, may prove useful. Additional assessments for swallowing, speech, auditory, ophthalmologic, and neuropsychiatric problems can also be helpful. For FXTAS, MRI can be a powerful diagnostic tool. Cerebellar atrophy with hyperintensity of the middle cerebellar peduncle on T2 Flair and other white matter hyperintensities are commonly found [24].

The most useful clinical tool for diagnosing hereditary ataxias is genetic testing. Clinical genetic testing is available for many inherited ataxias, including 25 of the 39 condition presented in Table 5.1. Due to the clinical overlap in symptoms between subtypes and within families, several genetic testing companies offer testing for hereditary ataxias in comprehensive panels, usually based on mode of inheritance or disease prevalence. Diagnosis and interpretation is based on presence of one or two pathogenic variants (based on mode of inheritance), and each of the ataxias caused by repeat expansions have their own normal, borderline, and pathogenic ranges associated with their respective conditions. It should be noted that at the present time, genetic testing with comprehensive panels is very expensive and may not be covered by insurance.

5.3 Treatment and Management

As with many inherited neurological conditions, no curative treatment currently exist, and therefore, clinical management for the SCAs, FRDA, and FXTAS remains symptomatic and supportive. The exception is AVED, which is responsive to high dose vitamin E treatment. Secondary disease manifestations in FRDA, such as cardiomyopathy, can be managed with anti-arrhythmic drugs, anticoagulants, and cardiac pacemaker or defibrillator implants. Diabetes can be managed through diet, appropriate exercise, and insulin when necessary. SCA patients with parkinsonian symptoms may benefit from amantadine/levodopa/dopamine agonists, baclofen/tizanidine/botulinum toxin for spasticity, or possibly deep brain stimulation for tremor [7]. All patients with ataxia can benefit from physical, occupational, and speech therapies, particularly including education about fall prevention. Falls are associated with both psychological and physical consequences, and are a high comorbidity for ataxias [28, 29]. Most patients with ataxia will benefit from the use of assistive ambulation devices and regular swallowing assessments to prevent choking and aspiration. Similarly psychological counseling may help to deal with the myriad of physical, social, and psychological challenges of these degenerative conditions.

Several potential therapies are under investigation for FRDA and the SCAs, including Coenzyme Q10 and vitamin E, Idebenone, lithium, acetyl-DL-leucine (Tanganil), and some have shown modest, statistical significant in clinical trials [30–33]. However, larger clinical trials with cohorts exhibiting greater and more consistent clinical efficacy are required before widespread recommendations will likely be made about their use for treating hereditary ataxias.

5.4 Genetics

5.4.1 SCAs

The prevalence of hereditary SCA is generally reported to be between 1 and 4/100,000, accounting for 25–89 % (most likely ~66 %) of all hereditary ataxias [1, 3, 4, 8, 9]. SCA3 is the most common inherited SCA, followed by SCA1, SCA2, SCA6, and SCA7 [6, 7, 9, 34]. The vast majority of SCAs are inherited in an autosomal dominant manner. They are caused by several types of genetic mutations (Table 5.1), including tri-, penta-, or hexa-nucleotide repeat expansions (SCA1, SCA2, SCA3, SCA6, SCA7, SCA8, SCA10, SCA12, SCA17, SCA31, SCA36), missense and frameshift point mutations (SCA5, SCA11, SCA13, SCA14, SCA19/22, SCA23, SCA26, SCA27, SCA28, SCA29, SCA35), deletions (SCA5, SCA15, SCA19/22), and duplications (SCA20). The majority of these mutations occur in the coding region of their associated genes (exonic mutations), though some are intronic (noncoding) regions (SCA8, SCA10, SCA12, SCA31, SCA36) [5, 8].

A few clinical symptoms show genotype–phenotype correlations with a specific subtype of SCA [17]. Several, such as SCA7, present with visual acuity problems. SCA17 can present with chorea and overlap HD. In SCAs that are due to repeat expansions, the length of the expansion has been reported to inversely correlate with the age of disease onset (though repeat length cannot be used to predict age of onset) [8, 17, 35]. In certain SCAs, repeat length may also inversely correlate with disease progression and severity [36, 37].

5.4.2 FRDA

FRDA is the most common form of autosomal recessive ataxia, with a reported prevalence between 2 and 4/100,000 [13, 38]. It is caused by a noncoding GAA trinucleotide repeat expansion in intron 1 of the *FXN* (alternate name is *X25*) gene located at chromosome 9q13 that encodes the protein frataxin. A homozygous polyglutamate expansion within this gene is found in approximately 96–98 % of patients [38–41]. The remaining patients carry a GAA expansion on one allele and an inactivating mutation in the coding region of the other allele.

Penetrance in the SCAs and FRDA is thought to be complete, though mode of inheritance, clinical variability, and age of onset (impacted by anticipation, in some cases) may mask the appearance of complete penetrance in some families. Genetic anticipation and mutation transmission instability caused by repeat expansions are hallmark features of the SCAs (aside from SCA6), particularly in the polyglutamine (CAG or CAA) trinucleotide repeat expansion disorders. Anticipation is seen more often in paternal than maternal transmission (particularly in SCA1, SCA2, and SCA7), often resulting from gonadal mosaicism [10]. In instances of anticipation, age of onset becomes earlier with each successive generation. Because FRDA is inherited in an autosomal recessive manner, and in some instances due to one allele with a point mutation, anticipation is not seen in this condition.

5.4.3 FXTAS

FXTAS is due to a premutation in the *FMR1* gene on the X chromosome. A premutation range between 50 and 200 CGG repeats results in a toxic effect of the CGG-repeat mRNA, perhaps by preventing RNA binding proteins from functioning properly [24]. Penetrance of FXTAS is age dependent, with about 40 % in males and about 16 % of females over 50 years of age developing symptoms. Symptoms are generally less severe in women. Female carriers tend to develop less dementia, but more autoimmune problems and hypertension.

5.5 Genetic Counseling Issues

(Ataxia video clip Part 2)

Except for recessive and mitochondrial ataxias that usually have childhood onset, the majority of hereditary ataxias are slowly progressive conditions with onset in mid to late adulthood. Genetic counseling and risk assessment for family members will depend on the patient's specific subtype of ataxia. Even in typically adult onset ataxias, genetic anticipation may lead to childhood onset in offspring of still healthy parents. Determining a diagnosis of SCA in a child with asymptomatic parents may consequently diagnose one of the parents or possibly raise issues of non-paternity.

If a familial pathogenic mutation has been identified, presymptomatic testing of at-risk family members is possible. When presymptomatic testing for an at-risk adult is requested, a protocol including a clinical neurological assessment and appropriate genetic counseling should be followed [42]. Counseling should include discussion about privacy laws (HIPAA) and genetic discrimination legislation (GINA) with particular attention paid to long-term care, disability, and life insurance coverage. Genetic testing of asymptomatic children age (<18 years) for most hereditary ataxias is not considered appropriate, particularly without established effective treatment. Exceptions exist for subtypes where symptomatic intervention may prevent or ameliorate disease progression (i.e., sibs of a proband with AVED).

Hereditary ataxias can have a profound impact on families and family dynamics. For many individuals with SCAs, emotional control can be problematic. Inappropriate social responses, uncontrolled outbursts, and lack of a "filter" when speaking can sometimes be the confusing, first symptoms of disease. Unfortunately, it is rarely recognized as such, particularly when individuals are unaware of the disease in their family. Patients presenting in clinic may already have strained relationships or unstable employment because of the psychiatric symptoms. Genetic counselors

genetic testing of stored DNA samples from her deceased son, Max. Prior to Max's death, he had been evaluated at several medical centers across the country, but none had been able to give the family a specific diagnosis. Mrs. H hoped that another clinical team's review of Max's medical records might result in consideration of alternative diagnoses. It had been approximately 1 year since Max passed away, and it was troubling to the family that they still did not have a genetically confirmed diagnosis of his condition. The family traveled over 2,000 miles to get to the clinic appointment.

At age 8 Max presented to the family's pediatrician with concentration problems and "clumsiness." Upon evaluation, the family's pediatrician found no evidence for concern, and reassured the family that their observations were typical of many 8-year-olds. The doctor attributed the clumsiness to a growth spurt, and assured the family that he would keep an eye out for further signs of "ADHD-like" behavior. After additional complaints and concerns from the family over a 9-month period, Max was referred to a local pediatric neurology clinic for further evaluation. He showed subtle signs of gait ataxia and was followed continuously thereafter by a neurologist. No family history of childhood-onset ataxias, movement disorders, or dementia was noted.

During the time of Max's evaluations, the H's also found out they were pregnant with Ellie. Max's condition continued to progress slowly, and by age 11 Max was found to have progressive ataxia, dysarthria, dysphagia, and cerebellar degeneration on MRI. Though Max's neurologist felt confident that his symptoms fit the diagnosis of childhood onset ataxia, genetic testing for Friedreich ataxia (FRDA) and ataxia telangiectasia (AT) were both negative. At age 12, subsequent genetic testing for a panel of spinocerebellar ataxias (SCAs) was also negative. Max's condition was treated with symptom management and palliative care, and rapidly progressed until he passed away at age 13. Since he never received a genetically confirmed diagnosis before his death, the family requested that tissue, blood, and brain samples be collected on autopsy, and DNA from Max be extracted and stored.

Upon first meeting the family in clinic, it was clear to the genetic counselor that Mrs. H was not only concerned about finding a diagnosis for Max's condition but was also concerned about the potential for her daughters to develop the same problems. Even though Mrs. H reportedly felt that both girls were currently asymptomatic, Lauren was 7½ years old at the appointment, and Max began showing symptoms at age 8. Prior to the formal clinical review and evaluation with the neurogenetics multidisciplinary team, the genetic counselor had Mr. and Mrs. H sign institution-specific consent forms related to the use of their son's specimens. While doing so, the genetic counselor noticed that Mr. H had a moderate hand tremor and slight dysmetria when touching the pen to the signature line.

The genetic counselor decided that, even though a family history had been collected in the past at an outside medical center, it was worth repeating. A very different family history began to emerge from the one included in Max's medical records. Mr. H's father was 78 years old and was in relatively good health. Mr. H's mother died suddenly at age 49 in a car accident during inclement weather, but did not have any known chronic health conditions prior to her death. However, several of Mr. H's maternal cousins (ages 35–69) had mild slurred speech. Two other maternal cousins needed a walking stick because they were "unsteady." Another cousin never lived on his own, even in adulthood, because he just wasn't "savvy enough" to handle his own finances or hold a job for a prolonged period of time. This cousin was not very "active" and seemed "shaky" when he moved around, though he had never undergone a formal medical or psychiatric evaluation for his issues. Most of Mr. H's maternal family members proudly consider this the 'wacky' side of the family. Mr. and Mrs. H continue to describe erratic, impulsive, adventurous (but mostly harmless) behavior in several of the cousins.

Through the conversation, Mr. and Mrs. H became aware of the genetic counselor noting different symptoms and behaviors on the pedigree. They realized that some of these family "quirks" were symptoms they never would have recognized as related to Max's condition. Though they had not previously discussed Mr. H's health, both Mr. and Mrs. H told the genetic counselor that recently they had also begun to notice some "odd" things happening to him, similar to some of the issues seen with Mr. H's cousins. For example, Mr. H had recently asked his cousin where to buy a good walking stick because he had been feeling a little unsteady on his feet. In fact, recently Mr. H had fallen off of a ladder while doing some repair work around the house. Mr. H also reported that he frequently become "tongue-tied" and felt like his head was "cloudy" at work because putting thoughts together was becoming more difficult. Mr. H stated that he felt frustrated and a little embarrassed, like he has been "failing in some way" because it has been taking him longer than usual to complete his work duties. In fact, Mr. and Mrs. H had argued about the increasing amount of time he was spending at work, even though his work load had not increased. Mrs. H also told the genetic counselor that she had felt embarrassed a few weeks ago because Mr. H had yelled loudly at a waitress when she brought him the wrong soft drink. Since Mr. H generally had a "laid back, easy-going" personality, Mrs. H thought this was quite out of character. After Mrs. H told the story, Mr. H stated that he did not remember doing this.

After finishing the family history, the genetic counselor briefly presented the information to the rest of the multidisciplinary neurogenetics team, and everyone proceeded to meet with the family. Since both Mr. and Mrs. H were already concerned about Lauren (and to a lesser degree, Ellie), and were growing increasingly concerned about some of Mr. H's recent difficulties, the neurogeneticist performed a clinical evaluation of Lauren, Ellie, and Mr. H. It was determined that Mr. H was showing some mild clinical symptoms of dysarthria, ataxia, and dysmetria. The clinical team recommended that Mr. H have an MRI. The team discussed the SCAs in great detail with the H's, including the possibility that Mr. H could be showing symptoms of Max's condition. Abbreviated neurological examinations were also performed on Lauren and Ellie, which were both normal. Neither showed evidence of ataxia, dysarthria, dysphagia, or memory trouble. Their drawings appeared to be age appropriate dysmetria.

The genetic counselor reviewed the panel of SCAs that Max had had 3 years previously, and discovered a more comprehensive SCA panel that had not been clinically available during Max's lifetime. The genetic counselor also reviewed autosomal dominant inheritance and trinucleotide repeat expansions, but since the H's had already been through testing for the SCAs with Max, they felt comfortable with the information and did not have any additional questions. The family decided to send extracted DNA from Max's autopsy for further testing. Mr. H also decided to provide a blood sample for DNA extraction and storage at the clinic's laboratory, in the event a diagnosis was determined using Max's sample and testing could be performed on him. Since the H's lived so far away, they wanted to make sure that the clinical team would have all of the necessary specimens and information to order further genetic testing on Mr. H, should the need arise. The genetic counselor arranged the genetic testing with the family. The H's and the genetic counselor made a follow-up plan to receive the genetic test results by phone in approximately 8 weeks.

Discussion questions:

- What are ways in which a genetic counselor can address difficult anniversaries for their patients? How might this differ between past patients and current patients? In the case of the H's, both the anniversary of their son's passing and the anniversary of their daughter arriving at the age at which their son became symptomatic coincide. How much do you think these types of anniversaries influence a patient's motivations to seek medical evaluation, genetic testing, or support? What other factors may have a similar influence?
- Working with long-distance patients presents its own set of challenges. What are some strategies genetic counselors can put in place to ensure that both the patient's time and the clinical team's time is well spent? What potential problems do you see arising when working with long-distance patients and what are ways to mitigate some of these issues?
- In general, in-person results disclosure for genetic testing is preferable (but not always possible). Are there certain types of genetic test results that you would not consider returning by phone? What information should genetic counseling "contracting" or anticipatory guidance include when both parties are agreeing to distance-based results disclosure?
- When counseling and evaluating for genetic conditions where new variations of the disease are consistently continuing to be discovered or testing technologies continually improving, how confident can you be in a negative test result that was performed greater than 3–5 years ago? How about 10 years ago? What are the risks, benefits, limitations, or concerns of retesting a gene(s) that was tested previously?

Several weeks later, genetic test results on Max's sample showed a deleterious trinucleotide repeat expansion in the *TBP* gene, diagnostic for SCA17. The genetic counselor arranged a telephone call with the H's to disclose the results. At first, the H's were very excited and said they were thankful and relieved to finally have a diagnosis for their son. The H's said that this was the "end of a long road" and that having an answer might help them "move on" in the wake of their son's death. After a few minutes, however, their concern naturally turned to Mr. H. After speaking with the H's about Max's results, reviewing the testing information, and obtaining consent, Mr. H's sample was also sent for genetic testing for SCA17. A few weeks later, Mr. H's results also came back positive for SCA17, with a smaller number of trinucleotide repeats. The H's were saddened by this news, but stated that they were expecting the diagnosis. Several months had passed since the family's initial clinic appointment and Mr. H had continued to exhibit symptoms. Mr. H was now seeing a neurologist regularly and had been started on antidepressants due to a developing mood disorder.

About 3 months after Mr. H's genetic test results came back positive, Mrs. H began calling the genetic counselor "to talk" at regular intervals. Initially, Mrs. H was experiencing anxiety due to uncertainty for the future, and wanted both Lauren and Ellie to testing. The genetic counselor discussed with Mrs. H the issues surrounding predictive testing in minors, including the current recommended genetic testing and counseling protocols. Mrs. H ended the conversation agreeing that she had a lot to think about before proceeding with testing. When she called back 4 weeks later, Mrs. H said that she was trying not to worry so much about her daughters. Since the H's had been counseled together, this was a good opportunity to speak with Mrs. H alone and assess her psychological wellbeing and support system. Mrs. H told the genetic counselor that she had strong family support and her circle of close friends. However, she had been growing increasingly concerned about her husband, and worried about her ability to care for him. The genetic counselor acknowledged these challenges and concerns, and praised Mrs. H's ability to seek the necessary help from her family and friends. She also provided Mrs. H with some information on local support groups and additional resources, and suggested that Mrs. H consider reaching out to a local psychologist to help her cope with her current life stressors. Mrs. H seemed amenable to the suggestion.

Nine months later Mrs. H called back and again requested that Lauren be tested (but not Ellie). Mrs. H was now convinced that Lauren was becoming symptomatic. Lauren was now 9 years old, and had started forgetting her books at school once or twice per week, and seemed withdrawn. When asked if Lauren had seen a doctor recently, Mrs. H said that her examination by her primary care provider last month had been normal. The genetic counselor asked if Lauren's forgetfulness had been similar to the early signs of Max's condition. Mrs. H gave a noncommittal answer, stating that some things seemed similar, but that might not look the same. She stated that she did not believe Lauren's exam had been normal, and again stated that she just "knew something was wrong." Mrs. H said that Lauren recently asked her if she was going to "get what Max had," and told her mother that she was sad because her dad did not play with her as often. The genetic counselor empathized with Mrs. H about how difficult that conversation must have been, and also asked if Mrs. H had talked to anyone about her fears. Mrs. H mentioned that she had begun seeing a psychiatrist who was treating her for depression and situational anxiety.

After conferring with the clinical team, the genetic counselor called Mrs. H and offered the opportunity for the family to come back to clinic to reevaluate Lauren. Though hesitant, the clinical team and genetic counselor also agreed to meet with the family and begin a series of counseling sessions for predictive testing. The uncertainty was causing the family (and Mrs. H, in particular) distress and anxiety. The long-distance trip to the clinic was a huge financial strain on the family, so the genetic counselor suggested that Lauren could be seen by another pediatric neurologist and genetic counselor closer to the family's home; however, Mrs. H said that they felt most comfortable with this clinical team and did not want to "start over." The H's were going to look into other funding to finance the trip back.

Three months later, Mrs. H called the genetic counselor again. Mrs. H had taken Lauren to the family's local neurologist to be evaluated. Though no obvious clinical symptoms were present upon exam, Mrs. H's request for testing and reports of Lauren's forgetfulness persuaded the physician to order the test without going through the recommended presymptomatic genetic counseling protocol. Mrs. H had received a call from the neurologist yesterday saying that Lauren's results had come back diagnostic for SCA17. After sharing the news with Lauren, Mrs. H was devastated. She was worried that the genetic counselor would be upset because she did not go through the recommended process to get Lauren's testing. However, Mrs. H stated that she needed to talk to someone who would understand the results, and was calling to seek further advice and counseling.

Discussion questions:

- What are the genetic counselor's obligations to continue to follow-up with Mrs. H and her family? What is the best way to do this, while also trying to transition them to a local care team even when the family seems resistant to the change?
- What are some coping strategies for dealing with a patient when you disapprove of their actions? What are ways for genetic counselors to help manage their own feelings of anger, disappointment, sadness, or shock?
- How much weight should a medical professional place on a "gut feeling" when weighing the risks and benefits of testing a patient?
- Genetic testing of minors for adult-onset genetic conditions is a complicated issue, particularly since the testing affects not only the child but also the parent (s). When discussing predictive testing with parents, how much emphasis should be placed on autonomy and the child's "right not to know" versus the potential benefit of early diagnosis and potential alleviation of parental anxiety?

5.6.2 Case History 2

Mr. M, a 67-year-old man with a 5-year history of a progressive gait disorder and more recent cognitive problems, presented to a movement disorders clinic. His wife and two adult children, Samantha and Luke, accompanied him. After a complete evaluation, Mr. M's diagnosis was still unclear. Despite the lack of family history, the physician suspected a genetic etiology, and asked the genetic counselor to meet with the family for a more complete family history and a discussion of genetic testing for the SCAs and GSS, a familial prion disease.

The genetic counselor introduced the purpose of the meeting, and proceeded to take a three-generation family history, which was negative for any neurological or psychiatric condition. She then asked about the fourth generation. Samantha, age 34, was newly married and had no children. Luke, age 38, had two sons who were 3 and 1, and were both healthy. Mr. M had two sisters and a brother, all of whom were healthy. His brother had three healthy children. One sister was childless, and the other had two adopted children. Mrs. M commented that both sisters had had fertility problems. The genetic counselor thanked them for the history, and said she wished to consult with the neurologist and would be back shortly.

Upon finding the neurologist, the counselor shared the family history findings, and suggested that Mr. M be tested for FXTAS because of his sisters' fertility problems. The neurologist agreed. The counselor returned to the M family and explained her concerns. She discussed the symptoms of FXTAS. Though Mr. M did not have a significant tremor, he had the other hallmark features of FXTAS, cerebellar ataxia, cerebellar hyperintensities on MRI, and cognitive impairment. The family history of premature ovarian failure was consistent with the diagnosis. She explained the genetics of FXTAS, including the nature of the triple repeat expansion, the difference between a premutation and a full mutation, and the ramifications for other family members. The family became very quiet. Luke commented that he already had children. The counselor reassured him that neither he nor his children would carry the premutation. However, if Mr. B were found to be a premutation carrier, Samantha would be at 50 % risk for being a carrier. Samantha understood her risk and felt that Mr. B should be tested. She said that she was already 34 and would want to try to get pregnant immediately.

Mr. B's *FMR1* testing revealed a CGG repeat of 127, thus confirming his diagnosis of FXTAS. At the result session, the genetic counselor first addressed the patient and asked him how he felt about knowing the diagnosis. Mr. B became quite agitated as he understood that he had a genetic disease that his children could also have. The genetic counselor acknowledged his feelings, but reminded him that even the neurologists hadn't figured it out. He had no way of knowing that he carried the gene and had now empowered his daughter to protect her children. The counselor then turned to Samantha, who had remained very quiet. She asked if Samantha had thoughts about what she would do with the information. She said that she wanted to be tested and then would want a referral for prenatal counseling. The genetic counselor agreed to facilitate both.

Discussion questions:

- How does genetic counseling specialty training help with the analysis of family history?
- How does a pleiotropic effect of a gene (in this case FXTAS, POF, and Fragile X syndrome) impact genetic counseling and the effect of genetic diagnosis?
- Although Mr. B was the patient, Samantha became the focus of genetic counseling. Should a genetic counseling session be divided between family members?

5.7 Resources for Patients

National Ataxia Foundation (**NAF**)
2600 Fernbrook Lane, Suite 119
Minneapolis, MN 55447
Phone: (763) 553-0020
E-mail: naf@ataxia.org
Web site: http://www.ataxia.org
International Network of Ataxia Friends (**INTERNAF**)
E-mail: internaf-owner@yahoogroups.com
Web site: www.internaf.org
Worldwide Education And Awareness For Movement Disorders (**WE MOVE**)
204 West 84th Street
New York, NY 10024
Phone: (212) 875-8312
E-mail: wemove@wemove.org
Web site: www.wemove.org
National Organization for Rare Disorders, Inc. (**NORD**)
55 Kenosia Avenue
P.O. Box 1968
Danbury, CT 06813-1968
Phone: (800) 999-6673
Web site: http://www.rarediseases.org
Friedreich's Ataxia Research Alliance (**FARA**)
533W. Uwchlan Ave
Downingtown, PA 19335
Phone: (484) 879-6160
E-mail: info@cureFA.org
Web site: www.curefa.org
National Fragile X Foundation
1615 Bonanza St. Suite 202
Walnut Creek, CA 94596
www.fragilex.org

References

1. Joo, B. E., Lee, C. N., & Park, K. W. (2012). Prevalence rate and functional status of cerebellar ataxia in Korea. *Cerebellum, 11*(3), 733–738.
2. Coutinho, P., Ruano, L., Loureiro, J. L., Cruz, V. T., Barros, J., Tuna, A., et al. (2013). Hereditary ataxia and spastic paraplegia in Portugal: A population-based prevalence study. *JAMA Neurology, 70*(6), 746–755.
3. Erichsen, A. K., Koht, J., Stray-Pedersen, A., Abdelnoor, M., & Tallaksen, C. M. (2009). Prevalence of hereditary ataxia and spastic paraplegia in southeast Norway: A population-based study. *Brain, 132*(Pt 6), 1577–1588.

4. Klockgether, T. (2008). The clinical diagnosis of autosomal dominant spinocerebellar ataxias. *Cerebellum, 7*(2), 101–105.
5. Jayadev, S., & Bird, T. D. (2013). Hereditary ataxias: Overview. *Genetics in Medicine, 15*(9), 673–683.
6. Verbeek, D. S., & van de Warrenburg, B. P. (2011). Genetics of the dominant ataxias. *Seminars in Neurology, 31*(5), 461–469.
7. Manto, M. U. (2005). The wide spectrum of spinocerebellar ataxias (SCAs). *Cerebellum, 4*(1), 2–6.
8. Durr, A. (2010). Autosomal dominant cerebellar ataxias: Polyglutamine expansions and beyond. *Lancet Neurology, 9*(9), 885–894.
9. van de Warrenburg, B. P., Sinke, R. J., Verschuuren-Bemelmans, C. C., Scheffer, H., Brunt, E. R., Ippel, P. F., et al. (2002). Spinocerebellar ataxias in the Netherlands: Prevalence and age at onset variance analysis. *Neurology, 58*(5), 702–708.
10. Stevanin, G., Dürr, A., & Brice, A. (2000). Clinical and molecular advances in autosomal dominant cerebellar ataxias: From genotype to phenotype and physiopathology. *European Journal of Human Genetics, 8*(1), 4–18.
11. Globas, C., du Montcel, S. T., Baliko, L., Boesch, S., Depondt, C., DiDonato, S., et al. (2008). Early symptoms in spinocerebellar ataxia type 1, 2, 3, and 6. *Movement Disorders, 23*(15), 2232–2238.
12. Paulson, H. L. (2007). Dominantly inherited ataxias: Lessons learned from Machado-Joseph disease/spinocerebellar ataxia type 3. *Seminars in Neurology, 27*(2), 133–142.
13. Bidichandani, S. I., & Delatycki, M. B. (1998). Friedreich ataxia. In R. A. Pagon, M. P. Adam, T. D. Bird, C. R. Dolan, C. T. Fong, & K. Stephens (Eds.), *Source GeneReviews™ [Internet* (pp. 1993–2013). Seattle, WA: University of Washington. Updated 2012 Feb 02.
14. Durr, A., Cossee, M., Agid, Y., Campuzano, V., Mignard, C., Penet, C., et al. (1996). Clinical and genetic abnormalities in patients with Friedreich's ataxia. *The New England Journal of Medicine, 335*, 1169–1175.
15. Harding, A. E. (1981). Friedreich's ataxia: A clinical and genetic study of 90 families with an analysis of early diagnostic criteria and intrafamilial clustering of clinical features. *Brain, 104*, 589–620.
16. Klockgether, T., Zühlke, C., Schulz, J. B., Bürk, K., Fetter, M., Dittmann, H., et al. (1996). Friedreich's ataxia with retained tendon reflexes: Molecular genetics, clinical neurophysiology, and magnetic resonance imaging. *Neurology, 46*(1), 118–121.
17. Durr, A., & Brice, A. (2000). Clinical and genetic aspects of spinocerebellar degeneration. *Current Opinion in Neurology, 13*(4), 407–413.
18. Coppola, G., De Michele, G., Cavalcanti, F., Pianese, L., Perretti, A., Santoro, L., et al. (1999). Why do some Friedreich's ataxia patients retain tendon reflexes? A clinical, neurophysiological and molecular study. *Journal of Neurology, 246*, 353–357.
19. De Michele, G., Filla, A., Cavalcanti, F., Di Maio, L., Pianese, L., Castaldo, I., et al. (1994). Late onset Friedreich's disease: Clinical features and mapping of mutation to the FRDA locus. *Journal of Neurology, Neurosurgery and Psychiatry, 57*(8), 977–979.
20. Gates, P. C., Paris, D., Forrest, S. M., Williamson, R., & Gardner, R. J. (1998). Friedreich's ataxia presenting as adult-onset spastic paraparesis. *Neurogenetics, 1*, 297–299.
21. Berciano, J., Combarros, O., De Castro, M., & Palau, F. (1997). Intronic GAA triplet repeat expansion in Friedreich's ataxia presenting with pure sensory ataxia. *Journal of Neurology, 244*, 390–391.
22. Hanna, M. G., Davis, M. B., Sweeney, M. G., Noursadeghi, M., Ellis, C. J., Elliot, P., et al. (1998). Generalized chorea in two patients harboring the Friedreich's ataxia gene trinucleotide repeat expansion. *Movement Disorders, 13*, 339–340.
23. La Pean, A., Jeffries, N., Grow, C., Ravina, B., & Di Prospero, N. A. (2008). Predictors of progression in patients with Friedreich ataxia. *Movement Disorders, 23*, 2026–2032.
24. Hagerman, R., & Hagerman, P. (2013). Advances in clinical and molecular understanding of the FMR1 premutation and fragile X-associated tremor/ataxia syndrome. *Lancet Neurology, 12*(8), 786–798.

25. Leehey, M. A. (2009). Fragile X-associated tremor/ataxia syndrome: Clinical phenotype, diagnosis, and treatment. *Journal of Investigative Medicine, 57*(8), 830–836.
26. Almeida-Silva, U. C., Hallak, J. E., Júnior, W. M., & Osório Fde, L. (2013). Association between spinocerebellar ataxias caused by glutamine expansion and psychiatric and neuropsychological signals—A literature review. *American Journal of Neurodegenerative Disease, 2*(2), 57–69.
27. Klockgether, T., & Paulson, H. (2011). Milestones in ataxia. *Movement Disorders, 26*, 1134–1141.
28. Van de Warrenburg, B. P. C., Steijns, J. A., Munneke, M., Kremer, H. P., & Bloem, B. R. (2005). Falls in degenerative cerebellar ataxias. *Movement Disorders, 20*, 497–508.
29. Fonteyn, E. M., Schmitz-Hübsch, T., Verstappen, C. C., Baliko, L., Bloem, B. R., Boesch, S., et al. (2010). Falls in spinocerebellar ataxias: Results of the EuroSCA fall study. *Cerebellum, 9* (2), 232–239.
30. Hart, P. E., Lodi, R., Rajagopalan, B., Bradley, J. L., Crilley, J. G., Turner, C., et al. (2005). Antioxidant treatment of patients with Friedreich ataxia: Four-year follow-up. *Archives of Neurology, 62*, 621–626.
31. Strupp, M., Teufel, J., Habs, M., Feuerecker, R., Muth, C., van de Warrenburg, B. P., et al. (2013). Effects of acetyl-DL-leucine in patients with cerebellar ataxia: A case series. *Journal of Neurology, 260*, 2556–2561.
32. Perroud, B., Jafar-Nejad, P., Wikoff, W. R., Gatchel, J. R., Wang, L., Barupal, D. K., et al. (2013). Pharmacometabolomic signature of ataxia SCA1 mouse model and lithium effects. *PLoS One, 8*(8), e70610.
33. Di Prospero, N. A., Baker, A., Jeffries, N., & Fischbeck, K. H. (2007). Neurological effects of high-dose idebenone in patients with Friedreich's ataxia: A randomised, placebo-controlled trial. *Lancet Neurology, 6*(10), 878–886.
34. Schöls, L., Bauer, P., Schmidt, T., Schulte, T., & Riess, O. (2004). Autosomal dominant cerebellar ataxias: Clinical features, genetics, and pathogenesis. *Lancet Neurology, 3*(5), 291–304.
35. Basu, P., Chattopadhyay, B., Gangopadhaya, P. K., Mukherjee, S. C., Sinha, K. K., Das, S. K., et al. (2000). Analysis of CAG repeats in SCA1, SCA2, SCA3, SCA6, SCA7 and DRPLA loci in spinocerebellar ataxia patients and distribution of CAG repeats at the SCA1, SCA2 and SCA6 loci in nine ethnic populations of eastern India. *Human Genetics, 106*(6), 597–604.
36. Hernandez-Castillo, C. R., Alcauter, S., Galvez, V., Barrios, F. A., Yescas, P., Ochoa, A., et al. (2013). Disruption of visual and motor connectivity in spinocerebellar ataxia type 7. *Movement Disorders, 28*, 1708–1716.
37. Lebre, A. S., & Brice, A. (2003). Spinocerebellar ataxia 7 (SCA7). *Cytogenetic and Genome Research, 100*(1–4), 154–163.
38. Delatycki, M. B., Williamson, R., & Forrest, S. M. (2000). Friedreich ataxia: An overview. *Journal of Medical Genetics, 37*, 1–8.
39. Campuzano, V., Montermini, L., Molto, M. D., Pianese, L., Cossee, M., Cavalcanti, F., et al. (1996). Friedreich's ataxia: Autosomal recessive disease caused by an intronic GAA triplet repeat expansion. *Science, 271*(5254), 1423–1427.
40. Cossee, M., Durr, A., Schmitt, M., Dahl, N., Trouillas, P., Allinson, P., et al. (1999). Friedreich's ataxia: Point mutations and clinical presentation of compound heterozygotes. *Annals of Neurology, 45*(2), 200–206.
41. Lodi, R., Cooper, J. M., Bradley, J. L., Manners, D., Styles, P., Taylor, D. J., et al. (1999). Deficit of in vivo mitochondrial ATP production in patients with Friedreich ataxia. *Proceedings of the National Academy of Sciences of the United States of America, 96*, 11492–11495.
42. McKinnon, W. C., Baty, B. J., Bennett, R. L., Magee, M., Neufeld-Kaiser, W. A., Peters, K. F., et al. (1997). Predisposition genetic testing for late-onset disorders in adults. A position paper of the National Society of Genetic Counselors. *The Journal of the American Medical Association, 278*(15), 1217–1220.

Part II
The Dementias

Chapter 6
Overview of the Dementias

Jill S. Goldman

The dementias are a group of conditions that are usually progressive and often neurodegenerative. Diagnosis is made on the basis of the patient's clinical history, neurological examination, neuroimaging (MRI, PET, SPECT), neuropsychological testing, and standard laboratory testing. The laboratory testing is performed to rule out reversible causes of dementia including vitamin deficiency, thyroid dysfunction, liver function (i.e., Wilson's disease), markers of infection or inflammation (i.e., HIV, autoimmune diseases), and paraneoplastic disease. Additionally several cerebrospinal fluid (CSF) biomarkers may increase or decrease the risk of various dementia diagnoses (refer to Chap. 8 for complete description of testing).

In the new *Diagnostic and Statistical Manual of Mental Disorders (DSM-5)*, the term dementia has been replaced by "major neurocognitive disorder." Criteria for this diagnosis include impairment in any of the domains of cognitive function (cognitive domains include memory, language, visual/spatial function, executive functioning including reasoning, judgment, and planning, and behavior/personality/mood) resulting in impairment in the activities of daily living (ADL's) at home, at work, or in social activities to the extent that independence is compromised [1]. Additionally this condition cannot be explained by delirium or a psychiatric condition. As mentioned above, dementias can be reversible or irreversible. The most common causes of irreversible dementia include Alzheimer disease, vascular dementia, and dementia with Lewy bodies (DLB, related to Parkinson's disease). All types of dementia may have associated motor disorders that can develop before or after the cognitive dysfunction. Initial symptoms usually dictate which specialist is consulted when the patient first enters the diagnostic process. Entry areas include the neurological specialties of memory disorders, movement disorders, neuromuscular disorders, and stroke, as well as psychiatry.

J.S. Goldman (✉)
Taub Institute, Columbia University Medical Center, 630 W. 168th St., Box 16, New York, NY 10032, USA
e-mail: jg2673@cumc.columbia.edu

J.S. Goldman (ed.), *Genetic Counseling for Adult Neurogenetic Disease*,
DOI 10.1007/978-1-4899-7482-2_6

This chapter will cover several primary neurodegenerative dementias. Dementia with Lewy Bodies is discussed with Parkinson's disease (Chap. 3) and CADASIL will be discussed in the chapter on stroke (Chap. 11). Many metabolic genetic diseases can result in secondary dementia (e.g., leukodystrophies, adult Tay Sachs disease, Kufs disease, mitochondrial diseases). Although these diseases are not be discussed in this book, many of the dementia counseling issues may apply to them as well.

6.1 Genetic Counseling Issues for All Dementia

Dementia presents several unique issues for genetic testing and counseling. Because these issues apply to all types of dementia, they are discussed here rather than in each section:

1. *Purpose of diagnostic genetic testing:* The motivation for genetic testing may be to attain information for the family or to confirm diagnosis during the patient's lifetime. However, in most cases, this clarification will not alter treatment and cannot be said to be medically necessary. Therefore, insurance may not pay for genetic testing.
2. *Presymptomatic genetic testing:* For relatives interested in predictive testing, it is recommended that in all but a few exceptional cases, mutations be identified first in an affected family member before testing an unaffected individual. Several reasons lead to this recommendation:

    - Symptoms overlap considerably across all dementia diagnoses. Without confirmation of a mutation in an affected family member, a negative presymptomatic result could be due to testing the wrong genes.
    - A great portion of dementia is not autosomal dominant. Familial clustering is common, especially for late-onset Alzheimer disease, and is probably due to a combination of genetic susceptibility genes and epigenetic factors that are not yet understood.
    - The finding of variants of unknown significance is common in these genes, and will become even more common when testing is performed using whole genome or exome sequencing. Thus, to determine whether such variants have clinical meaning, the mutation should be seen to segregate with the disease in the family.

    When presymptomatic testing is an option, clinicians should follow the Huntington Disease protocol that includes several genetic counseling sessions, clinical evaluation by a neurologist, neuropsychologist, and/or a psychiatrist, and a face-to-face result counseling session with a support person [2]. Although this protocol may be seen as paternalistic, most patients are compliant and many choose to forego testing after going through the protocol. Thus, although most patients who choose to proceed cope well with their results, the great majority of people at risk for these diseases opt not to test because they feel the results would negatively impact their lives [3, 4]. When treatment trials are available for mutation carriers, it is likely that more people will choose to be tested.

3. *Testing an affected individual:* Capacity to consent is an essential element of genetic testing for dementia. The genetics of these diseases and implications for family members are quite complex and demand significant cognitive ability. As a result, a family member or person authorized to make health care decisions should be present during the pretest discussion of genetic testing, the signing of the informed consent, and the posttest result session. Regardless of the family's wishes, testing of the patient should not be coercive. Additionally relatives helping with the decision may actually be at as much as a 50 % risk, and, therefore, have their own agenda for recommending or discouraging testing. Thus, reasons for testing need to be explored prior to actual testing [5].
4. *Determining what type of genetic testing to do.* As next generation sequencing (NGS) panels and whole exome sequencing become more common and less expensive, ordering these tests rather than single gene sequencing and small disease-specific panels will be tempting. However, the amount of the genome being tested influences the complexity of results. Finding gene variants in several genes may lead to more, not less, diagnostic confusion for the physician, counselor, and patient. When the clinical presentation is clear, single gene or disease-specific panels may still be the first line of action, reflexing to an NGS panel as necessary. For example, presentation of an autosomal dominant rapidly progressive dementia should result in testing *PRNP* not in NGS. However, if a patient presents late in a disease course with symptoms that could overlap FTD and AD, a full dementia panel more be more efficacious.

6.2 Family History Questions Pertinent to Dementia

Targeted questions about family history can help determine if a condition is hereditary and assist with diagnosis. A pedigree consisting of 3 or more generations should always be taken and include documentation of any neurological or psychiatric condition with age of onset and age of death. When taking the pedigree, the patient and informant should be asked the following questions:

- Did anybody have dementia, senility, or memory loss?
- Did anybody have a change in personality or behavior?
- Did anybody have a mental illness including chronic depression? Did anyone have a nervous breakdown?
- Was anyone in a nursing home or mental institution? If so, why?
- Was anyone an alcoholic or drug addict?
- Were there any suicides in the family?
- Did anyone have a neurological disease such as Parkinson's disease or ALS? Did anyone have a tremor or trouble walking?

- Did anyone have migraines?
- Did anyone have a language or speech problem?
- Did anyone have hypertension, stroke, or cardiovascular problem?

If the answer to any of these questions is affirmative, age of onset and details of symptoms should be explored and documented.

References

1. American Psychiatric Association. (2013). *Diagnostic and statistical manual of mental disorders*. 5th Edition: DSM-5.
2. HDSA. (1994). *Guidelines for genetic testing*. New York, NY: The Huntington's Disease Society of America.
3. Quaid, K. A. (2011). Genetic counseling for frontotemporal dementias. *Journal of Molecular Neuroscience, 45*(3), 706–709.
4. Fortea, J., Lladó, A., Clarimón, J., Lleó, A., Oliva, R., Peri, J., et al. (2011). PICOGEN: Five years experience with a genetic counselling program for dementia. *Neurología, 26*(3), 143–149.
5. Hedera, P. (2001). Ethical principles and pitfalls of genetic testing for dementia. *Journal of Geriatric Psychiatry and Neurology, 14*(4), 213–221.

Chapter 7
Alzheimer Disease

Jill S. Goldman

With a prevalence of 5.2 million people in the USA, Alzheimer disease (AD) is the most common dementia and the most common of all neurodegenerative diseases. It is estimated that the incidence will double by 2050 [1]. Although AD is more common among women, this difference is largely due to length of life. The disease is found around the world in all ethnic groups. In the USA, African-Americans and Hispanics are at greater risk for AD, probably because of their increased risk of other diseases such as hypertension and diabetes [1].

Of those people with AD, approximately 200,000 are under the age of 65. It is this group with early-onset AD that is more likely to have a familial form of the disease. Although the genetic burden of AD is likely to be quite large, overall less than 1 % of all AD is due to autosomal dominant genes. Regardless of the cause, the definitive diagnosis of AD is made at autopsy [1].

7.1 Clinical Presentation

Alzheimer disease typically has an insidious onset with forgetfulness demonstrated by repeating conversation and questions, misplacing items, forgetting events, getting lost, having trouble with calculations such as making correct change or balancing a checkbook, and having word-finding problems. However, diagnostic criteria for Alzheimer disease are in a state of flux largely due to advances in

Electronic supplementary material Supplementary material is available in the online version of this chapter at 10.1007/978-1-4899-7482-2_7. Videos can also be accessed at http://www.springerimages.com/videos/978-1-4899-7481-5.

J.S. Goldman (✉)
Taub Institute, Columbia University Medical Center, 630 W. 168th St., Box 16, New York, NY 10032, USA
e-mail: jg2673@cumc.columbia.edu

J.S. Goldman (ed.), *Genetic Counseling for Adult Neurogenetic Disease*,
DOI 10.1007/978-1-4899-7482-2_7

neuroimaging and CSF biomarkers, as well as in clinical and pathological assessment. Atypical presentations of AD have been described where patients demonstrate relatively preserved memory but autopsy reveals AD pathology. Whereas the existing diagnosis of AD required impairment in memory and another cognitive domain, the proposed revised criteria state that there must be a gradual onset of symptoms with progression to cognitive impairment in any domain which impairs the activities of daily living, and that other forms of dementia are largely ruled out [2–4]. Atypical AD presentations include mood/behavior change, language impairment resulting in a progressive aphasia, or cortically derived vision problems resulting from posterior cortical atrophy. About a third of people with early-onset AD have atypical features [5].

As AD progresses, all areas of cognitive function will be affected. In early to middle stages of the disease, short-term memory is primarily affected. Later, long-term memory will become impaired. Eventually the ability to recognize faces, including family, will be lost. People with middle to late stage AD may have psychiatric symptoms such as depression, agitation, delusions, and hallucinations. They will have poor judgment, may become disoriented to time and place, lose language and the ability for self-care, and become incontinent. Many people develop parkinsonian features that can lead to an increased risk of falling. Myoclonus and seizures also can develop. Ultimately, patients will be bedridden. Disease duration is variable with the mean being approximately 12 years from onset (6 years from clinical presentation) [6]. The ultimate cause of death is likely to be an unrecognized infection, aspiration pneumonia, or dehydration.

People with AD and their caregivers often become progressively isolated. The need for maintaining a good quality of life for both patient and caregivers should be addressed by healthcare providers including genetic counselors, and appropriate resources should be given.

7.2 Diagnosis

In addition to the neurological history, AD is diagnosed by meeting the clinical criteria and ruling out infection, paraneoplastic disease, hormonal, and metabolic causes of dementia through routine laboratory testing and lumbar puncture. A quick neuropsychological screen that can be performed during a clinical visit is the Mini Mental Status Exam (MMSE). However, much more extensive neuropsychological testing is necessary to reveal the type and extent of cognitive impairment. Additionally, the diagnostic process includes neuroimaging, neuropsychological testing, and often a lumbar puncture to test the CSF markers, β-amyloid and tau proteins. In typical AD, MRIs show reduced hippocampal volume and temporal–parietal atrophy. Functional imaging shows reduction in metabolism and blood flow in the temporal–parietal cortex [3]. PET imaging using amyloid staining can assist with diagnosis, but as of this writing, has limited availability and is very expensive. The CSF biomarker profile increasing the likelihood of an AD diagnosis is low amyloid

β_{42} and high total tau and phosphorylated tau. Neuroimaging and biomarkers as well as the neuropsychological profile help to improve diagnostic confidence, but are not foolproof. The finding of amyloid deposition in the brains of some elderly people who do not develop AD demonstrates how even amyloid neuroimaging is not 100 % predictive [4, 7]. Definitive diagnosis is autopsy with the pathological findings of amyloid plaques and neurofibrillary tangles composed of hyperphosphorylated tau protein.

7.3 Treatment and Management

Treatment for Alzheimer disease is largely symptomatic. Although there are many clinical trials, at the present time available treatments include cholinesterase inhibitors ((donepezil, rivastigmine, galantamine) and an NMDA receptor antagonist, memantine. These compounds slightly improve cognition and function in some patients and may slow the rate of disease, but do not stop or cure it. Yet other patients gain no benefit from these medications and complain of side effects including gastrointestinal complications and sleep disorder [8]. Additionally, symptoms such as depression and agitation can be treated through antidepressants and antipsychotics.

Non-pharmacological treatment includes behavior modification, cognitive retraining, and stimulation activities. As social isolation is a problem for patients and their caregivers, support groups, daycare centers, and cultural programs designed for families living with dementia can be helpful. Organizations, such as the Alzheimer Association, run workshops for families on essential topics such as legal issues and handling difficult behaviors.

7.4 Genetics

Three genes have been linked to autosomal dominant AD: Presenilin 1 (*PSEN1*) at 14q24.3, Presenilin 2 (PSEN2) at 1q31-q42, and the amyloid precursor protein gene (*APP*) at 21q21.2. Of these, approximately 50 % of autosomal dominant AD has been attributed to *PSEN1*. Whereas several cases of asymptomatic *PSEN2* gene carriers have been reported, *PSEN1* and *APP* are thought to be 100 % penetrant (see Table 7.1).

Over 180 mutations have been described in *PSEN1*. Genotype/phenotype correlations exist for some mutations; however, phenotypic variation can be significant, even within families. Age of onset is usually in the 40s or 50s, although cases have been reported as young as the 20s and possibly as old as 70. Yet onset after 60 is highly unusual. In addition to typical Alzheimer type dementia, which begins with memory loss and/or visual/spatial problems, all areas of cognition can be affected including behavior, mood, executive function and language. Aphasia and

Table 7.1 Genetic risk factors for Alzheimer disease

Gene	Chromosome	Inheritance	Penetrance	Age of onset
PSEN1	14q24.3	Autosomal dominant	100 %	24–65 (AAO 45)
PSEN2	1q31-q42	Autosomal dominant	<100 %	39–75 (AAO 54)
APP	21q21.2	Autosomal dominant	100 %	40s–60s
APOE	19q13.2	Autosomal dominant	Dosage related risk factor	Highly variable

AAO average age of onset

behavioral/psychiatric symptoms are relatively common. Additionally parkinsonism, ataxia, myoclonus, seizures, and spastic paraparesis have all been reported [9, 10].

APP accounts for 10–15 % of autosomal dominant AD. Approximately 25 point mutations and duplications have been found in this gene [11]. In addition to cognitive impairment, the *APP* phenotype can include autonomic failure, seizures, behavioral changes, intracerebral hemorrhage, and cerebral amyloid angiopathy found on autopsy [12, 13].

PSEN2 mutations are very rare. Approximately 15 mutations have been found in families of Volga German, Italian, and Spanish descent [14]. Age of onset is quite variable, and reduced penetrance has been reported. Seizures are also relatively common. Autopsy often reveals Lewy Body pathology (associated with Parkinson's disease) in addition to amyloid plaques and tau tangles, which accounts for occurrence of hallucinations [15].

Whereas less than 1 % of AD is due to these autosomal dominant genes, a significant portion is thought to involve genetic susceptibility factors. Heritability of AD is estimated at 58–79 % [16]. Through GWAS studies, numerous loci have been associated with risk. Of all the identified genes, only the apolipoprotein E gene (*APOE*) repeatedly shows a significant effect on risk.

APOE has 3 alleles, e2, e3, and e4. The e4 allele is associated with increased Alzheimer risk in a dose dependent manner, while the e2 allele is thought to be protective. A single e4 allele increases risk 2–3 times, whereas individuals with an e4/e4 genotype have about a 15-fold increase in lifetime risk [17, 18]. Risk is age-dependent and in e4/e4 individuals is about 50 % in males and 60 % in women by age 85. Individuals with e3/e4 have a 23 % (males)—30 % (females) risk by age 85 [18].

The significant increased risk conferred by this locus has led to interest in predictive testing. However, practice guidelines and position statements have not supported the use of *APOE* testing whether for diagnostic or predictive reasons [19]. This gene is neither necessary nor sufficient for developing AD. However, the REVEAL study has demonstrated that the select group of research patients who opt to hear their *APOE* status after genetic counseling generally cope well with their results. Yet a small minority (9 %) experienced depression up to a year after receiving results. Additionally the study showed that genetic counseling helped to reduce anxiety, perhaps by focusing on the difference between perceived risk and objective risk [20]. *APOE* disclosure in the study group resulted in some behavioral change of *APOE* e4 positive as compared to negative individuals. Individuals testing positive were 4.75 times more likely to increase their use of vitamins and supplements (for which there is no good scientific basis), but not to increase exercise (which has been shown to be beneficial) [21]. Likewise, those testing positive were more likely to buy long-term care insurance [22]. Long-term care insurance is beneficial; however, since it is not covered by GINA, it should be purchased before testing to avoid any claim of insurance fraud or discrimination. *APOE* testing is available through DTC with or without counseling; thus, healthcare professionals may be asked questions about the implications of testing after it has already been performed.

In addition to *APOE*, other loci in combination contribute approximately 35 % to AD risk [23]. Of these, replication studies have confirmed *PICALM*, *BIN1*, *CLU*, *CR1*, where others including *SORL1*, *CD33*, *EPHA1*, *ABCA7* have been replicated in some populations [23–25]. More recent GWAS studies are concentrating on specific endophenotypes, such as age of onset or psychotic features, to increase significance of findings. Additionally, ethnic differences are being studied. The *ABCA7* gene seems to double the risk of AD in African-Americans [26]. Identification of these genes is important for a better understanding of Alzheimer disease pathways, even though testing for predictive purposes will not be productive.

7.5 Genetic Counseling Issues

Since interventions are not currently available, genetic testing for Alzheimer disease lacks clinical utility. Yet for some individuals or families, testing provides a better understanding of the family disease and closure to uncertainty. Genetic testing of an affected individual reveals the risk of disease for other family members, and therefore, the possibility of taking action on one's own risk. For many individuals, having this option increases anxiety. Thus, an important job of the genetic counselor is to prepare the family for possible backlash from extended family members. For many families, discussions prior to testing can prevent this backlash. Other families feel that they do not want to raise family anxiety until necessary or decide not to share results with others.

As mentioned in the introduction to this section, the genetic counselor should understand who and what is driving the interest in testing. If there is not family consensus and the patient is not fully competent, the genetic counselor can attempt a family meeting to reach consensus. Additionally, the family should be provided alternatives to testing, such as DNA banking and autopsy. If consensus cannot be reached, the counselor must accept the wishes of the legal power for healthcare decisions or next of kin.

In families for whom a mutation is unknown, the process of testing a person with AD is complicated by the existence of the three autosomal dominant genes as well as *APOE*. The strategy for testing is driven largely by whether insurance will cover testing, as well as the ages of onset of family members. If cost is not an issue, the autosomal dominant AD panel can be ordered. If cost is of concern, testing should be done sequentially: first *PSEN1*, then *APP* (point mutations then duplications), and lastly, *PSEN2* (unless the family is of Volga German origin in which case *PSEN2* should be first). While whole exome or genome testing will expedite this process, results of unknown significance must be taken into account. The family needs to understand that a possible negative result for all three genes would reduce, but not eliminate, the risk of autosomal dominant inheritance. Testing for *APOE* is not recommended for diagnostic purposes. Although an *APOE* e4/e4 genotype might explain early onset and family clustering, this conclusion is not definitive. Likewise, in an autosomal dominant family, if the AD genes are negative, consideration should be given to testing for frontotemporal degeneration (FTD) and prion disease.

Once a mutation has been found in the family, other family members are eligible for testing, at which time the Huntington Disease protocol should be followed. As stated above, guidelines do not advocate *APOE* testing. However, patients may wish to proceed anyway. Genetic counseling should be offered, followed by testing at the physician's discretion. Some patients may present for counseling after DTC testing. These patients need to understand that carrying an e4 allele does not mean that they will definitely develop the disease, and conversely, that even if they do not carry an e4 allele, but have a positive family history, their risk only decreases slightly. They may wish to prepare for the possibility of developing AD.

7.6 Alzheimer Disease Case History (Fig. 7.1)

Mrs. L was a 59-year-old woman with a 3-year history of progressive cognitive impairment starting with memory loss. A complete neurological evaluation resulted in a diagnosis of probable Alzheimer disease. At the time of her initial evaluation, Mrs. L's Mini Mental Status Exam (MMSE) score was 24/30. Although she was very forgetful and had word-finding problems, she was still working. Yet, because of anxiety, she was having more problems at work. When the neurologist discussed applying for disability, she became agitated. The neurologist then referred Mr. and Mrs. L for genetic counseling about early-onset Alzheimer disease.

They presented at clinic with their 30-year-old daughter Maria. The counselor began the session by asking the family to explain the reason for referral. They understood that their doctor was concerned about hereditary AD. The family, especially the patient, seemed quite anxious during the initial discussion. A review of family history revealed that Mrs. L had 2 older sisters and a younger brother. Her oldest sister, now 62, developed memory problems at age 57. Their father, 2 out of 4 paternal uncles, and paternal grandmother died in their 70s with dementia. Mrs. L had been the primary caregiver to her father since her mother had died several years before his death. Mr. L reported that when Mrs. L started having symptoms, she

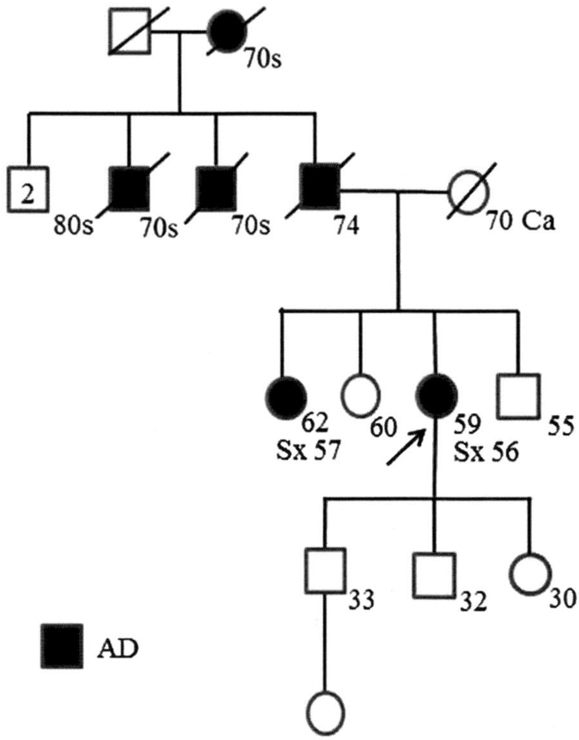

Fig. 7.1 AD case history pedigree

became terrified that she would deteriorate to her father's state, and had refused evaluation until now. Mrs. L and her daughter both cried during this discussion.

The genetic counselor acknowledged how scary it is to be part of a family with a hereditary disease, especially when one has watched the dementia process. She asked Mrs. L if she wished to learn more about the inheritance of the disease and the possibility of testing for it. Mrs. L nodded yes. The counselor then discussed AD genetics and used Mrs. L's family tree to demonstrate autosomal dominant inheritance. She explained that it was possible to test for the 3 known autosomal dominant AD genes, and that if a mutation were found in any of them, it would prove the cause of the dementia in the family. Mr. L asked whether it would make any difference to her diagnosis or treatment. The counselor told him that testing would confirm diagnosis, but not change treatment. The discovery of a mutation would provide information for the children and other family members who might wish to find out whether they carry the mutation. It would also allow family members to enroll in a national research study looking at the earliest markers for the disease and/or a drug trial only open to families with a known mutation (DIAN-Dominantly Inherited Alzheimer Network). However, if no mutations were found, or the result was a variant of unknown significance, presymptomatic testing would not be possible. Maria said that she was newly engaged and would not want to discover her status at this time, but perhaps would in the future. She added that her oldest brother already had a child and had disengaged himself from his mother and would not want to receive any information, but her other brother had gotten married recently and might be interested in results for reproductive options. At this point, Mrs. L became very agitated. When the counselor asked whether she was worried about her children, she cried that she did not want them or her husband to have to care for her, and she was terrified that they too would get the disease.

Again, the genetic counselor acknowledged Mrs. L's fears, but also asked her to consider how much research is being done on AD and how the world might be very different in 20 years. Both women nodded their heads and grinned. Maria said that she thought it was important for the family to find out everything they could. Mr. L agreed, but raised concerns about insurance discrimination. The counselor said that testing Mrs. L would not further affect her insurance since she was already diagnosed. She discussed GINA and suggested that anyone in the family who was interested in presymptomatic testing consider long-term care and/or life insurance prior to testing. She then asked whether the family would communicate results to other family members. She suggested asking people if they wished to know Mrs. L's results before any testing took place so that the family could honor the right not to know. However, she also discussed the difficulty of keeping family secrets. Once again Mrs. L became agitated because she feared her older son would get mad at her. Mr. L stepped in and said that he would handle it. The plan was to have a family meeting to discuss the genetic testing.

Discussion Questions

- How does diminished capacity influence a genetic counseling session and informed consent for genetic testing?
- How should consenting for AD testing take place in light of family disagreement?
- How do family secrets influence decisions to test?
- How much should a genetic counselor challenge optimism? Should hope for future treatment and prevention be a part of counseling?

Mr. and Mrs. L returned a month later, this time with their younger son, David. The men stated that they wanted Mrs. L to have genetic testing to provide information to this son and his wife, and perhaps to his sister, for future reproductive decisions. They said that the older son was not interested in testing, nor in learning the results, and that they would respect his choices. Mrs. L still seemed upset, and when asked if she wanted to be tested said, "I guess so." The counselor reminded her that testing was voluntary, and asked what was upsetting her. She said that she would test for David, but was scared that her children would get the disease. The counselor emphasized that knowledge of the genetic result would not alter her children's risk, but rather provide information enabling them to have choices. Mrs. L agreed to sign the consent and blood was drawn. Because she was found to be competent by a physician, no other signatures were necessary. Mr. and Mrs. L and David returned for results, which were positive for a *PSEN1* mutation. David said that he would like to arrange an appointment with the genetic counselor.

Several months later David contacted the counselor for an appointment. He and his wife were going to try to get pregnant so he wanted presymptomatic testing. The counselor suggested that both come for the appointment. In the office she reviewed Mrs. L's result and what it implied for David. She explored David's motivation for testing, which was largely for reproductive reasons. She then asked David whether he thought much about his risk. He denied being very concerned, saying that he was generally an optimistic guy. She asked him to imagine getting a positive result and how he would feel. Once again he reacted unemotionally, saying he would be fine. His wife, however, became tearful. When the question was addressed to her, she said she would be sad and scared about the future, but added that she thought David could cope with the information and that she could as well. Finally, she concluded that she would also want to have children sooner rather than later. The counselor reminded the couple that presymptomatic genetic testing would tell them if David carried the mutation, but not when he would develop symptoms. The family's average age of onset was in their 50s, which would, therefore, be the most likely age of onset for him as well. She also spoke about whether he would inform his relatives of his result. He said that he would not; that telling his mom would destroy her, and he did not want to burden his sister or father. They also spoke about the possibility of non-disclosing PGD and obtaining long-term care insurance prior to testing. David said that he would work to obtain the insurance.

The genetic counselor made several follow-up calls to David who continued to say he was pursuing long-term care insurance. On the second call he informed the counselor that he and his wife were expecting. He participated in the DIAN study and found the neuropsychological testing very stressful and then began to worry about his own cognitive ability. He never called back.

Discussion Questions

- What is the responsibility of a genetic counselor to follow up with patients who are considering testing? Does follow-up lead to pressure?
- Can giving "an out" like getting insurance be a good way for a genetic counselor to give a patient a legitimate excuse for not testing?
- How does a pregnancy influence the choice to get predictive testing for a late-onset disease?
- How does participation in a genetic family study influence the choice for clinical testing?

7.7 Resource for Patients

Alzheimer Association: www.alz.org/
Family Caregiver Alliance: www.caregiver.org
Alzheimer Disease Education & Referral Center (National Institute on Aging) www.nia.nih.gov/Alzheimers/

References

1. Alzheimer's Association. (2013). 2013 Alzheimer's disease facts and figures. *Alzheimer's & Dementia, 9*(2), 208–245.
2. American Psychiatric Association. (2000). *Diagnostic and statistical manual of mental disorders* (4, text rev.th ed.). Washington, DC: American Psychiatric Association.
3. McKhann, G., Drachman, D., Folstein, M., Katzman, R., Price, D., & Stadlan, E. M. (1984). Clinical diagnosis of Alzheimer's disease: Report of the NINCDS-ADRDA Work Group under the auspices of Department of Health and Human Services Task Force on Alzheimer's Disease. *Neurology, 34*(7), 939–944.
4. McKhann, G. M., Knopman, D. S., Chertkow, H., Hyman, B. T., Jack, C. R., Jr., Kawas, C. H., et al. (2011). The diagnosis of dementia due to Alzheimer's disease: Recommendations from the National Institute on Aging-Alzheimer's Association workgroups on diagnostic guidelines for Alzheimer's disease. *Alzheimers Dement, 7*(3), 263–269.
5. Balasa, M., Gelpi, E., Antonell, A., Rey, M. J., Sánchez-Valle, R., Molinuevo, J. L., et al. (2011). Clinical features and APOE genotype of pathologically proven early-onset Alzheimer disease. *Neurology, 76*(20), 720–725.
6. Roberson, E. D., Hesse, J. H., Rose, K. D., Slama, H., Johnson, J. K., Yaffe, K., et al. (2005). Frontotemporal dementia progresses to death faster than Alzheimer disease. *Neurology, 65*(5), 719–725.
7. Devanand, D. P., Mikhno, A., Pelton, G. H., Cuasay, K., Pradhaban, G., Dileep Kumar, J. S., et al. (2010). Pittsburgh compound B (11C-PIB) and fluorodeoxyglucose (18F-FDG) PET in patients with Alzheimer disease, mild cognitive impairment, and healthy controls. *Journal of Geriatric Psychiatry and Neurology, 23*(3), 185–198.
8. Massoud, F., & Léger, G. C. (2011). Pharmacological treatment of Alzheimer disease. *Canadian Journal of Psychiatry, 56*(10), 579–588.
9. Bird, T. D. (1993). Internet. In R. A. Pagon, T. D. Bird, C. R. Dolan, & K. Stephens (Eds.), *GeneReviews*. Seattle, WA: University of Washington. 1999 Sep 24 [updated 2010 Dec 23].
10. *Alzheimer Disease & Frontotemporal Dementia Mutation Database*. http://www.molgen.ua.ac.be/ADMutations/
11. McNaughton, D., Knight, W., Guerreiro, R., Ryan, N., Lowe, J., Poulter, M., et al. (2012). Duplication of amyloid precursor protein (APP), but not prion protein (PRNP) gene is a significant cause of early onset dementia in a large UK series. *Neurobiology of Aging, 33*(2), 426.e13–21.
12. Basun, H., Bogdanovic, N., Ingelsson, M., Almkvist, O., Näslund, J., Axelman, K., et al. (2008). Clinical and neuropathological features of the arctic APP gene mutation causing early-onset Alzheimer disease. *Archives of Neurology, 65*(4), 499–505.
13. Wu, L., Rosa-Neto, P., Hsiung, G. Y., Sadovnick, A. D., Masellis, M., Black, S. E., et al. (2012). Early-onset familial Alzheimer's disease (EOFAD). *Canadian Journal of Neurological Sciences, 39*(4), 436–445.
14. Tanzi R. E. (2012). The genetics of Alzheimer disease. *Cold Spring Harbor Perspectives Medicine, 2*(10), doi 2:a006296.
15. Jayadev, S., Leverenz, J. B., Steinbart, E., Stahl, J., Klunk, W., Yu, C. E., et al. (2010). Alzheimer's disease phenotypes and genotypes associated with mutations in presenilin 2. *Brain, 133*(Pt 4), 1143–1154.
16. Gatz, M., Reynolds, C. A., Fratiglioni, L., Johansson, B., Mortimer, J. A., Berg, S., et al. (2006). Role of genes and environments for explaining Alzheimer disease. *Archives of General Psychiatry, 63*(2), 168–174.
17. Farrer, L. A., Cupples, L. A., Haines, J. L., Hyman, B., Kukull, W. A., Mayeux, R., et al. (1997). Effects of age, sex, and ethnicity on the association between apolipoprotein E genotype and Alzheimer disease. A meta-analysis. APOE and Alzheimer Disease Meta Analysis Consortium. *JAMA, 278*(16), 1349–1356.

18. Genin, E., Hannequin, D., Wallon, D., Sleegers, K., Hiltunen, M., Combarros, O., et al. (2011). APOE and Alzheimer disease: A major gene with semi-dominant inheritance. *Molecular Psychiatry, 16*(9), 903–907.
19. Goldman, J. S., Hahn, S. E., Catania, J. W., LaRusse-Eckert, S., Butson, M. B., Rumbaugh, M., et al. (2011). Genetic counseling and testing for Alzheimer disease: Joint practice guidelines of the American College of Medical Genetics and the National Society of Genetic Counselors. *Genetics in Medicine, 13*(6), 597–605. Erratum in: *Genet Med,* 2011. 13(8), 749.
20. Ashida, S., Koehly, L. M., Roberts, J. S., Chen, C. A., Hiraki, S., & Green, R. C. (2010). The role of disease perceptions and results sharing in psychological adaptation after genetic susceptibility testing: The REVEAL Study. *European Journal of Human Genetics, 18*(12), 1296–1301.
21. Vernarelli, J. A., Roberts, J. S., Hiraki, S., Chen, C. A., Cupples, L. A., & Green, R. C. (2010). Effect of Alzheimer disease genetic risk disclosure on dietary supplement use. *American Journal of Clinical Nutrition, 91*(5), 1402–1407.
22. Zick, C. D., Mathews, C. J., Roberts, J. S., Cook-Deegan, R., Pokorski, R. J., & Green, R. C. (2005). Genetic testing for Alzheimer's disease and its impact on insurance purchasing behavior. *Health Affairs (Millwood), 24*(2), 483–490.
23. Naj, A. C., Jun, G., Beecham, G. W., Wang, L. S., Vardarajan, B. N., Buros, J., et al. (2011). Common variants at MS4A4/MS4A6E, CD2AP, CD33 and EPHA1 are associated with late-onset Alzheimer's disease. *Nature Genetics, 43*(5), 436–441.
24. Hollingworth, P., Harold, D., Sims, R., Gerrish, A., Lambert, J. C., Carrasquillo, M. M., et al. (2011). Common variants at ABCA7, MS4A6A/MS4A4E, EPHA1, CD33 and CD2AP are associated with Alzheimer's disease. *Nature Genetics, 43*(5), 429–435.
25. Seshadri, S., Fitzpatrick, A. L., Ikram, M. A., DeStefano, A. L., Gudnason, V., Boada, M., et al. (2010). Genome-wide analysis of genetic loci associated with Alzheimer disease. *JAMA, 303*(18), 1832–1840.
26. Reitz, C., Jun, G., Naj, A., Rajbhandary, R., Vardarajan, B. N., Wang, L. S., et al. (2013). Variants in the ATP-binding cassette transporter (ABCA7), apolipoprotein E $\epsilon 4$, and the risk of late-onset Alzheimer disease in African Americans. *JAMA, 309*(14), 1483–1492.

8.1 Clinical Presentation

(FTD video clip Part 1).

Early symptoms of FTD are variable, however, unlike Alzheimer disease, memory is usually relatively preserved at the onset of the disease. FTD generally presents with changes in personality and behavior (behavioral variant FTD, bvFTD) or with language dysfunction, primary progressive aphasia (PPA), as demonstrated by word finding problems and nonfluent speech (primary nonfluent aphasia, PNFA), or with a loss of semantic meaning (semantic dementia). Although not every patient will display all symptoms, diagnostic criteria for bvFTD include the following:

- Behavioral disinhibition (saying or doing inappropriate things such as "boy, are you fat" or touching someone's breasts in public).
- Loss of insight (the patient does not realize that anything is unusual).
- Loss of empathy (the patient does not identify the emotional needs of others).
- Blunted affect (the patient does not express facial emotion, similar to what occurs in Parkinson's disease).
- Apathy (loss of interest in normal activities, even family).
- Ritualistic behavior (repetitive behaviors and/or speech).
- Hyperorality or changes in eating (overeating to the point of large weight gains or ritualistic eating patterns).
- Aberrant motor behavior (a need to walk or pace).
- Speech changes (perseverative speech, echolalia)

Diagnosis is often quite delayed because the patient may be unaware of symptoms and the family often blames changes on depression, stress, or "midlife crisis." Even when a physician is consulted, a psychiatric diagnosis is common. Alternatively, when the patient appears to have memory problems (usually because of executive dysfunction), a diagnosis of Alzheimer disease may be made. This diagnostic delay is extremely stressful to families that are trying to understand what is happening [2, 5].

As the disease progresses, symptoms change, and other parts of the brain become affected. In addition to cognitive dysfunction, some patients develop parkinsonism and/or motor neuron disease, even full-blown ALS. These motor features increase the difficulty of caring for the patient, and usually shorten the disease duration. Additionally, 2 parkinsonism diseases, progressive supranuclear palsy (PSP) and cortical basal degeneration (CBD), are closely related pathologically to FTD-tau. Both diseases can include FTD-like dementia. Ultimately the course of FTD is similar to AD, but the duration tends to be shorter (6–10 years).

FTD is a devastating disease for families. Like early-onset AD, children may still live at home. They may have a hard time understanding the emotional absence of their parent or why their parent does bizarre and embarrassing things. Additionally, not only can the family lose a breadwinner, but also the person with FTD may deplete family savings through poor judgment or compulsive buying. The mental and physical health of the well spouse is also at risk.

8.2 Diagnosis

An FTD diagnosis is made through a careful clinical history in which both the patient and a knowledgeable informant are interviewed. The presence of the informant is essential since the patient may have little insight into the problem. As with AD, a thorough neurological examination, neuropsychological testing, neuroimaging, and routine laboratory tests are used to rule out other diagnoses. Typical neuroimaging findings that increase the likelihood of an FTD diagnosis are atrophy of the frontal and/or temporal lobes (either symmetrical or not) on MRI, and decrease metabolism or blood flow in these areas on functional imaging. Neuropsychological testing may find impaired executive function and/or language impairment with relatively preserved memory. However, both imaging and neuropsychological findings are variable, and can overlap with those of other dementias. To investigate this overlap further, a lumbar puncture may be performed to measure levels of CSF amyloid and tau. Currently there are no specific biomarkers for FTD.

8.3 Treatment and Management

Currently treatment for FTD is symptomatic. Selective serotonin re-uptake inhibitors (SSRIs) are the first choice of medication, as FTD is thought to cause a serotonin deficit unlike AD, which causes a depletion of acetylcholine. Different symptoms may respond to different SSRIs. Antipsychotics may also be used, though with caution because of potential side effects. Although the anticholinesterase inhibitors are not effective treatments for FTD, some doctors will try them in case the underlying cause is actually AD. FTD drug trials for specific inherited forms of FTD will soon be under way. Because of the different FTD pathologies, it is highly unlikely that any one drug will treat all forms of FTD [2, 6].

8.4 Genetics

Depending on the population, 30–50 % of FTD cases have some family history of dementia or related neurological disease. Of these, approximately 25 % demonstrate autosomal dominant inheritance [1, 7]. With 3 relatively common genes, and 4 rare ones, autosomal dominant FTD is quite heterogeneous. The first common genes to be linked to FTD, *MAPT* and *PGRN (GRN)*, are both on chromosome 17p, and each causes approximately 8–9 % of familial FTD [6]. Additionally, *PGRN* mutations have been found in about 3 % of sporadic FTD [8].

MAPT encodes the tau protein. *MAPT*'s more than 40 mutations are 100 % penetrant, but show both intrafamilial and interfamilial phenotypic variability of onset, symptoms, and duration. Behavioral variant FTD (including the old diagnosis of Pick's disease) is the most common presentation, however, PPA, and the related parkinsonism diseases, PSP and CBD, are all possible diagnoses with *MAPT*' mutations. The average age of onset is in the 50s with a range from the 30s to 70s. The duration is about 9 years from symptom onset with a range of 5–20 years [2]. Tau pathology is found on autopsy in all cases [3].

Like *MAPT*, *PGRN* mutations are highly penetrant (although some sporadic cases have had *PGRN* mutations which may indicate reduced penetrance in the parent) and have highly variable presentations. While bvFTD, particularly with apathy, and PNFA are the most common presenting symptoms, corticobasal syndrome (CBS) with parkinsonism and even memory dysfunction are not unusual. CBS caused by PGRN mutations will have TDP-43 pathology, not the tau pathology seen in pathological CBD. Neuroimaging may reveal that the parietal lobe, as well as the temporal and frontal lobes, is involved [1, 9]. Again, age of onset is variable with the average being around 60 years of age and ranging from the 30s to 80s, thus slightly older than cases with *MAPT* mutations. Mean duration is 8 years with a range of 3–22 [1]. The pathological hallmark of *PGRN* mutations is neuronal intranuclear inclusions of TDP-43 [3].

The 2011 discovery of a hexanucleotide (GGGGCC) intronic expansion in the *C9orf72* gene changed the face of FTD and ALS genetics. This expansion has been found in the great majority of families that have a history of both FTD and ALS. In addition it appears to account for the greatest portion of familial FTD. *C9orf72* is responsible for 12–24 % of familial and 6 % of sporadic FTD, as well as 23–39 % of familial and 4 % of sporadic ALS [10–12].

Once again, intra- and inter-familial variation is common. Some individuals will have only FTD clinically, some only ALS, and some a combination. Typically ALS reduces life expectancy greatly. The mean age of onset is approximately 55 years with a range from 34 to 76 years. Duration averages 6 years with a range from 1 to 22 years. Presenting symptoms can be bvFTD or memory dysfunction, with PPA less common. However, these cases may also present with motor weakness, parkinsonism, or ataxia. Hallucinations, delusions, and psychosis occur much more frequently than with other FTD mutations. In fact, a psychiatric prodrome may occur before the onset of classic FTD symptoms [13–15]. Autopsy reveals TDP-43 pathology with ubiquitin and p62 positive, TDP-43 negative neuronal cytoplasmic and intranuclear inclusions, particularly in the cerebellum, hippocampus and dentate gyrus [16].

A hexanucleotide expansion in *C9orf72* results in an increase from under 30 repeats to hundreds, even thousands. It is unclear whether the number of repeats influences symptoms or age of onset, or if anticipation occurs [13]. At the time of this writing, much is still unknown about penetrance and anticipation [14, 15]. The expansion is very unstable, and repeat numbers can differ between tissue types of the same individual. Thus, as of now, presymptomatic testing is very difficult.

In addition to *MAPT*, *PGRN*, and *C9orf72*, genetic etiology for FTD has been attributed to mutations in five rare genes. Mutations in the *VCP* gene are associated with inclusion body myopathy, Paget's disease of the bone, and FTD (IBMPFD). Approximately 35 % of patients in these families develop FTD. Without a family history of the other two findings, testing for *VCP* would be unlikely to reveal a mutation [17].

The *CHMP2B* gene is a very rare cause of FTD and results in bvFTD with other cognitive dysfunction, parkinsonism, dystonia, and myoclonus. It has only been reported in two Danish families [17]. Unlike the other genes, ubiquitin positive, tau and TDP-43 negative staining distinguish *CHMP2B* mutation carrier autopsies.

The *TARDBP* and *FUS* genes are each responsible for about 5 % of the familial ALS cases. Extraordinarily rare cases of FTD have been reported with these gene mutations [18, 19]. Families with another ALS gene, *UBQLN2*, may also develop FTD [20] (Table 8.1).

Several GWAS studies have indicated the possibility of susceptibility loci for FTD. However, none have yet to be associated with enough risk to warrant genetic testing.

As is obvious from this discussion of the heterogeneous nature of FTD genetics, autopsy can greatly help guide genetic testing. Thus, particularly when families are hesitant to test during life, autopsy should be encouraged to narrow diagnosis and freeze tissue for later testing if needed. A close examination of presenting clinical symptoms may also assist genetic testing [4] (see Fig. 8.1).

Table 8.1 Autosomal dominant genes causing FTD [21–25]

Gene	Age of onset	FTD characteristics	Percent of familial FTD
MAPT	50s (30s–70s)	bvFTD, PPA parkinsonism, CBD, PSP	5–20 %
PGRN (GRN)	60 (30s–80s)	bvFTD, PPA, memory impairment CBS (parkinsonism)	5–20 % ~1–5 % sporadic FTD
C9orf72	55 (34–76)	bvFTD, ALS (MND), PPA (less frequent), memory impairment, parkinsonism, ataxia, psychosis	~12–24 % ~6 % sporadic FTD
CHMP2B	51(43–68)	bvFTD, MND (rare) parkinsonism, dystonia, myoclonus	Rare
VCP	~55 for FTD	bvFTD, IBMPFD, ALS	Rare
TARDBP	≥25	bvFTD, ALS	Very rare
FUS	55 (43–68)	bvFTD, CBS, ALS	Very rare
UBQLN2	Late teens-30s	bvFTD, ALS,PLS	Very rare

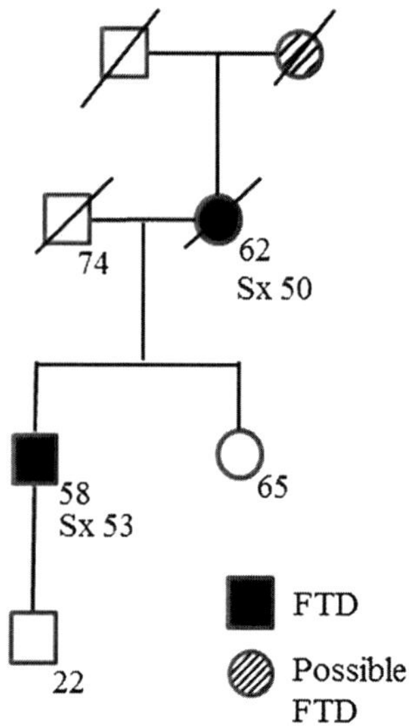

Fig. 8.1 FTD case history pedigree

8.5 Genetic Counseling Issues

(FTD video clip Part 2).

Treatments for FTD are not yet available, thus, like Alzheimer's disease, genetic testing for FTD lacks clinical utility. However, family members may want genetic information for reproductive options or future planning. Since FTD is heterogeneous, testing an affected individual is necessary before presymptomatic testing should be offered. A cardinal feature of FTD is the loss of insight. Therefore, the affected individual may not be aware of symptoms and may not agree to testing. In this situation, the genetic counselor can raise the alternatives of DNA banking or autopsy. No matter how frustrating it is to family members, genetic testing should not occur against a patient's will. In the same vein, family members may be aware of a relative's early symptoms and ask for genetic testing as evidence. Once again, testing should only occur with the patient's consent or assent, even if he is declared incompetent. If indeed the individual is in early stages, a clinical diagnosis can be made as the disease progresses. Other genetic counseling issues such as family consensus and communication are similar to the issues raised with AD (see Chaps. 6 and 7).

A careful study of clinical symptoms and family history can sometimes assist the determination of which FTD genes to test, particularly if an autopsy has been obtained on a family member. However, for many individuals, it will be necessary to send for a panel. Additionally, if an autosomal dominant FTD panel is negative, consideration should be given to testing for AD and prion disease.

Once a mutation has been found in the family, other relatives may wish to have presymptomatic testing, and the Huntington Disease protocol should be followed (see Chap. 2). However, accurate prediction of age of onset and symptoms cannot be given to the mutation carrier.

FTD is a very painful and difficult disease for the patient's spouse and children. It typically strikes at a young age, is often difficult to diagnose, and changes the personality. The genetic counselor can play a key role in educating the family about the disease, validating their feelings, and supporting them through referrals to therapists, support groups, and resources such as the Association for Frontotemporal Degeneration.

8.6 FTD Case History (Fig. 8.1)

Mr. P was a 58-year-old man who presented at the Memory Disorders Center with his older sister, Anna. Over the previous 5-years he had exhibited odd behavior and, recently, had problems with the law. Mr. P was an established businessman who owned 12 retail stores in the Midwest. He had been married and divorced twice. The most recent divorce had taken place two years prior, when the ex-wife had discovered that Mr. P had spent half of their bank account on a "get rich quick" scheme in the Caribbean. He had also become emotionally remote and uninterested in his previous hobbies of golf and travel. Mr. P's sister was forced to get involved when he was arrested after reneging on business loans. As a result, his business was lost and he was in bankruptcy. Anna knew that something was terribly wrong with him, and first sought out a psychiatric assessment. The psychiatrist treated him for bipolar disease, but his condition began to decline further. He lost his ability to use the computer and even the TV remote. The psychiatrist referred him for a neurological evaluation at an academic medical center.

On initial screening, Mr. P scored 27/30 on the MMSE, losing 1 point for recall, 1 for repetition, and 1 for WORLD backwards. He was a large man who appeared slightly disheveled. He was apathetic and unengaged in the conversation, and while admitting to having financial problems, he seemed unconcerned and took no responsibility for these problems. He was very annoyed, however, that his computer was not working, preventing him from buying things on favorite websites. He repeated this complaint obsessively.

Anna reported that she was very concerned that Mr. P might have the same disease as their mother, who died of a dementing condition called Pick's disease. The neurologist agreed that this was a possibility and referred her to the genetic counselor. An MRI revealed significant frontal atrophy and some mild atrophy in the temporal and parietal lobes. A complete neuropsychological evaluation found significant deficits in attention and executive function; language, visuospatial function, and memory were in the low normal range, which was below his premorbid ability. Analysis of illness history and test results led to the diagnosis of bvFTD.

Anna came to see the genetic counselor alone. She gave a family history that revealed that her mother had started acting strangely around 50 years of age, but that everyone assumed that she was depressed and was having symptoms due to menopause. Her behavior included pacing, and despite this constant movement, a 30 pound weight gain due to hoarding food and eating what ever was near her, including other people's food. Over time she became more docile and apathetic, and eventually mute. She died at age 62. Anna said that her mother was an only child and little was known about her family history except that the mother's mother had been institutionalized in a mental hospital. The other significant piece of family history was that Mr. P had a 22-year-old son from his first marriage, but had been totally uninvolved in his upbringing and hadn't been in touch with him since the divorce. The counselor reviewed the genetics of FTD and how both Anna and Mr. P's son were at 50 % risk of inheriting the same gene. Anna was not concerned about herself since, at 65, she was older than either her mother or brother had been when developing symptoms. However, she felt a commitment to provide genetic information to her estranged nephew. The counselor asked how she could know whether he would even want the information, and Anna said she didn't, but would want to have the testing just in case. The counselor told her that Mr. P could be tested, but that it would be extremely expensive since both *MAPT* and *PGRN* (this case was before the discovery of *C9orf72*) would need to be tested. She said that this could be done sequentially, but also suggested that if there was resistance from her brother, that she consider autopsy to narrow down pathology and, therefore, testing. Anna said that she would think about it.

Anna called several months later to say that she was extremely frustrated because Mr. P had refused to be tested. The counselor said that they would not test against a patient's wishes, even if that person was demented. She reinforced that, if he did not change his mind, testing would be possible from autopsy tissue, and put Anna in touch with the Brain Donation Program's nurse.

Discussion Questions:

- Who is "the patient", Mr. P or Anna? How does defining "the patient" impact genetic counseling?
- How does genetic testing on autopsy tissue differ from testing during life?

Four years later, the nurse informed the counselor that Mr. P had died, and that an autopsy had been performed. The autopsy confirmed the FTD diagnosis and revealed TDP-43 pathology, thus eliminating *MAPT* as the cause of the family disease. The nurse said that when the autopsy report was given, Anna said that she was still interested in genetic testing for *PGRN*. The genetic counselor called and informed her that, in the interim since they had last talked, another gene causing TDP-43 pathology had been discovered so that there were still two major genes to test and several other very rare ones to test if those two were negative. The counselor asked whether she had contacted her nephew. She hadn't, but intended to do so after testing. The counselor encouraged her to start the process before results came back to provide him with the right not to know. They also discussed whether Anna would consider her own testing. She said no as she had no children.

She had already purchased long-term care insurance, had given legal authority for healthcare and financial decisions to her best friend, and would simply live whatever life was in store for her.

Genetic testing of Mr. P's autopsy tissue was arranged so that *PGRN* was to be tested first, reflexing to *C9orf72* if negative. When results came back, the genetic counselor informed Anna that a *PGRN* mutation was discovered. She asked whether Anna had reached her nephew. She said that she had contacted his mother who would not inform her son, as she felt her son had just started his life and she did not wish to disrupt the chosen path. Anna said she tried to get her to understand that he should have the option of knowing, but she refused. The counselor acknowledged her frustration, but told her that this reaction was not uncommon, and that she had still provided them with information for the future.

Discussion Questions:

- In many families, one person seems to take responsibility for everyone else. Why does this dynamic occur, and how can it help or hinder the genetic counseling process?
- In this scenario, had Mr. P tested for *PGRN* during life and it was found to be negative, what responsibility would the counselor have had about informing Anna that a second gene was now available for testing?

8.7 Resources for Patients

Association for Frontotemporal Degeneration:
www.theaftd.org
866-507-7222

References

1. Seelaar, H., Rohrer, J. D., Pijnenburg, Y. A., Fox, N. C., & van Swieten, J. C. (2011). Clinical, genetic and pathological heterogeneity of frontotemporal dementia: a review. *Journal of Neurology, Neurosurgery, and Psychiatry, 82*(5), 476–486.
2. Rabinovici, G. D., & Miller, B. L. (2010). Frontotemporal lobar degeneration: epidemiology, pathophysiology, diagnosis and management. *CNS Drugs, 24*(5), 375–398.
3. Josephs, K. A., Hodges, J. R., Snowden, J. S., Mackenzie, I. R., Neumann, M., Mann, D. M., et al. (2011). Neuropathological background of phenotypical variability in frontotemporal dementia. *Acta Neuropathologica, 122*(2), 137–153.
4. Goldman, J. S., Rademakers, R., Huey, E. D., Boxer, A. L., Mayeux, R., Miller, B. L., et al. (2011). An algorithm for genetic testing of frontotemporal lobar degeneration. *Neurology, 76*(5), 475–483.

5. Rascovsky, K., Hodges, J. R., Knopman, D., Mendez, M. F., Kramer, J. H., Neuhaus, J., et al. (2011). Sensitivity of revised diagnostic criteria for the behavioural variant of frontotemporal dementia. *Brain, 134*(Pt 9), 2456–2477.
6. Manoochehri, M., & Huey, E. D. (2012). Diagnosis and management of behavioral issues in frontotemporal dementia. *Current Neurology and Neuroscience Reports, 12*(5), 528–536.
7. Rohrer, J. D., Guerreiro, R., Vandrovcova, J., Uphill, J., Reiman, D., Beck, J., et al. (2009). The heritability and genetics of frontotemporal lobar degeneration. *Neurology, 73*(18), 1451–1456.
8. Le Ber, I., van der Zee, J., Hannequin, D., Gijselinck, I., Campion, D., Puel, M., et al. (2007). Progranulin null mutations in both sporadic and familial frontotemporal dementia. *Human Mutation, 28*(9), 846–855.
9. Pickering-Brown, S. M., Rollinson, S., Du Plessis, D., Morrison, K. E., Varma, A., Richardson, A. M., et al. (2008). Frequency and clinical characteristics of progranulin mutation carriers in the Manchester frontotemporal lobar degeneration cohort: comparison with patients with MAPT and no known mutations. *Brain, 131*(Pt 3), 721–731.
10. Majounie, E., Renton, A. E., Mok, K., Dopper, E. G., Waite, A., Rollinson, S., et al. (2012). Frequency of the C9orf72 hexanucleotide repeat expansion in patients with amyotrophic lateral sclerosis and frontotemporal dementia: a cross-sectional study. *Lancet Neurology, 11* (4), 323–330.
11. Dejesus-Hernandez, M., Mackenzie, I. R., Boeve, B. F., Boxer, A. L., Baker, M., Rutherford, N. J., et al. (2011). Expanded GGGGCC hexanucleotide repeat in noncoding region of C9ORF72 causes chromosome 9p-linked FTD and ALS. *Neuron, 72*(2), 245–256.
12. Le Ber, I., Camuzat, A., Guillot-Noel, L., Hannequin, D., Lacomblez, L., Golfier, V., et al. (2013). C9ORF72 repeat expansions in the frontotemporal dementias spectrum of diseases: a flow-chart for genetic testing. *Journal of Alzheimer's Disease, 34*(2), 485–499.
13. Hsiung, G. Y., DeJesus-Hernandez, M., Feldman, H. H., Sengdy, P., Bouchard-Kerr, P., Dwosh, E., et al. (2012). Clinical and pathological features of familial frontotemporal dementia caused by C9ORF72 mutation on chromosome 9p. *Brain, 135*(Pt 3), 709–722.
14. Simón-Sánchez, J., Dopper, E. G., Cohn-Hokke, P. E., Hukema, R. K., Nicolaou, N., Seelaar, H., et al. (2012). The clinical and pathological phenotype of C9ORF72 hexanucleotide repeat expansions. *Brain, 135*(Pt 3), 723–735.
15. Boeve, B. F., Boylan, K. B., Graff-Radford, N. R., DeJesus-Hernandez, M., Knopman, D. S., Pedraza, O., et al. (2012). Characterization of frontotemporal dementia and/or amyotrophic lateral sclerosis associated with the GGGGCC repeat expansion in C9ORF72. *Brain, 135* (Pt 3), 765–783.
16. Mann, D. M., Rollinson, S., Robinson, A., Bennion Callister, J., Thompson, J. C., Snowden, J. S., et al. (2013). Dipeptide repeat proteins are present in the p62 positive inclusions in patients with frontotemporal lobar degeneration and motor neurone disease associated with expansions in C9ORF72. *Acta Neuropathologica Communications, 1*(1), 68.
17. Kimonis, V. E., Fulchiero, E., Vesa, J., & Watts, G. (2008). VCP disease associated with myopathy, Paget disease of bone and frontotemporal dementia: review of a unique disorder. *Biochimica et Biophysica Acta, 1782*(12), 744–748.
18. Gydesen, S., Brown, J. M., Brun, A., Chakrabarti, L., Gade, A., Johannsen, P., et al. (2002). Chromosome 3 linked frontotemporal dementia (FTD-3). *Neurology, 59*(10), 1585–1594.
19. Benajiba, L., Le Ber, I., Camuzat, A., Lacoste, M., Thomas-Anterion, C., Couratier, P., et al. (2009). TARDBP mutations in motoneuron disease with frontotemporal lobar degeneration. *Annals of Neurology, 65*(4), 470–473.
20. Van Langenhove, T., van der Zee, J., Sleegers, K., Engelborghs, S., Vandenberghe, R., Gijselinck, I., et al. (2010). Genetic contribution of FUS to frontotemporal lobar degeneration. *Neurology, 74*(5), 366–371.
21. Vengoechea, J., David, M. P., Yaghi, S. R., Carpenter, L., & Rudnicki, S. A. (2013). Clinical variability and female penetrance in X-linked familial FTD/ALS caused by a P506S mutation in UBQLN2. *Amyotroph Lateral Scler Frontotemporal Degener, 14*(7–8), 615–619.

22. Rademakers, R., Neumann, M., & Mackenzie, I. R. (2012). Advances in understanding the molecular basis of frontotemporal dementia. *Nature Reviews. Neurology, 8*(8), 423–434.
23. Nalbandian, A., Donkervoort, S., Dec, E., Badadani, M., Katheria, V., Rana, P., et al. (2011). The multiple faces of valosin-containing protein-associated diseases: inclusion body myopathy with Paget's disease of bone, frontotemporal dementia, and amyotrophic lateral sclerosis. *Journal of Molecular Neuroscience, 45*(3), 522–531.
24. Synofzik, M., Born, C., Rominger, A., Lummel, N., Schöls, L., Biskup, S., et al. (2013). Targeted high-throughput sequencing identifies a TARDBP mutation as a cause of early-onset FTD without motor neuron disease. *Neurobiol Aging*.
25. Huey, E. D., Ferrari, R., Moreno, J. H., Jensen, C., Morris, C. M., Potocnik, F., et al. (2012). FUS and TDP43 genetic variability in FTD and CBS. *Neurobiology of Aging, 33*(5), 1016.e9–17.

Chapter 9
Prion Disease

Jill S. Goldman

Prion diseases are rare conditions occurring in both animals and humans. The animal diseases include chronic wasting disease in deer, scrapie in sheep, and bovine spongiform encephalitis in cows (also known as mad cow disease) [1]. The three main forms of human prion disease that occur in 1–2/1,000,000 persons are Creutzfeldt–Jakob disease (CJD), Gerstmann–Sträussler–Scheinker disease (GSS), and fatal familial insomnia (FFI) [2]. Although 85–90 % of human prion disease occurs sporadically, 10–15 % is familial. Additionally, there are rare iatrogenic sources including contaminated human growth hormone, brain electrodes, corneal transplant, and the variant CJD (vCJD) caused by consuming contaminated brain tissue (mad cow disease). In fact, the first prion disease to be discovered was Kuru in Papua New Guinea. The disease resulted from cannibalistic funeral rituals of eating the dead, and was more common in women and children who prepared the bodies [3].

This group of diseases causing transmissible spongiform encephalopathy results from the conversion of normal prion protein (PrP^{c}) from an alpha helix form to the pathogenic beta sheeted scrapie form, PrP^{sc}. Whether due to spontaneous conversion of normal protein, an abnormal protein structure caused by a mutation, or the introduction of iatrogenic abnormal protein, the initial misfolded protein acts as a template for conversion of PrP^{c} to PrP^{sc}. A domino effect is produced, which causes a rapidly progressive disease [4]. Both intraspecies and interspecies transmission can occur. There are two main strains of mutant protein that form PrP^{sc}, Type 1 and 2. The type of mutant protein and a polymorphism at codon 129 are contributing factors to the phenotype that is expressed both in sporadic and genetic forms of the disease [5]. Prion protein is highly protease resistant. Therefore, special precautions need to be taken when handling tissue from an individual with suspected prion

J.S. Goldman (✉)
Taub Institute, Columbia University Medical Center, 630 W. 168th St., Box 16, New York, NY 10032, USA
e-mail: jg2673@cumc.columbia.edu

J.S. Goldman (ed.), *Genetic Counseling for Adult Neurogenetic Disease*,
DOI 10.1007/978-1-4899-7482-2_9

disease and equipment that has been used on them. Recently a very rare third strain that is protease sensitive has been identified. This strain leads to a distinct pathology and longer disease duration [6].

The average age of onset for sporadic CJD (sCJD) is 67 with a range of 17–90. Disease duration averages 4 months and is usually less than 1 year. Variant CJD usually occurs in the late teens or 20s and lasts about 1.5 years. Familial CJD has an average age of onset of less than 55 with a range from the 20s to 80s and disease duration of 1–5 years. GSS also usually occurs before 55 (range 20s to 60s) and has a duration of 2–10 years. FFI's age of onset is about 48 (range 25–61) and duration is about 1 year [4].

9.1 Clinical Presentation

The three major prion disease forms have different clinical presentations. CJD can present with psychiatric or personality changes (especially depression), confusion, memory loss, vision problems, hallucinations, insomnia, headache, weight loss, or neurological symptoms (including myoclonus, hyperreflexia, eye movement problems, ataxia, neuropathy, chorea, parkinsonism, and cortical blindness). Both cognitive and neurologic symptoms progress rapidly.

GSS is extremely rare (1–10/100,000,000) and always familial [7]. It usually presents with motor symptoms including ataxia and parkinsonism. However, cognitive and behavioral changes can also be seen. The disease course is appreciably longer than CJD, typically about 5 years or longer. As is obvious in the name, FFI usually begins with several months of insomnia followed by a movement disorder and then cognitive impairment [8]. Though usually inherited, rare sporadic cases have occurred [9].

9.2 Diagnosis

A neurological evaluation may reveal any of the above symptoms. In addition to routine laboratory testing, CSF from a lumbar puncture may be assayed for elevated 14:3:3 protein and tau protein. These findings, which indicate neuronal death, are relatively nonspecific. Diffusion weighted MRI is the best method for detecting the classic findings of cortical ribboning and hyperintensities in the basal ganglia [4, 6]. Additionally an EEG may be abnormal with periodic biphasic or triphasic complexes. A brain biopsy will reveal pathogenic prion protein, but is invasive and expensive to perform. If there is a family history of neurological disease (especially when it is rapidly progressive), genetic testing for *PRNP* should be considered. The brain biopsy analysis for prion protein, 14:3:3 testing, and gene sequencing are performed at the National Prion Surveillance Laboratory at Case Western University.

9.3 Treatment and Management

Management of prion disease is completely symptomatic. Despite several drug trials, no treatment has been found to slow progression of or cure the disease. Psychiatric symptoms such as depression and agitation can be treated pharmacologically with SSRIs and antipsychotics. Some of the movement disorders may respond to appropriate medication.

Families of people with CJD need significant support. They are faced with such a rapidly progressive disease that they often feel as if they cannot swim to the surface. They must obtain diagnosis, manage financial and legal concerns, and take care of end-of-life issues almost at the same time. The healthcare team should refer to support services and the CJD Foundation.

9.4 Genetics

The genetic form of human prion disease is due to mutations in the prion gene (*PRNP*) on chromosome 20. Inheritance always follows an autosomal dominant pattern and mutations are nearly fully penetrant, but expression is variable. Over 30 mutations have been reported [10]. Certain mutations exhibit consistent genotype/phenotype correlations, while others are more unpredictable. In some cases, phenotype is influenced by a polymorphism in codon 129 of this gene. This polymorphism is also thought to play a part in the risk for sporadic CJD and new variant CJD (mad cow disease). Codon 129 can code for methionine (Met) or valine (Val). Homozygosity (Met/Met or Val/Val) is a risk factor for sCJD and Met/Met is also a risk factor for variant CJD as found in cases exposed to Mad Cow [11]. This genotype also predicts a more rapid progression of sCJD. Other polymorphisms may also contribute to phenotypic variability of familial forms [4]. Additionally the genotype at codon 129 may influence the strain of PrP^{Sc} produced in familial CJD, with cis M to the mutation associated with type 1 and cis V associated with Type 2 [5].

Point mutations and octapeptide repeat deletion/insertion mutations in *PRNP* have been found to cause human prion disease [5]. The most common mutation is E200K that causes CJD with variable presentation, but very rapid decline (duration averaging just 5 months). In comparison, an octapeptide repeat insertion causes a slowly progressive disease beginning with personality and psychiatric changes and dementia. Not only does phenotype differ between mutations, but pathology does as well.

The most common mutation causing GSS is the P102L mutation. This mutation often causes a progressive cerebellar disease resembling spinocerebellar ataxia (SCA). In fact, for patients with ataxia for whom SCA testing has been negative, *PRNP* testing should be considered. Particularly interesting is the D178N mutation which, when coupled in cis with codon 129 M, causes FFI, but, when in cis with 129 V, causes CJD [5]. Since 60 % of inherited prion disease cases lack family history of similar neurological disease, genetic etiology is not always considered. Whether *de novo* mutations occur is unknown. Family history may be lacking because of lost information, misdiagnosis, premature death, false paternity, or undisclosed adoption. Thus, counseling about penetrance is compromised [12].

9.5 Genetic Counseling Issues

The issues confronting genetic counseling for prion disease should be divided into counseling about diagnostic testing and counseling individuals interested in presymptomatic testing. This discrepancy is due to the often urgent need for diagnostic testing. CJD is characterized by a rapid decline in clinical status. In early stages of the disease, the family is focused on getting a diagnosis, and when they do, are left reeling from its implication and how to best care for the patient. To insert the possibility of a genetic etiology is often too much for the family to comprehend and handle. Yet at the same time, if a family history indicates the possibility of hereditary CJD, a positive genetic test from a blood sample can confirm the diagnosis and eliminate the need for a brain biopsy. Having the patient and family together at the hospital presents the perfect time for genetic counseling and obtaining the blood sample. However, the ease of doing so must be weighed against the emotional impact and ability to absorb the information.

Counseling for diagnostic testing may also be complicated by the lack of family history or misdiagnoses. As stated above, about 60 % of inherited prion disease cases lack family history of similar neurological disease. Since most mutations have high penetrance, a lack of family history may be due to lost family members, early death from unrelated causes, false paternity, undisclosed adoption, or *de novo* mutations. Even when there is a family history of neurological disease, diagnoses of Alzheimer disease, ataxia, or Parkinson disease can be attributed to cases of GSS that have a long duration and can present as memory disorders or with ataxia or parkinsonism. Thus, families may be unwilling to accept the possibility of hereditary prion disease.

As with all dementia genetic counseling, the proband may not be sufficiently cognizant for informed consent. Thus, a durable power of attorney or next of kin must be present. Agitation is a common symptom of moderate to late prion disease and may be exacerbated in stressful situations. Cooperation from the patient may be impossible. In this situation, genetic testing should be delayed in favor of testing of autopsy tissue (when possible).

Presymptomatic genetic counseling for prion disease is similar to that for other dementias. A modified HD protocol should include genetic counseling sessions as well as a psychiatric evaluation. Because of the lack of a prodromal syndrome, and depending on the proximity to the average age of onset in the family, a neurological and neuropsychological evaluation may be unnecessary. The patient should, however, expect to bring a support person, at least to the result session.

The presymptomatic patient needs to understand that testing will reveal a mutation, but age of onset and presentation are not predictable. The variability of phenotype is dependent not only on the specific mutation and the codon 129 genotype, but also on the strain of PrP that will eventually arise. The patient may have experienced a particular presentation in a family member, but must be prepared for these ambiguities. Yet, although certain mutations (such as E200K) are slightly less than 100 % penetrant, the patient must expect that he will eventually develop the disease.

9.6 Prion Disease Case History (Fig. 9.1)

Mr. B was a 72-year-old man with a 2-month history of a rapidly progressive cognitive and movement disorder. His wife and daughter accompanied him to the Memory Disorders Clinic. Mr. B's first symptoms were balance problems and dizziness. Within a month, he developed insomnia, depression, and short-term memory loss. More recently, gait problems, slurred speech, worsening cognition, confusion, behavior changes, and paranoia were noted. On examination he was found to have ataxic gait and speech and right arm dystonia. The neurologist ordered a full blood workup including B-12 level, a paraneoplastic panel, and HIV testing. Neuropsychological testing, an EEG, and a diffusion weighted MRI were also ordered. Neuropsychological testing done three weeks later showed a 5 point decline in the MMSE and multi-domain cognitive problems. The MRI

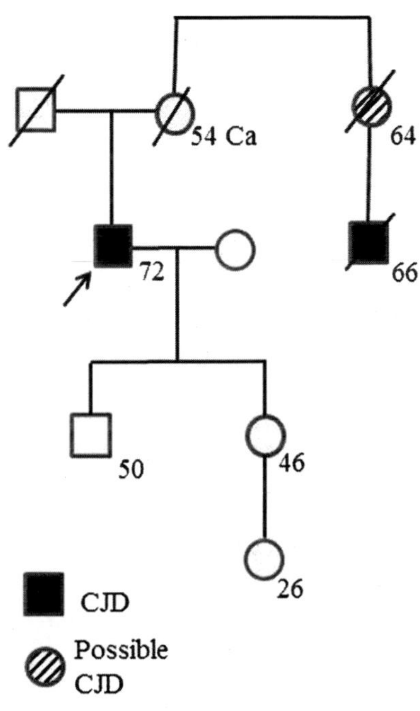

Fig. 9.1 CJD case history pedigree

revealed frontotemporal atrophy, dilated ventricles, and some mild cortical ribboning. The EEG was normal, as were all blood test measures. The neurologist suspected that the patient had CJD. He scheduled a lumbar puncture to draw CSF for 14-3-3 analysis. By the time the patient returned, he was extremely agitated. The physician met with the family to discuss his diagnostic suspicion. That same day, the family had received a call from a distant relative saying that they should ask about CJD because another relative had died recently from the disease and had similar symptoms. The neurologist called the genetic counselor to meet with the family to discuss genetic testing for *PRNP*.

Upon entering the room, it was obvious to the counselor that the family was in shock. Not only had they learned that their loved one had an incurable disease and would die within months, but that this disease was probably genetic. At the same time, the counselor felt a sense of urgency from the doctor to obtain a blood sample for genetic testing. The patient was recovering from the LP and was not in the room. The counselor first acknowledged the family's shock and sorrow. She reviewed the family pedigree and what the family had learned about other relatives with CJD. It appeared that the patient's mother had died of cancer in her 50s, but a maternal aunt had died in her 60s of a mysterious disease and her son had recently died in his 60s of CJD. His family had agreed on genetic testing at autopsy from the National Prion Surveillance Laboratory. The result revealed a genetic etiology. Documentation of an E200K mutation was obtained at a later date.

The family had little understanding of genetics. The genetic counselor reviewed CJD and its genetics, including autosomal dominant inheritance, and discussed how the patient's mother was probably a carrier of the gene, but died before it was expressed. She discussed implications for the patient's children and grandchildren were a genetic mutation found. She then attempted to discuss the informed consent for testing. The family was clearly distressed and could not absorb the information or confront the testing at that time. The genetic counselor asked if they would prefer to take the informed consent home and discuss testing at a later date. They said yes.

Discussion Questions

- Once the genetic counselor assessed the situation, should formal genetic counseling been immediately delayed to another time? Why or why not?
- How do you think the genetic counselor's directive to obtain the blood sample influence her actions?
- What role should the neurologist have played in preparing the family for the blood test?

Approximately a week later, the counselor spoke with the son, Evan, on the phone. He had many questions concerning penetrance, and felt that he and his sister were in disagreement about the testing as he might want to know his own status and she would not. His mother was having a very hard time with the realization that she might lose her children, as well as her husband, to the disease. The counselor reinforced that learning the cause of his father's illness did not necessitate testing any other family member, and that that was a very personal decision. She also reminded him that if he were to eventually test himself, the test would not reveal the age of onset of the disease, as demonstrated by the family history. She told him that she would be glad to speak to his sister on the phone or have another family meeting. Evan said that he would encourage his sister to call. However, a week later, the nurse who directed brain donations for the university called to say that Mr. B was in hospice and the family wished to complete paperwork for genetic testing to be done on brain tissue. The counselor prepared the paperwork without further communication with the family. Mr. B died later that week.

Discussion Questions

- To what extent should the genetic counselor become involved with family disputes about genetic testing?
- Once a family member contacts the counselor for consultation, should that person then be considered a patient?
- In this case, the person being considered for genetic testing cannot give informed consent. His wife is his healthcare proxy, but is not at risk for inheriting the gene. If she rejects testing, should her children be able to obtain testing for themselves despite guidelines to test the affected first? Try to consider this question in the absence of a known family history or autopsy.
- Discuss whether growing up with the knowledge of a genetic disease in the family versus finding out late in a disease stage would change perspective on genetic testing.

Three months later the family returned for a meeting with the doctor and genetic counselor to discuss autopsy and genetic testing results. Mrs. B, her son and daughter, their spouses, and her daughter's daughter, Carol age 26, attended. They were told that the autopsy confirmed CJD caused by a mutation in the prion gene. The mutation was the same as the cousin's, E200K, and had the same codon 129 polymorphism. However, the species of prion differed between the two cases. At the present time, there was no explanation for the cause of different prion types or the difference in age of onset of family members.

The counselor reviewed much of the previous discussion about the genetics of prion disease. Evan's sister repeatedly asked if onset could be later than her father's or even never happen. The counselor acknowledged how scary it is to think of the future, and reiterated that onset was unpredictable, but that it would usually occur within the range of the ages of onset in the family, and that it was highly unlikely that the gene would not be expressed if a person lived to be elderly. Evan told his sister that "everyone must die of something," and that "they just needed to go on living as usual." Mrs. B's granddaughter, Carol, remained silent through the discussion. The genetic counselor discussed how, since there was a known mutation, reproductive options, such as PGD, were available. Carol nodded but did not participate.

Carol called the counselor for an appointment by herself. She said she wished to be tested without having her family know. Exploration into her motivation revealed that she was in a significant relationship and expected to marry. She felt it was only fair to her boyfriend to have full knowledge of her genetic status for life planning purposes as well as reproductive options. She said that she had discussed this with her boyfriend who said that he wanted to continue together regardless, but thought it was important to understand where they were headed. However, she had not discussed testing with her family and had no intention of doing so.

Discussion Questions

- How do you respond to someone who does not want to hear that a gene is fully penetrant and that they have a 50 % chance of dying of their relative's devastating disease?
- What does a counselor do when she knows that the consultand is seeing the counselor against her family's wishes and will not discuss testing or its outcome with the family?
- Should the counselor have referred Carol to another counselor because of the existing relationship with the family?
- If Carol tests positive, she will automatically have knowledge of her mother's genetic status. How does the counselor deal with this fact?

After a second discussion with Carol and her boyfriend, the counselor concluded that Carol had legitimate reasons for testing. She had reflected on what it would mean for herself personally, for them as a supportive couple, and for their relationship with her family. Carol was determined to go ahead with testing and to keep the results from her family. The counselor referred them to the neurogeneticist for final counseling, psychiatric evaluation, and testing. Carol was found not to have the family mutation.

9.7 Patient Resources

CJD Foundation

341W. 38th Street, Suite 501 New York, NY 10018
212-719-5900, 1-800-659-1991
http://www.cjdfoundation.org
National Prion Surveillance Laboratory
216-368-0587
http://www.cjdsurveillance.com
UCSF Memory and Aging Center Web site:
www.memory.uscf.edu

References

1. Safar, J., Roller, P. P., Gajdusek, D. C., & Gibbs, C. J., Jr. (1993). Conformational transitions, dissociation, and unfolding of scrapie amyloid (prion) protein. *Journal of Biological Chemistry, 268*(27), 20276–20284.
2. Collinge, J. (2001). Prion diseases of humans and animals: their causes and molecular basis. *Annual Review of Neuroscience, 24*, 519–550.
3. Lee, H. S., Brown, P., Cervenáková, L., Garruto, R. M., Alpers, M. P., Gajdusek, D. C., et al. (2001). Increased susceptibility to Kuru of carriers of the PRNP 129 methionine/methionine genotype. *Journal of Infectious Diseases, 183*(2), 192–196.
4. Brown, K., & Mastrianni, J. A. (2010). The prion diseases. *Journal of Geriatric Psychiatry and Neurology, 23*(4), 277–298.
5. Capellari, S., Strammiello, R., Saverioni, D., Kretzschmar, H., & Parchi, P. (2011). Genetic Creutzfeldt-Jakob disease and fatal familial insomnia: insights into phenotypic variability and disease pathogenesis. *Acta Neuropathologica, 121*(1), 21–37.
6. Sikorska, B., Knight, R., Ironside, J. W., & Liberski, P. P. (2012). Creutzfeldt-Jakob disease. *Advances in Experimental Medicine and Biology, 724*, 76–90.
7. Liberski, P. P. (2012). Gerstmann-Sträussler-Scheinker disease. *Advances in Experimental Medicine and Biology, 724*, 128–137.
8. Gambetti, P., Parchi, P., Petersen, R. B., Chen, S. G., & Lugaresi, E. (1995). Fatal familial insomnia and familial Creutzfeldt-Jakob disease: clinical, pathological and molecular features. *Brain Pathology, 5*(1), 43–51.
9. Montagna, P., Gambetti, P., Cortelli, P., & Lugaresi, E. (2003). Familial and sporadic fatal insomnia. *Lancet Neurology, 2*(3), 167–176.
10. Beck, J. A., Poulter, M., Campbell, T. A., Adamson, G., Uphill, J. B., Guerreiro, R., et al. (2010). PRNP allelic series from 19 years of prion protein gene sequencing at the MRC Prion Unit. *Human Mutation, 31*(7), E1551–E1563.
11. Bishop, M. T., Pennington, C., Heath, C. A., Will, R. G., & Knight, R. S. (2009). PRNP variation in UK sporadic and variant Creutzfeldt Jakob disease highlights genetic risk factors and a novel non-synonymous polymorphism. *BMC Medical Genetics, 10*, 146.
12. Dagvadorj, A., Petersen, R. B., Lee, H. S., Cervenakova, L., Shatunov, A., Budka, H., et al. (2002). Spontaneous mutations in the prion protein gene causing transmissible spongiform encephalopathy. *Annals of Neurology, 52*(3), 355–359.

Part III
Stroke

Chapter 10
Overview of Cerebrovascular Disease and Stroke Risk Factors

Heather Workman

Stroke is the fourth leading cause of death in the USA. The term "stroke" is used to describe an interruption of blood and oxygen flow to the brain, without which brain cells begin to die within minutes. If blood supply is not restored, permanent damage will occur. About 795,000 Americans suffer from a stroke every year, and 137,000 will die because of the stroke. Thus on average, a person dies from a stroke every 4 min.

Medical literature often refers to a stroke as a cerebral vascular accident (CVA). The majority of CVAs are due to ischemic stroke (80–90 %), with the remainder due to hemorrhagic stroke (10–20 %). Ischemic stroke is caused by a complete blockage of a cerebral artery, blocking the flow of blood and oxygen to the brain. The blockage is commonly caused by artherosclerosis, which is the narrowing of the arteries due to cholesterol deposits. If the narrowing is too great, blood cells can accumulate and develop a blood clot. Another cause of ischemic stroke is a clot that forms in the heart (sometimes as a result of atrial fibrillation) and travels through a blood vessel until it becomes lodged and obstructs blood flow. Individuals may also experience TIAs (transient ischemic attacks), which are often referred to as "mini strokes." A TIA is a minor clot that typically resolves in a short period of time without lasting damage. TIAs can be a precursor to ischemic stroke.

Hemorrhagic stroke is caused by sudden rupture of a brain vessel. The rupture occurs in the presence of a weakened blood vessel resulting from an aneurysm or arterial venous malformation. A ruptured vessel can occur within the brain (intracerebral hemorrhage) or surrounding the outside of the brain (subarachnoid hemorrhage) [1].

H. Workman (✉)
Department of Medical Genetics, Dayton Children's Hospital, 1 Children's Plaza, Dayton, OH 45404, USA
e-mail: workmanh@childrensdayton.org

J.S. Goldman (ed.), *Genetic Counseling for Adult Neurogenetic Disease*,
DOI 10.1007/978-1-4899-7482-2_10

10.1 Clinical Presentation

Warning signs of a stroke include weakness in face, hands or feet, headache, sudden confusion, abnormal speech, or visual problems in one or both eyes. Some people may have trouble with balance and walking. Others will experience a sudden, extreme headache. The effects of stroke largely depend on the area and amount of the brain affected. Common after effects include weakness, paralysis, and problems with speech and cognitive skills. The acronym F.A.S.T. has been adopted by the American Stroke Association to educate the public on the warning signs of a stroke. F.A.S.T. stands for F—face droop; A—arm weakness; S—speech difficulty; T—time to call 9-1-1.

10.2 Diagnosis

Medical history, a neurological exam, blood flow testing, and imaging studies confirm a suspected diagnosis of a stroke. MRI is used to look for brain and blood vessel abnormalities that suggest damage from a stroke. An EEG (encephalogram) may show unusually slow brain waves that are suggestive of a stroke. Blood flow tests are usually guided by ultrasound to look for vessels that have blockage (carotid and vertebral arteries).

10.3 Treatment and Management

For ischemic stroke, the FDA-approved drug, tissue plasminogen activator (tPA) may be able to dissolve the blockage; however, it must be administered within a few hours of stroke onset. An endovascular procedure, using a catheter to remove the blood clot from the blocked vessel, may be used alone or in conjunction with tPA. For an ischemic stroke, a coil is placed near the aneurysm or arteriovenous malformation (AVM) to prevent rupture of the artery. In certain cases, endovascular procedures may also be used for hemorrhagic stroke. However, hemorrhagic stroke due to an aneurysm may require surgery to place a clip to stop the bleeding.

After a stroke, individuals will need varying levels of personal care assistance as well as physical, occupational, and speech therapy. Many individuals will develop personality changes, persistent cognitive processing difficulties, and depression. Aphasia is a common side effect of stroke, and is characterized by difficulty in both verbal and written expressive language and possibly semantic understanding of language.

10.4 Genetics

Many factors can affect an individual's risk for stroke. Genetic syndromes make up a relatively small percentage (around 1 %). Common risk factors for ischemic stroke include age, gender and ethnicity. Some medical conditions, including hypertension, smoking, and diabetes, increase the risk of stroke. However, it is important to keep in mind that many of the risk factors for stroke include a hereditary component in themselves: hypertension, high cholesterol, artherosclerosis, and obesity are some examples [2].

Family studies and twin studies show that stroke is heritable. Twin studies demonstrate that concordance rates are 65 % greater in identical than in fraternal twins. Cohort and case–control studies have showed that having a family history of stroke increases the odds of stroke by about 30–75 %. When stroke occurs before the age of 70, these studies suggest an even stronger genetic component. After adjusting for age, sex, hypertension, diabetes, cholesterol, smoking, and obesity, having a family history of stroke increases the odds of developing stroke by 38 % [3]. Women have a greater risk for ischemic stroke than men [4].

African Americans also have an increased susceptibility to stroke, perhaps because of a higher incidence of conditions that can increase stroke risk including smoking, diabetes, high blood pressure and obesity. This population also has a greater risk for first time stroke and a higher risk for complications and mortality [5].

Several monogenic syndromes include stroke as a symptom of the condition, including: sickle cell disease, Fabry disease, Hereditary Hemorrhagic Telangiectasia, Homocystinuria, MELAS, CADASIL, and connective tissue disorders. Stroke is also a known complication of hereditary cardiomyopathies, dysrhythmias, hemoglobinopathies, coagulopathies, dyslipidemias, and vasculopathies. CADASIL will be discussed in the following chapter as an example of an autosomal dominant stroke disorder (Table 10.1).

Sickle cell disease is an autosomal recessive condition affecting 1 in 300–500 individuals of African American descent. It is characterized by vaso-occlusive events that lead to chronic pain and inflammation. A common feature in infants is dactylitis (pain and swelling of the hands and feet). Ischemic stroke can occur in up to 11 % of children and young adults with sickle cell disease. Approximately 22–35 % of individuals will develop silent cerebral infarcts. Though individuals are typically asymptomatic at the time the infarcts are noted, they may be a precursor to ischemic stroke.

Fabry disease is an X-linked condition that has a significant clinical course in males, with many women carriers also developing symptoms. The condition occurs from a deficiency of the enzyme α-galactosidase (α-GAL A), which leads to a buildup of globotriaosylceramide (GL-3). The first manifestations of the condition include angiokeratomas (cutaneous lesions) and acroparesthesias (periodic severe pain in the extremities). Specific eye changes are also present in both males and females, and are noted as cornea verticillata and "Fabry cataracts." Adults with the

Table 10.1 Mendelian stroke syndromes

Syndrome	Gene	Inheritance	Symptoms
CADASIL	*Notch3*	AD	Recurrent stroke; migraines; depression; cognitive impairment; dementia; white matter lesions on brain MRI
EDS, Vascular	*COL3A1*	AD	Vascular complications, uterine and intestinal rupture; uncommon cause of stroke in young adults
Fabry disease	*GLA*	X-linked	ESRD; TIAs/stroke, acroparesthesias, angiokeratomas, cardiovascular disease
Hereditary Hemorrhagic Telangiectasia	*ENG, ACVRL1, SMAD4*	AD	Mucocutaneous Telangiectasias, AVMs, recurrent nosebleeds
Homocystinuria	*CBS*	AR	Developmental delay, lens dislocation, thromboembolism
MELAS	*MT-TL1*	Mitochondrial	Seizures, dev delay, stroke-like episodes, diabetes, elevated lactate and pyruvate
Pseudoxanthoma Elasticum	*ABCC6 (MRP6)*	AR	Skin papules, angioid streaks on eye, retinal hemorrhage, arteriole narrowing

condition may develop progressive end-stage renal disease (ESRD), as well as left ventricular hypertrophy, conduction abnormalities, and stroke/TIAs or frank cerebral hemorrhage. Stroke or TIAs have been noted in up to 13 % of individuals with Fabry disease, and is a significant cause of morbidity and mortality.

Hereditary Hemorrhagic Telangiectasia (HHT) is an autosomal dominant condition that is characterized by cutaneous and mucosal telangiectasias and epitaxis, which are frequent nosebleeds. Arteriovenous malformations (AVMs) are another common feature and may occur in the brain, GI tract, lung, and liver. AVMs are at risk for bleeding, and this leads to the increased risk for brain bleeds. In addition, pulmonary AVMs may lead to TIAs.

Homocystinuria is a rare autosomal recessive condition that is caused by a cystathionine β-synthase (CBS) deficiency. Features of the condition include developmental delay and intellectual disability, Marfanoid habitus, severe myopia and lens dislocation. Individuals have an increased risk for blood clots due to an increase in plasma homocysteine levels. The risk of blood clots puts individuals at increased risk for stroke, and is a major cause of morbidity and mortality in homocystinuria.

MELAS, Mitochondrial Encephalopathy, Lactic Acidosis, and Stroke-like episodes, is a syndrome that includes seizures, developmental delay, and elevated lactate and pyruvate levels. Seizures have been reported in conjunction with stroke-like episodes. Symptoms of the stroke-like episodes include paralysis/weakness on one side of the body (hemiparesis), altered vision, and possible change in consciousness. Although symptoms can occur any time in life, typically affected individuals have a period of normal development followed by the onset of symptoms between the ages of 2 and 10. MELAS is a mitochondrial condition with most affected individuals having one of 3 common mutations in the *MT-TL1* gene.

Autosomal dominant polycystic kidney disease (ADPKD) is caused by mutations in the *PKD1* and *PKD2* genes. It is mainly characterized by bilateral renal cysts, as well as cysts in other organs such as the liver. There is a risk for intracranial and arterial aneurysm. Intracranial aneurysms occur in approximately 10 % of individuals with ADPKD and may be asymptomatic.

Pseudoxanthoma Elasticum (PXE) is an autosomal recessive condition that is associated with skin papules, and retinal complications including angioid streaks of the retina and retinal hemorrhage. Vascular manifestations are rare but can be related to arterial narrowing significant enough to cause claudication (a problem with blood flow which can cause pain and fatigue) in the arms or legs, myocardial infarction, intestinal angina, and stroke.

10.5 Genetic Counseling Issues

There is currently no genetic testing for idiopathic stroke. An individual who presents with a family history of ischemic stroke may be looking for screening tools and methods to decrease their own risk. Genetic counselors should involve a physician to discuss manageable environmental risk factors, such as high cholesterol, hypertension, and diabetes. Hereditary factors that can predispose to blood clots, such as Factor V Leiden, prothrombin, and protein C deficiency, should also be explored.

The hereditary clotting factors conditions, factor V Leiden, prothrombin, and protein C deficiencies, are all autosomal dominant conditions that carry varying risks of thrombosis. The association of these disorders with the risk of stroke in both adults and children is controversial, but bears consideration [6].

If the individual has a family history of hemorrhagic stroke, the genetic counselor should screen for possible hereditary explanations, such as connective tissue disorders and hereditary hemorrhagic telangiectasia.

10.5.1 Family History Questions for Stroke

When taking a family history in the context of stroke, it is important to keep in mind known risk factors such as age and ethnicity. A three-generation family history should include the type of stroke in affected individuals and age of onset. Also be mindful of medical findings that are suggestive of an underlying syndrome (i.e., nosebleeds and AVM are associated with HHT; renal disease and TIAs are

history of the condition as well as autosomal dominant inheritance. The counselor states that genetic testing is available, and asks if Mr. B is interested in discussing this further. He and Mrs. B are very interested in hearing more about testing and what it might tell them. The genetic counselor also gently discusses that should a mutation be identified then his 2 siblings would be at risk for the condition as well. At this point, Mr. B becomes angry and states that his brother and sister are ignorant, and wouldn't do anything with the information even if he did share it with them.

The counselor discusses how genetic testing for HHT involves looking for mutations in 3 different genes. The risks and benefits of the testing are reviewed. Mr. B states that it would be helpful to have a tangible answer for his own risk as well as his father's history. The genetic counselor also discussed that if a mutation were found, then Mr. B. could undergo routine screening for cerebral AVMs and other AVMs, and that he could be followed in a nearby HHT multidisciplinary clinic.

Since the couple is pregnant, the genetic counselor also broaches a discussion of prenatal testing for HHT. The couple is adamant that they are not interested in prenatal testing/screening of any kind and do not want information on available options.

At the end of the visit, Mr. B. consents to genetic testing for HHT. A follow up appointment is made to discuss the results in person. Mr. B and his wife are encouraged to come to the appointment together. Mrs. B. is concerned about missing work since she has just started a new job, so the counselor makes arrangements for them to come late in the day.

Genetic testing reveals that Mr. B carries a pathogenic mutation in the *ACVRL1* gene. Mr. and Mrs. B both start crying. The genetic counselor acknowledges that they must be anxious about the implications of the result. However, Mr. and Mrs. B both state they are relieved to not only have an explanation for Mr. B's father's death, but to also have a name for the condition and a plan of action. Mr. B wants to be seen in the local HHT multidisciplinary clinic, and a referral is made for him that day.

Again, the genetic counselor discusses the positive result and implications for other family members. At this point the couple gives each other a knowing look. Mrs. B states that they discussed at length what to do about his siblings. In the end, Mr. B decided it would be best to contact them since he has nieces and nephews and is concerned about how this would affect them. Mrs. B had even gone so far as to find Mr. B's sister on Facebook and has a plan to contact her after this appointment.

The genetic counselor makes a call to the couple a month after the results appointment. Mr. B is not available, but the counselor speaks with Mrs. B who states that Mr. B. has his appointment with the HHT clinic the following week, and they are looking forward to the information. She states that the genetic test results have given them a sense of relief and optimism. Mrs. B also says that she had reached out to Mr. B's sister on Facebook, but has not gotten a response. The genetic counselor commends Mrs. B for attempting to notify her in-laws of the test results. The genetic counselor also notes that there is no guarantee that other relatives would be as eager to act on the information. Mrs. B comments that her sister-in-law's silence only further confirms Mr. B's feelings that his estranged family is "ignorant." Mrs. B feels that she may have done more harm than good by trying to contact Mr. B's sister. The genetic counselor says that they have a right to know if they wish to, and that she had acted appropriately. She offers to speak to any family member who might like more information.

Discussion Questions:

- How did the couple's knowledge of the expected baby influence the genetic counseling referral?
- How did the couple react to learning that there could be a genetic explanation for Mr. B's father's death?
- How should the counselor handle Mr. B's reaction to sharing genetic information with his siblings?
- What are possible reasons for why the couple was not interested in prenatal testing options?
- What is the genetic counselor's role in guiding notification of at-risk family members?
- What impact has attempting to contact estranged family members had on Mr. and Mrs. B?

References

1. Alg, V. S., Sofat, R., Houlden, H., & Werring, D. J. (2013). Genetic risk factors for intracranial aneurysms: A meta-analysis in more than 116,000 individuals. *Neurology, 80*(23), 2154–2165.
2. Biffi, A., Anderson, C. D., Falcone, G. J., Kissela, B., Norrving, B., Tirschwell, D., et al. (2013). Novel insights into the genetics of intracerebral hemorrhage. *Stroke, 44*(6 Suppl 1), S137.
3. Gelfand, A. A., Croen, L. A., Torres, A. R., & Wu, Y. W. (2013). Genetic risk factors for perinatal arteriol ischemic stroke. *Pediatric Neurology, 48*(1), 36–41.
4. Jerrard-Dunne, P., Evans, A., McGovern, R., Hajat, C., Kalra, L., Rudd, A. G., et al. (2003). Ethnic differences in markers of thrombophilia: Implications for the investigation of ischemic stroke in multiethnic populations: The South London Ethnicity and Stroke Study. *Stroke, 34*(8), 1821–1826.
5. Touzé, E., & Rothwell, P. M. (2007). Heritability of ischaemic stroke in women compared with men: A genetic epidemiological study. *Lancet Neurology, 6*(2), 125–133. Erratum in: (2008) *Lancet Neurol*, 7(1), 25.
6. J, V. J., & Howard, P. (2013). Reasons underlying racial differences in stroke incidence and mortality. *Stroke, 44*(6 Suppl 1), S126–S128.

Chapter 11
CADASIL

Jamie C. Fong

Cerebral autosomal dominant arteriopathy with subcortical infarcts and leukoencephalopathy, known as CADASIL, is the most common inherited cause of stroke and vascular dementia in adults. First described in 1955, this hereditary condition of small cerebral arteries was eventually mapped to a locus on chromosome 19q12 [1]. Linkage studies that followed refined the genetic interval, culminating in the identification of the *NOTCH3* gene as harboring pathogenic mutations [2, 3].

Since 1996, CADASIL has been reported in more than 500 families worldwide, though its overall prevalence remains unknown. Despite increasing awareness of the condition, it likely remains underdiagnosed. The estimated prevalence of the disease is 4.14 per 100,000, and about 0.05 % of individuals with lacunar stroke carry a *NOTCH3* gene mutation [3]. However, when considering individuals with both lacunar stroke and white matter abnormalities on neuroimaging, *NOTCH3* gene mutations are responsible for about 2 % of disease with onset by age 65 years, and about 11 % of disease with onset by age 50 years.

In contrast to sporadic ischemic stroke and vascular dementia of the elderly, CADASIL usually occurs in the absence of traditional vascular risk factors. Nonetheless, many of the clinical manifestations of CADASIL, as well as its cognitive profile and neuroimaging abnormalities, overlap with that of sporadic small artery diseases with subcortical ischemic vascular dementia. While sporadic small artery diseases in the elderly are frequently associated with Alzheimer-type neuropathology, CADASIL is not associated with amyloid plaques and neurofibrillary tangles. Consequently, in contrast to sporadic disease, clinical-pathological correlations are not confounded in CADASIL; thus this relatively rare monogenic disorder serves as a model for the more common, sporadic forms of ischemic stroke and vascular dementia.

J.C. Fong (✉)
Department of Neurology, Memory and Aging Center, University of California, MC:1207, 675 Nelson Rising Lane, Suite 190, San Francisco, CA 94158, USA
e-mail: jfong@memory.ucsf.edu

J.S. Goldman (ed.), *Genetic Counseling for Adult Neurogenetic Disease*,
DOI 10.1007/978-1-4899-7482-2_11

11.1 Clinical Presentation

The clinical presentation and age of onset of CADASIL are variable. Despite intra- and inter-familial variability, CADASIL has several key features: migraine with aura; subcortical ischemic events, including ischemic stroke and transient ischemic attacks (TIA); cognitive impairment with progression to dementia; and mood problems or other psychiatric disturbances. Approximately 5–10 % of patients have epileptic seizures, but rarely as the presenting symptom [4, 5].

About 20–40 % of patients with CADASIL experience migraine with aura. Though affecting fewer than half of all patients, migraine with aura occurs at a four- to five-fold greater frequency among individuals with CADASIL than in the general population [6]. When present, migraine with aura is often the first symptom, with mean onset in the late 20s (age range 6–48 years) [4, 6]. Auras are usually characterized by visual or sensory disturbances, but motor or speech problems may also occur. Visual aura symptoms frequently include blind spots with flickering or shimmering light traveling in a zigzag pattern across the visual field (scintillating scotomas); impaired vision involving half of a visual field of both eyes (lateral homonymous hemianopia); or blurred vision. Sensory symptoms usually include numbness or tingling. Migraine accompanied by atypical features affects more than half of CADASIL migraineurs and include basilar headache, aura without headache, or prolonged aura [7–9]. The clinical picture prior to onset of ischemic disease may not be different from that of other migraineurs in the general population.

Ischemic stroke and TIA are predominant features of CADASIL, affecting about 60–85 % of patients [6]. In most families with CADASIL, stroke is the first recognized symptom of disease. Ischemic events usually begin in middle age, with mean onset in the middle to late 40s (age range 20–70 years), and often in the absence of conventional vascular risk factors [4, 6, 10]. They usually present as classic lacunar syndromes that yield motor or sensory symptoms [11]. However, some events are clinically silent, while others occur as mild or vague symptoms of fatigue, dizziness, or confusion. Still others occur abruptly as focal neurologic deficits: dysarthria with or without motor or sensory symptoms, weakness or abnormal sensations of a single limb, isolated gait impairment, or nonfluent aphasia [11]. These acute deficits may be associated with headache and, when transient, can mimic migraine with aura [7]. Ischemic events usually recur, with many patients experiencing two to five strokes over several years. As the strokes recur, deficits accumulate and lead to stepwise cognitive and functional decline.

Up to 90 % of patients have cognitive deficits characterized by deficits in attention, processing speed, and executive function [12, 13]. These deficits are observed prior to the onset of stroke or TIA, and begin as subtle changes in the middle 40s, possibly as early as in the late 20s; mutation carriers may not come to medical attention until faced with either significant disability or the onset of ischemic disease [12]. However, difficulty with tasks involving set-shifting, response inhibition, working memory, verbal fluency, and abstract reasoning can be detected by formal neuropsychological assessment well in advance of ischemic disease [13, 14]. These deficits are consistent with patients' subjective complaints of reduced mental efficiency, disorganization, and poor recall during the early stages of illness [15]. In contrast, episodic memory tends to be well preserved, even in later stages of illness [12]. Taken together, the cognitive profile of CADASIL is similar to that of sporadic subcortical ischemic vascular dementia, although impairment in CADASIL occurs at much younger ages. A dysexecutive syndrome is also observed in post-stroke patients with CADASIL, with deficits worsening not only in the presence of infarction [12], but also with age [4, 15]. Focal deficits in CADASIL eventually progress to diffuse impairment in multiple cognitive domains, with 60 % of patients older than 60 years of age meeting DSM-IV (*Diagnostic and Statistical Manual of Mental Disorders*, fourth edition) criteria for dementia [13]. About 10 % of patients have dementia in the absence of any other symptoms. In later stages of illness, patients with dementia frequently have gait impairment, urinary urgency with or without incontinence, and pseudobulbar palsy [11]. By the time of death, most patients are completely dependent and require assistance in performing activities of daily living [16].

Psychiatric disturbances are also prominent features of CADASIL. About 20–45 % of patients have a significant mood disorder, including major depression and major depressive episodes that alternate with periods of mania, the latter of which may be mistaken for bipolar disorder rather than features of a CADASIL prodrome [4, 10, 11, 17, 18]. Though age of onset varies, mood disorders often present concurrently with cognitive impairment and/or ischemic disease. Families characterize early signs of illness by the presence of mild depression and changes in patients' behavior or personality, including new or increased irritability, as well as decreased motivation and interest in home and work life. In addition to mood lability and apathy, sleep disturbances are frequently observed in patients with CADASIL. Few patients experience delusions or hallucinations, and few have histories of attempted suicide [17, 18].

In summary, despite CADASIL's variability, some generalizations about the disorder's temporal course are possible. CADASIL becomes evident in young or middle adulthood with migraine, if present, or with an ischemic event. The mean age of onset is approximately 37 years. Subtle cognitive impairment and psychiatric disturbances can appear in early stages of disease, though they may be overlooked until functional decline is disabling, or a stroke or TIA occurs. Functional disability before age 40 is rare, but its incidence increases rapidly with age. Frank dementia, frequently associated with motor problems, is usually apparent after age 60, and nearly 40 % of patients are unable to walk without assistance by age 65. The mean duration of disease is about 20 years, and mean age at death is 65 years among men and 70 years among women. Pneumonia with or without aspiration is the most frequent cause of death [4, 10, 16].

11.2 Diagnosis

Clinical history and neurologic exam are used in the clinical confirmation of CADASIL. Subcortical infarcts and leukoencephalopathy of CADASIL are best detected by magnetic resonance imaging (MRI). In addition to neuroimaging, skin biopsy is used with limitations. Skin biopsy immunostaining using a NOTCH3 antibody is highly sensitive (96 %) and specific (100 %) for a diagnosis of CADASIL [23]. However, the gold standard for diagnosis of CADASIL is molecular analysis of the *NOTCH3* gene.

Widespread diffuse white matter hyperintensities on MRI are the imaging hallmarks of CADASIL. The white matter lesions first appear between ages 20 and 30 years, preceding the onset of ischemic disease by about 10–15 years [8, 19]. Little is known about the presence of hyperintensities in individuals under age 20 years, as they have not been extensively studied, but all mutation carriers have evident leukoencephalopathy by age 35 [8]. With age, the punctate lesions become more diffuse and symmetric. These neuroimaging findings, while not pathognomonic, are highly suggestive of CADASIL. White matter hyperintensities may occur in the basal ganglia and thalamus, distinguishing CADASIL from multiple sclerosis, which can mimic CADASIL [8, 19, 20]. The brainstem and corpus callosum may also be affected. By contrast, orbitofrontal and occipital white matter are usually spared.

Lacunar infarcts typically appear at age 40–50 years in the same areas as white matter hyperintensities [19]. Microbleeds are also observed in about one-third of patients with CADASIL, frequently after age 50 years. However, they are not unique to the disorder, and, in addition to the extent of white matter hyperintensities and lacunar infarction, are associated with hypertension and poor glucose control [19].

Although brain atrophy may be a better marker of disease progression, MRI studies show a positive correlation between leukoencephalopathy burden and/or lacunar infarct volume in CADASIL and the extent of cognitive impairment and functional disability [21, 22].

11.3 Treatment and Management

There is currently no cure for CADASIL. Treatment involves secondary prevention, although no medication with proven efficacy exists. Prophylactic treatment of migraine with aura may be needed depending on the frequency of attacks. Patients with frequent migraines may benefit from antiepileptic medications or beta blockers. A few case studies and a preliminary report suggest that acetazolamide is effective [24]. Patients in need of symptomatic treatment of migraine should avoid vasoconstrictors including ergot derivatives and triptans, and should instead use nonsteroidal anti-inflammatory analgesics [24, 25].

Although empiric data are sparse, prevention of ischemic events in patients with CADASIL is based on the treatment of sporadic, non-cardioembolic ischemic stroke. For example, patients should use antiplatelet agents instead of anticoagulants like warfarin because of the latter's associated risk of hemorrhage.

Cognitive symptoms are difficult to treat in CADASIL. The only randomized, placebo-controlled clinical trial investigated the impact of donepezil in patients with a broad range of cognitive impairments [26]. While the study demonstrated improvement on certain measures of executive function, it failed to achieve the primary goal of improved performance on a subscale of the vascular Alzheimer disease assessment scale. The clinical significance of these findings is unclear, and administration of donepezil in CADASIL would constitute off-label use, as is the case for sporadic subcortical ischemic vascular dementia.

11.4 Genetics

CADASIL is caused by mutations in the *NOTCH3* gene. The *NOTCH3* gene encodes a single-pass transmembrane receptor that is primarily expressed in vascular smooth muscle cells. About 200 mutations have been reported. The *NOTCH3* gene has 33 exons, but most CADASIL-associated mutations occur in exons 2–24. More than 70 % of CADASIL patients carry a mutation in either exon 3 or 4 [27]. Genotype-phenotype correlations in CADASIL are weak [28]. *De novo* mutations have been reported, although their exact frequency is not known [29]. Homozygous state *NOTCH3* mutations have been reported and appear indistinguishable from those in heterozygous mutation carriers [30].

11.5 Genetic Counseling Issues

Genetic testing is appropriate for patients with a characteristic clinical syndrome, distinct neuroimaging, and a family history of stroke or dementia in at least one first-degree relative before age 60. The additional presence of migraine with aura and the absence of cardiovascular risk factors in the proband increase the likelihood of detecting an underlying *NOTCH3* mutation, although the opposite scenarios do not preclude the presence of a mutation. Genetic testing may also be considered for patients with characteristic white matter burden and cognitive impairment, even in the absence of a clear family history [31]. Genetic testing lacks clear benefit if the patient only has migraine with aura, a few hyperintensities on neuroimaging, and a negative family history.

As with other neurodegenerative conditions, genetic counseling for CADASIL raises unique issues about diagnostic and predictive testing. Family history should be assessed thoroughly, with specific focus on relatives with a history of migraine with or without aura, stroke or TIA, dementia, epilepsy, and/or psychiatric

NOTCH3 mutation. The patient was glad to finally have a definitive diagnosis, but was saddened about her future and the potential burden she placed on her family. She planned to work through these negative ruminations with her therapist, and hoped that her husband would also consider talking to someone about his concerns. She planned to write a letter to her daughter, who still had no desire to know the patient's genetic status. The patient and her husband intended to share information with their son, but had not yet thought about how best to do so. The son was vaguely aware of family history of dementia. They were counseled to be honest with their son in an age-appropriate manner. The couple was given the information about "CADASIL, Together We Have Hope," a national source and advocacy organization for families with CADASIL.

Discussion Questions

- How do ambiguous or nonspecific symptoms in a child raise ethical concerns about genetic testing of minors?
- How does the possibility of detecting hallmark neuroimaging features warrant caution when considering the clinical evaluation of minors with ambiguous or nonspecific symptoms?

11.7 Patient Resources

CADASIL, Together We Have Hope
http://cadasilfoundation.org/

References

1. Tournier-Lasserve, E., Joutel, A., Melki, J., Weissenbach, J., Lathrop, G. M., Chabriat, H., et al. (1993). Cerebral autosomal dominant arteriopathy with subcortical infarcts and leukoencephalopathy maps to chromosome 19q12. *Nature Genetics, 3*(3), 256–259.
2. Ducros, A., Nagy, T., Alamowitch, S., Nibbio, A., Joutel, A., Vahedi, K., et al. (1996). Cerebral autosomal dominant arteriopathy with subcortical infarcts and leukoencephalopathy, genetic homogeneity, and mapping of the locus within a 2-cM interval. *American Journal of Human Genetics, 58*(1), 171–181.
3. Dong, Y. B., Hassan, A., Zhang, Z. Y., Huber, D., Dalageorgou, C., & Markus, H. S. (2003). Yield of screening for CADASIL mutations in lacunar stroke and leukoaraiosis. *Stroke, 34*(1), 203–205.
4. Dichgans, M., Mayer, M., Uttner, I., Bruning, R., Muller-Hocker, J., Rungger, G., et al. (1998). The phenotypic spectrum of CADASIL: Clinical findings in 102 cases. *Annals of Neurology, 44*(5), 731–739.
5. Velizarova, R., Mourand, I., Serafini, A., Crespel, A., & Gelisse, P. (2011). Focal epilepsy as first symptom in CADASIL. *Seizure, 20*(6), 502–504.
6. Herve, D., & Chabriat, H. (2010). CADASIL. *Journal of Geriatric Psychiatry and Neurology, 23*(4), 269–276.

7. Vahedi, K., Chabriat, H., Levy, C., Joutel, A., Tournier-Lasserve, E., & Bousser, M. G. (2004). Migraine with aura and brain magnetic resonance imaging abnormalities in patients with CADASIL. *Archives of Neurology, 61*(8), 1237–1240.
8. Chabriat, H., Tournier-Lasserve, E., Vahedi, K., Leys, D., Joutel, A., Nibbio, A., et al. (1995). Autosomal-dominant migraine with MRI white-matter abnormalities mapping to the CADASIL locus. *Neurology, 45*(6), 1086–1091.
9. Verin, M., Rolland, Y., Landgraf, F., Chabriat, H., Bompais, B., Michel, A., et al. (1995). New phenotype of the cerebral autosomal dominant arteriopathy mapped to chromosome 19: Migraine as the prominent clinical feature. *Journal of Neurology, Neurosurgery, and Psychiatry, 59*, 579–585.
10. Desmond, D. W., Moroney, J. T., Lynch, T., Chan, S., Chin, S. S., Shungu, D. C., et al. (1998). CADASIL in a North American family—clinical, pathologic, and radiologic findings. *Neurology, 51*(3), 844–849.
11. Chabriat, H., Vahedi, K., Iba-Zizen, M. T., Joutel, A., Nibbio, A., Nagy, T. G., et al. (1995). Clinical spectrum of CADASIL: A study of 7 families. Cerebral autosomal dominant arteriopathy with subcortical infarcts and leukoencephalopathy. *Lancet, 346*(8980), 934–939.
12. Amberla, K., Walijas, M., Tuominen, S., Almkvist, O., Poyhonen, M., Tuisku, S., et al. (2004). Insidious cognitive decline in CADASIL. *Stroke, 35*(7), 1598–1602.
13. Buffon, F., Porcher, R., Hernandez, K., Kurtz, A., Pointeau, S., Vahedi, K., et al. (2006). Cognitive profile in CADASIL. *Journal of Neurology, Neurosurgery, and Psychiatry, 77*(2), 175–180.
14. Peters, N., Opherk, C., Danek, A., Ballard, C., Herzog, J., & Dichgans, M. (2005). The pattern of cognitive performance in CADASIL: A monogenic condition leading to subcortical ischemic vascular dementia. *The American Journal of Psychiatry, 162*(11), 2078–2085.
15. Peters, N., Herzog, J., Opherk, C., & Dichgans, M. (2004). A two-year clinical follow-up study in 80 CADASIL subjects: Progression patterns and implications for clinical trials. *Stroke, 35* (7), 1603–1608.
16. Opherk, C., Peters, N., Herzog, J., Luedtke, R., & Dichgans, M. (2004). Long-term prognosis and causes of death in CADASIL: A retrospective study in 411 patients. *Brain, 127*(Pt 11), 2533–2539.
17. Reyes, S., Viswanathan, A., Godin, O., Dufouil, C., Benisty, S., Hernandez, K., et al. (2009). Apathy: A major symptom in CADASIL. *Neurology, 72*(10), 905–910.
18. Leyhe, T., Wiendl, H., Buchkremer, G., & Wormstall, H. (2005). CADASIL: Underdiagnosed in psychiatric patients? *Acta Psychiatrica Scandinavica, 111*(5), 392–396.
19. van den Boom, R., Lesnik Oberstein, S. A., Ferrari, M. D., Haan, J., & van Buchem, M. A. (2003). Cerebral autosomal dominant arteriopathy with subcortical infarcts and leukoencephalopathy: MR imaging findings at different ages—3rd-6th decades. *Radiology, 229*(3), 683–690.
20. O'Riordan, S., Nor, A. M., & Hutchinson, M. (2002). CADASIL imitating multiple sclerosis: The importance of MRI markers. *Multiple Sclerosis, 8*(5), 430–432.
21. Liem, M. K., van der Grond, J., Haan, J., van den Boom, R., Ferrari, M. D., Knaap, Y. M., et al. (2007). Lacunar infarcts are the main correlate with cognitive dysfunction in CADASIL. *Stroke, 38*(3), 923–928.
22. Jouvent, E., Viswanathan, A., Mangin, J. F., O'Sullivan, M., Guichard, J. P., Gschwendtner, A., et al. (2007). Brain atrophy is related to lacunar lesions and tissue microstructural changes in CADASIL. *Stroke, 38*(6), 1786–1790.
23. Joutel, A., Favrole, P., Labauge, P., Chabriat, H., Lescoat, C., Andreux, F., et al. (2001). Skin biopsy immunostaining with a Notch3 monoclonal antibody for CADASIL diagnosis. *Lancet, 358*(9298), 2049–2051.
24. Donnini, I., Nannucci, S., Valenti, R., Pescini, F., Bianchi, S., Inzitari, D., et al. (2012). Acetazolamide for the prophylaxis of migraine in CADASIL: A preliminary experience. *Journal of Headache and Pain, 13*(4), 299–302.

Chapter 12
Overview of Motor Neuron Diseases

Alice B. Schindler

Motor neuron disorders (MNDs) are a clinically and pathologically heterogeneous group of sporadic and hereditary neurologic diseases characterized by progressive degeneration of motor neurons. Either or both of the following two sets of motor neurons can be affected:

- Upper motor neurons (UMNs, also called corticospinal neurons), which originate from the primary motor cortex of the cerebrum (precentral gyrus) and possess long axons forming corticospinal and corticobulbar tracts
- Lower motor neurons (LMNs), which originate in the brainstem (cranial nerve [CN] motor nuclei) and spinal cord (anterior horn cells) and directly innervate skeletal muscles

MNDs can be classified into those affecting primarily the UMNs, those affecting primarily the LMNs, and those affecting both, and the nomenclature is used accordingly. The patient's symptoms vary by the set of motor neurons involved.

The motor neuron diseases are progressive neurological disorders that destroy motor neurons, the cells that control voluntary muscle activity such as speaking, walking, breathing, and swallowing. Normally, messages from nerve cells in the brain (UMNs) are transmitted to nerve cells in the brain stem and spinal cord (LMNs) and from there to particular muscles. Upper motor neurons direct the lower motor neurons to produce movements such as walking or chewing. Lower motor neurons control movement in the arms, legs, chest, face, throat, and tongue.

When signaling disruptions occur between the lower motor neurons and the muscle, the muscles do not work properly; the muscles gradually weaken, may begin wasting away (*atrophy*), and develop uncontrollable twitching (*fasciculations*). When signaling disruptions occur between the upper motor neurons and the

A.B. Schindler (✉)
Neurogenetics Branch/NINDS/NIH, 10 Center Drive, Building 10 Room 5S-219, Bethesda, MD 20892-1671, USA
e-mail: schindlerab@mail.nih.gov

J.S. Goldman (ed.), *Genetic Counseling for Adult Neurogenetic Disease*,
DOI 10.1007/978-1-4899-7482-2_12

Chapter 13
Amyotrophic Lateral Sclerosis

Elisabeth McCarty Wood

Amyotrophic lateral sclerosis (ALS) is a progressive neurodegenerative disease characterized by involvement of both the upper and lower motor neurons. In the USA, ALS is more commonly known as Lou Gehrig's disease, while other countries primarily use the term "motor neuron disease." The prevalence of ALS ranges from 2.7 to 7.4 per 100,000 in European populations with a lifetime risk of 1 in 400. There is a slight increased rate of ALS in men, with a male-female ratio of 1.5 to 1 [1].

The onset of ALS is primarily seen in the sixth and seventh decades of life, with a median onset age of 65. Incidence markedly increases around age 40, peaks between ages 60 and 79, and then gradually declines at age 80 [2]. The one clinical feature that differs between genetic and non-genetic forms of ALS is a slight reduction in the average age of onset in genetic/familial forms of ALS [3]. However, genetic or not, the majority of ALS is adult-onset, with only 5 % classified as juvenile-onset (<30 years) [1].

Research on the molecular basis of ALS has provided considerable insight into the biology of this severely progressive neurodegenerative condition. Genetics has played an important role in furthering ALS research, as there are now 16 known ALS genes [4]. While environmental factors have long been thought to be involved in the pathogenesis of ALS, no environmental factor has been proven to play such a role. ALS is now considered to have a primarily multifactorial basis with complex genetic-environmental interactions [1]. Research is ongoing to further elucidate the role of environmental factors in ALS.

Electronic supplementary material Supplementary material is available in the online version of this chapter at 10.1007/978-1-4899-7482-2_13. Videos can also be accessed at http://www.springerimages.com/videos/978-1-4899-7481-5.

E. McCarty Wood (✉)
Center for Neurodegenerative Disease Research, University of Pennsylvania, 3rd floor Maloney Building, 3600 Spruce Street, Philadelphia, PA 19104, USA
e-mail: mccarty@upenn.edu

J.S. Goldman (ed.), *Genetic Counseling for Adult Neurogenetic Disease*,
DOI 10.1007/978-1-4899-7482-2_13

13.1 Clinical Presentation

ALS is a rapidly progressive disease with a median survival of 3 years, but a wide range of duration from only a few months to over 10 years [5]. The most common presenting symptom, seen in approximately two-thirds of cases, is asymmetric limb weakness presenting in either a lower limb, affecting gait and/or movement, or an upper limb, affecting strength and/or dexterity. About one-third of patients have initial onset of bulbar symptoms, such as dysarthria and dysphagia, and only a small subset present with respiratory weakness. The onset and progression of respiratory weakness are important prognostic features given that respiratory complications are the most common cause of death. Other classic features of ALS include muscle atrophy and cramps, fasciculations, and pseudobulbar affect (emotional lability). The disease spreads from the point of origin to other regions of the body. For limb-onset ALS, the typical disease course is to spread to the opposite limb and then elsewhere in the body, whereas bulbar onset typically first affects the upper limbs before spreading to the lower limbs.

While severely progressive muscle weakness and wasting are the hallmark clinical feature of ALS, a subset of patients also develop cognitive decline. Approximately 5 % of patients fulfill clinical criteria for frontotemporal degeneration (see Chap. 8), while 30–50 % have documented cognitive involvement, but do not meet clinical dementia criteria [6–8]. Though the overlap between motor neuron symptoms and dementia has been historically well documented, the molecular relationship between ALS and FTD has only been proven recently because of the advances in understanding the neuropathology and genetics of these conditions.

13.2 Diagnosis

Like many neurodegenerative conditions, the clinical diagnosis of ALS is dependent on ruling out other possible causes of the symptoms and meeting established clinical criteria; there is no diagnostic test that confirms an ALS clinical diagnosis. Clinical retrospective studies have shown that an average of 8–13 months pass between initial symptom onset and receiving a clinical diagnosis [9, 10]. This length of time is highly significant in a condition with an average duration of 3 years, affecting not only the provision of appropriate clinical care, but also eligibility for clinical trials looking to include patients with early stage of disease. In order to help standardize ALS clinical diagnoses for research purposes, the El Escorial criteria were established in 1994, and then revised in 2000 as the Airlie House criteria [11]. These criteria are used by many centers as the standard for documenting a clinical diagnosis of ALS. The criteria include the following:

- The presence of lower and upper motor neuron degeneration with documented progressive spread of symptoms, either within a region or to other regions

- The absence of electrophysiologic or pathologic evidence of other disease processes that could cause lower and/or upper motor neuron degeneration
- The absence of neuroimaging evidence of other disease processes that could explain the clinical and electrophysiologic signs

Based on these criteria, a clinical ALS diagnosis can be categorized as clinically definite ALS, clinically definite familial ALS, laboratory-supported ALS, clinically probable ALS, clinically probable laboratory-supported ALS, clinically possible ALS, and clinically suspected ALS.

In order to gather the clinical evidence to apply these criteria, an individual would typically undergo a diagnostic work-up that includes a neurological examination, an electromyogram (EMG), neuroimaging (MRI) of the brain and spinal cord, a spinal tap for cerebrospinal fluid analysis, and blood work. An EMG is often considered the most critical diagnostic tool for ALS, as it is able to identify loss of lower motor neurons, even in areas that are clinically unaffected. Neuroimaging of the brain and spinal cord, CSF analysis, and blood work are all conducted to rule out possible causes that could mimic ALS symptoms. A systematic approach to the clinical diagnosis of ALS is needed, as there are many ALS-mimic syndromes, such as cervical spondylosis, multiple sclerosis, and thyroid disorders. There are also closely related clinical phenotypes, including progressive muscular atrophy (PMA), primary lateral sclerosis (PLS), and progressive bulbar palsy (PBP), which can also complicate the clinical diagnosis of classic ALS.

A diagnosis can be confirmed postmortem by means of an autopsy focusing on the brain and spinal cord. Classic neuropathological features of ALS include degeneration of motor neurons in the anterior horns and motor nuclei of the cranial nerves VII, X, XI, and XII, as well as neuronal loss and gliosis in the primary motor cortex with associated axonal loss in the corticospinal tracts. Ubiquitinated inclusions are an associated hallmark to the degenerative changes of ALS pathology. An initial breakthrough in understanding the neuropathology of ALS came in 2006, with the discovery that TDP-43 was the major disease protein seen in inclusions in the overwhelming majority of ALS cases [12]. Interestingly, a minority of ALS patients had inclusion bodies and resultant neurodegeneration that were not composed of TDP-43. Many of these cases were proven to have mutations in *SOD1,* which, at the time, was the most common genetic cause of familial ALS. Subsequently, other disease proteins associated with genetic forms of ALS, such as FUS, OPTN, UBQLN2, and NEFH, have also been identified as inclusions in neuropathological studies of these TDP-43 negative cases of ALS [13]. For reasons that currently are uncertain, the newly discovered *C9orf72* pathogenic hexanucleotide expansions are associated with both ALS and FTD with TDP-43 inclusions [14, 15]. Thus over the past decade, neuropathological and genetic advances in ALS have gone hand in hand with those of FTD, as a new discovery in either field has provided insight and research direction for the other.

13.3 Treatment and Management

The treatment of ALS focuses primarily on the management of symptoms and provision of supportive care and resources to maximize a patient's quality of life. ALS is a complex disease, so it is not surprising that a multidisciplinary approach to treating ALS has been correlated with improved prognosis [16]. Many medical professionals are involved in ALS care and management, including neurologists, nurses, nutritionists, pulmonologists, social workers, genetic counselors, as well as therapists in speech, physical, occupational, respiratory, and mental health specialties.

There is currently only one FDA-approved medication that is considered a disease-modifying treatment for ALS: riluzole (brand name Rilutek), which delays progression of ALS by several months in some patients. Clinical trials have been conducted for many neuroprotective agents in both animal and human models, but to date there are no other medications for ALS-specific treatment. Given the considerable advances in understanding the molecular basis of ALS, as well as advances in the fields of gene- and stem cell-based therapies, there is considerable hope for future therapies specifically developed for the treatment of ALS [1, 17]. Medications and non-pharmacological treatments are currently used in the management of ALS symptoms, like muscle cramping, spasticity, excessive oral secretions, and emotional lability [18]. Patients with ALS also have secondary symptoms, such as fatigue, pain, and depression, which can be treated both pharmacologically and non-pharmacologically.

Nutrition is a concern as swallowing difficulties, limb weakness, depression, and constipation can all have a negative impact on food intake. While nutritional guidance and supportive therapies can help improve nutritional intake in early stages, many patients will eventually need to consider options for enteric feeding, such as a gastronomy tube. Progressive weakness typically leads to respiratory impairments, which should be closely monitored given that respiratory complications are the most frequent cause of death. Pharmacological treatments, as well as noninvasive ventilation by means of bilevel positive pressure device (biPAP), are used to ameliorate respiratory issues.

Assistive technologies play a significant role not only in the management of ALS, but also in improving quality of life. For example, a motorized wheelchair greatly improves the mobility of a patient who is no longer able to walk. Large electronic switches that require only a small amount of pressure ease the ability to control any electronic device in the home. Communication devices now range from simply amplifying an individual's voice to a computerized vocalization system controlled by the patient's eye movements. There are even assistive communication applications available for personal electronics, such as smartphones and tablets.

Due to the progressive nature of ALS, discussions of end-of-life care are important to include in the management plan. Advance directives provide patients with the autonomy to address their healthcare wishes and make their decisions known. Hospice care can provide expert management and care to both the patient

and family members during the final stages of ALS. Like any chronically progressive disease, there is a long-lasting impact on family members and caregivers from both a financial and psychological standpoint. Ideally, support for family members and caregivers should be provided in conjunction with a patient's care and management. Social workers, nurses, mental health professionals, and genetic counselors can all provide professional services to help address not only the needs of the patient, but also the concerns, questions, and anxieties of those close to the patient.

13.4 Genetics

ALS can be separated into familial ALS (FALS) and sporadic ALS (SALS) forms. For several decades, the rate of FALS was generally accepted to be 10 %, but careful review of clinical ALS cohorts has revised the actual FALS rate to approximately 5 % [19]. Because mutations in most ALS genes have been found in both SALS and FALS, there is suggested caution in using the term "sporadic," as this term typically identifies a non-genetic disease. Likewise, the FALS label does not exclude the possibility that non-Mendelian factors, such as environment or epigenetics, may also contribute to the cause of ALS within a family [4]. Furthermore, since two relatives within an extended pedigree could both have ALS by chance, there is concern that the generally accepted definition of familial as having one or more affected first- or second-degree relatives may not be specific enough to identify truly genetic cases of ALS [20].

As the clinical features of genetic and non-genetic ALS are indistinguishable, the assessment of family history may be the only clinical tool available to try to help guide genetic testing decisions. Criteria to define FALS pedigrees as definite, probable, and possible, in terms of the likelihood of a genetic cause, have been proposed as follows: "definite FALS" for kindred with three or more affected relatives and kindred with two or more affected relatives with gene positive co-segregation; "probable FALS" for kindred with one affected first- or second-degree relative; and "possible FALS" for either (1) ALS in a distant relative, (2) a known ALS gene mutation in a patient with apparently sporadic ALS, or (3) frontotemporal degeneration in a first-degree relative [20]. These criteria are still being tested in the ALS research community [21].

The incidence of juvenile-onset ALS (jALS) is 5 % or less of the ALS population. However, jALS is most strongly correlated with a possible genetic etiology, and the use of clinical genetic testing to establish a cause is more common. Identified genes associated with jALS are reviewed in Table 13.1.

Alsin, a protein abundant in motor neurons with known and unknown functions related to cell life, development, and transport, is the most common genetic cause of jALS thus far [22, 23]. As an autosomal recessive disorder, there is typically no known family history. The phenotype caused by ALS2 mutations ranges from infantile ascending hereditary spastic paraplegia (IAHSP) to juvenile-onset primary lateral sclerosis (jPLS) to jALS. The phenotypes of IAHSP and jPLS are closely linked; both are associated with onset within the first 2 years of life, present with

Table 13.1 Genetic factors for juvenile/young-onset ALS

Locus	Gene	Chromosome	Inheritance	Penetrance	Age of onset
ALS2	*ALSIN*	2q33.1	Autosomal recessive	Complete	Range from infant to 20 years, depending on phenotype
ALS4	*SEXT*	9q34.13	Autosomal recessive	Unknown	Range 8–17 years
ALS16	*SIGMAR1*	9p13.3	Autosomal recessive	Unknown	1–2 years

Source: http://alsod.iop.kcl.ac.uk/als—The Amyotrophic Lateral Sclerosis Online Database

upper motor neuron findings, and are slowly progressive into adulthood [22, 24]. In contrast, the jALS phenotype of ALS2 has a somewhat older age of onset, averaging 6 years, but ranging anywhere from 3 to 20 years. The phenotype of jALS due to ALS2 has been characterized by pseudobulbar affect with facial muscle spasticity and spastic gait. Muscle atrophy is not characteristic of ALS2-related jALS, but mild atrophy does occur [25].

ALS4 is associated with *SETX*, a gene that can cause a juvenile-onset form of ALS, as well as ataxia and oculomotor apraxia type 2. The gene encodes senataxin, a helicase protein with a possible role in RNA processing. Mutations in *SETX* are rare and associated with a slowly progressive disease course that allows some individuals to live a normal life-span [26].

Homozygous mutations in *SIGMAR1* were found to be the cause of jALS in a consanguineous family in Saudi Arabia. Onset was noted in the first 2 years of life with a slowly progressive course through childhood [27]. Other loci have been linked to jALS, but the causative genes have yet to be identified.

The first gene identified in FALS for adult-onset forms of ALS was discovered in 1993: *SOD1*, encoding superoxide dismutase [28]. For years, *SOD1* was the only gene associated with an autosomal dominant form of classic ALS. It accounts for about 20 % of FALS cases, as well as 3 % of SALS. Over 160 mutations have been identified in *SOD1* that are believed to cause a toxic gain of function leading to degeneration of the upper and lower motor neurons [13]. Mutations in *SOD1* cause misfolding of SOD1, a protein that typically protects cells from oxidative damage by metabolizing superoxide radicals. It has been hypothesized that the toxic gain of function relates to instability of the misfolded protein, leading to an increased propensity for self-aggregation [29].

Clinically, ALS due to *SOD1* mutations is similar to non-genetic ALS, but does tend to have fewer upper than lower motor neuron signs and is less often associated with FTD. There are several genotype-phenotype correlations in the *SOD1* literature. The most common mutation in North America, accounting for half of all *SOD1* positive cases, is A4V. The A4V mutation is associated with an extremely rapid course of disease, with an average survival of 1 year. G85S mutations are also associated with a rapid course of disease. Other mutations correlate with a slower, prolonged course of ALS, including D90A, G37R, G41D, G93C, and D11Y

[30]. The D90A mutation can be inherited in either an autosomal dominant or recessive fashion. The recessive form of ALS, caused by homozygosity for the D90A mutation, is known to have a predominantly lower motor neuron and lower limb weakness [13]. Overall, the average age of onset in *SOD1*-associated ALS is lower than in sporadic ALS, but this can vary even within families. Certain mutations, including L106V, G37R, and L38V, are associated with young-onset ALS. The neuropathology of SOD1-related ALS is similar to that of classic ALS, but an important distinction is the lack of positive staining for the TDP-43 protein.

In 2006, the protein TDP-43 (TAR DNA-binding protein-43) was found to be a significant component of the ubiquitinated inclusions of motor neurons seen in both SALS as well as non-*SOD1* FALS [12]. This neuropathological discovery quickly led to the analysis of the responsible gene, *TARDBP*. TDP-43 plays a role in gene expression and RNA activity. Other ALS-associated genes share a similar function, giving rise to new hypotheses regarding the molecular pathways of ALS pathogenesis.

Over 40 *TARDBP* mutations have been identified. While overall the rate of *TARDBP* mutations is rare, accounting for 1–4 % of FALS, one particular mutation, p.A382T, is found in one-third of ALS cases in Sardinia [31]. Clinically, the phenotype of *TARDBP*-mediated ALS does not differ significantly from the non-genetic forms of ALS or *SOD1*-mediated ALS. The neuropathology of ALS due to *TARDBP* mutations is similar to sporadic, non-genetic ALS.

FUS (fused in sarcoma) mutations were discovered to cause ALS in 2009 [32, 33]. Similar to TDP-43, the FUS protein plays a role in DNA and RNA metabolism. *FUS* mutations are seen in approximately 4–6 % of FALS, and rarely in SALS. *FUS* mutations have also been identified in jALS. Clinically, *FUS*-mediated ALS has lower ages of onset than other forms of FALS, with a reported average onset age of 44 years, and has been shown to be the most common cause of young-onset ALS (<40 years old) [34]. Neuropathological features of ALS due to *FUS* include motor neuron loss that is more severe in the spinal cord than the brain stem and mild-to-moderate upper motor neuron loss in the motor cortex. Unlike classic ALS, *FUS*-mediated disease rarely has ubiquitin-positive cytoplasmic inclusions in the anterior horn of the spinal cord, and overall is negative for TDP-43 pathology [32, 33].

The most recent and highly significant discovery in the field of ALS genetics is *C9orf72* (chromosome 9 open reading frame 72). In late 2011, two separate research groups published the identification of an expanded hexanucleotide repeat (GGGGCC) in a noncoding region of chromosome 9 as a cause of both ALS and FTD. *C9orf72* is now considered to be the most common genetic cause of both familial and sporadic ALS; a review of *C9orf72* population frequency data estimates that *C9orf72* accounts for approximately 34 % of FALS and 6 % of SALS [35]. While repeat size correlations are in the process of being defined, the value of 30 repeats has been used as the cutoff between normal ($\leq$30) and pathogenic (>30). However, some laboratories use 21 repeats as the top end of the normal zone, 22–30 as borderline, and greater than 30 as positive. Future research will likely further define the clinical significance of *C9orf72* repeat lengths. Currently, therefore, the cutoff value of 30 should be used with caution [35, 36]. Anticipation is also being investigated in *C9orf72*, as occurrence of earlier ages of onset in subsequent generations has been reported, but the significance has not been proven [37].

ALS due to *C9orf72* expansions is associated with a slightly younger age of onset (~56 years) and more rapid progression than sporadic, non-*C9orf72*-related ALS. There is also a higher rate of bulbar onset ALS seen among *C9orf72* positive carriers [38, 39]. The most notable clinical feature of *C9orf72*-associated ALS is the strong association with frontotemporal degeneration (FTD), as *C9orf72* expansions are also the most common genetic cause of familial FTD. Approximately 27 % of *C9orf72* positive ALS cases also exhibit symptoms of dementia [35]. Family histories can display great heterogeneity in clinical phenotypes, exhibiting ALS, FTD, and ALS/FTD with a range of symptoms, ages of onset, and severity. For families with both diseases in the pedigree, *C9orf72* is the most consistent cause.

The specific findings of *C9orf72* pathology are considered to be highly distinctive, even predictive of the presence of the hexanucleotide expansion. Neuropathological features of *C9orf72*-mediated ALS include the presence of both TDP-43 positive inclusions in the anterior horn neurons of the spinal cord and ubiquitin-positive, TDP-43 negative inclusions in other specific regions of the central nervous system, such as the hippocampus and cerebellum [13].

A number of rare ALS genes have been identified as either Mendelian causes of ALS or susceptibility factors. The following provides a brief review of distinguishing characteristics and facts to assist in genetic counseling and testing discussions.

- *VAPB* mutations are associated with an atypical ALS phenotype that is also known as spinal muscular atrophy (SMA) IV, or Finkel-type SMA. Phenotypic heterogeneity has been observed within families. ALS due to *VAPB* mutations is characterized by primarily lower motor neuron findings, but phenotypic heterogeneity has been observed within families including more classic ALS presentations [40].
- *ANG* mutations have primarily been described in patients of European ancestry with classic ALS, although bulbar onset is slightly more common. Mutations have been found in both FALS and SALS cases, as well as Parkinson disease (PD), and research is ongoing to better understand this gene's role as a risk factor for both ALS and PD [41].
- *FIG4* mutations were previously known to cause a recessive peripheral nerve disorder CMT4J. Research suggests that heterozygous *FIG4* mutations are risk factors for classic ALS as well as primary lateral sclerosis (PLS) [42].
- Both heterozygous and homozygous mutations in *OPTN* have been described in association with ALS. Reported ages of onset range from the third through sixth decades of life. These mutations are extremely rare, primarily described in kindreds of Japanese ancestry [43].
- *ATXN2* is known to cause spinocerebellar ataxia type 2 due to a CAG-trinucleotide expansion of $\geq$34 repeats. Repeats in the intermediate range (27–33) are considered a risk factor for ALS [44].

- *VCP* (ALS14) was first associated with inclusion body myopathy with Paget disease of bone and frontotemporal dementia (IBMPFD), a specific syndrome that fell under the spectrum of FTD. Further research showed that individuals with *VCP* mutations were also at risk for ALS, thus expanding the phenotype of IBMPFD [45].
- Mutations in *UBQLN2* cause an X-linked autosomal dominant form of classic ALS. This gene can also be associated with jALS, as the reported range in onset age spans from 16 to 71. ALS with dementia is also observed in cases due to *UBQLN2* mutations [46]. For individuals who test negative for *UBQLN2*, but present with an ALS phenotype in an X-linked pedigree pattern, clinicians should consider the differential diagnosis of spinal bulbar muscular atrophy (Kennedy's disease) (see Chap. 14).
- *PFN1* mutations were linked to autosomal dominant, adult-onset ALS and account for 1–2 % of FALS [47].
- *CHMP2B* mutations were first described as being a rare cause of FTD. Subsequent research has shown that they are also a rare cause of ALS, found in approximately 1 % of patients. ALS due to *CHMP2B* has predominant lower motor neuron degeneration. ALS with and without dementia has been reported [48] (Table 13.2).

13.5 Genetic Counseling Issues

Genetic counseling for ALS presents both scientific and psychological challenges. ALS is an extremely complex disease with multiple genetic contributions. It is also a severely debilitating disease, typically with a rapid course toward death and little that can be offered in terms of medical intervention. The possibility that such a condition can be inherited could understandably have psychological impacts on patients and families. The recent scientific advances in ALS are considerable and may lead to improved treatment options, and, hopefully, improved patient outcomes. It is more important than ever for clinicians and genetic counselors to stay educated and updated regarding the molecular basis of ALS in order to provide the highest level of patient care.

In the case of jALS due to autosomal recessive inheritance, the parents are obligate carriers and therefore have a 25 % recurrence risk. In this scenario, parents would likely benefit from genetic counseling services, not only for recurrence risk counseling and education on the cause of their child's condition, but also for psychological support because of feelings such as guilt or depression regarding their child's diagnosis. Siblings may require genetic counseling in the future regarding their two-thirds chance of being a mutation carrier. Any offspring of an individual with autosomal recessive jALS would have a 100 % chance of being a mutation carrier.

While mutations in many of the genes described have been found in SALS, the greatest risk of a genetic cause is in familial cases. An accurate family history is

Table 13.2 Genetic factors for adult-onset ALS

Locus	Gene	Gene name	Chromosome	Inheritance	Mutation prevalence
ALS1	*SOD1*	Cu/Zn superoxide dismutase 1	21q22.11	Majority autosomal dominant; rare autosomal recessive and *de novo* cases reported	20 % of FALS 3 % of SALS
ALS6	*FUS*	Fused in sarcoma	16p11.2	Autosomal dominant	4–6 % of FALS Rare in SALS
ALS8	*VAPB*	Vesicle-associated membrane protein-associated protein B	20q13.3	Autosomal dominant	Rare
ALS9	*ANG*	Angiogenin	14q11.1	Autosomal dominant risk factor	Rare
ALS10	*TARDBP*	TAR DNA-binding protein	1p36.22	Autosomal dominant	1–4 % of FALS≤2 % of SALS
ALS11	*FIG4*	FIG4 homolog	6q21	Autosomal dominant risk factor	Rare
ALS12	*OPTN*	Optineurin	10p13	Autosomal recessive or autosomal dominant	Rare
ALS13	*ATXN2*	Ataxin 2	12q23-q24.1	Autosomal dominant risk factor	Rare
ALS14	*VCP*	Valosin-containing protein	9p13	Autosomal dominant	<2 % of FALS
ALS15	*UBQLN2*	Ubiquilin 2	Xp11.21	X-linked dominant	Rare
ALS17	*CHMP2B*	Chromatin-modifying protein 2B	3p12.1	Autosomal dominant	1 %
ALS18	*PFN1*	Profilin 1	17p13.3	Autosomal dominant	1–2 %
ALS-FTD 2	*C9orf72*	Chromosome 9 open reading frame 72	9p21.2	Autosomal dominant	23–30 % of FALS 4–7 % of SALS

Source: http://alsod.iop.kcl.ac.uk/als—The Amyotrophic Lateral Sclerosis Online Database

vital for assessing this risk. A three-generation pedigree that includes first- and second-degree relatives of the patient (children, siblings, parents, aunt/uncles, and grandparents) should be collected. According to proposed ALS pedigree criteria, the greatest risk of a detectable genetic mutation exists in those pedigrees that have $\geq$3 family members with ALS, or pedigrees that contain parent-child affected pairs [20, 21].

Still, pedigree collection should not be limited to questions pertaining to classic ALS. Documentation of symptoms and diagnoses in family members must include other possible neurodegenerative disease symptoms (such as dementia and parkinsonism), late-onset psychological disorders (due to the possibility of misdiagnosed FTD or other dementia), other neurological diagnoses (such as ataxia), as well as bone or joint complaints (due to the Paget disease of bone and inclusion body myopathy associated with *VCP* mutations). If there are family members with any of these symptoms or diagnoses, medical and/or autopsy records should be requested whenever possible in order to provide a means of confirming the diagnosis or providing insight into possible differential diagnoses. This thorough approach to family history collection will best enable the genetic counselor or clinician to guide the patient regarding genetic testing decisions.

Given the large number of genes associated with ALS, it can be overwhelming to provide genetic counseling on all known causes of genetic ALS. Baseline genetic counseling should include information regarding the two most common genetic causes of ALS: *C9orf72* and *SOD1*, together accounting for over half of FALS cases. Then, when appropriate, the patient's own symptoms and the symptoms in their family members should be used to customize the genetic counseling session. For example, patients with symptoms or a family history of FTD/dementia may benefit from a more detailed conversation regarding *C9orf72* and its association with both ALS and FTD. Also, for patients with cognitive impairment, it will be necessary to include a patient advocate, such as a spouse or other family member, in the genetic counseling and testing decisions. For patients with a young age of onset (<40), a discussion of *FUS* may be appropriate given that it is more often seen in patients with younger onset. Given the rarity of juvenile ALS (jALS), genetic counseling should be offered to all jALS cases to review the known genetic causes and provide testing options.

The majority of sporadic ALS cannot be explained by known gene mutations and therefore, most SALS patients, if they pursue genetic testing, will receive negative results. However, a small percentage will have a positive test, and it is important for clinicians and genetic counselors to keep this possibility in mind when providing pre- and post-test counseling services. Patients and families with SALS should be educated about the chance that a genetic mutation could be found, despite the lack of other affected family members. While discussions of testing motivation should always be included in genetic counseling sessions, the reason a patient with non-familial ALS desires genetic testing may be less apparent than a patient with clearly familial disease. For example, there could be a misunderstanding regarding the purpose of genetic testing, such as a patient thinking that the test outcome will provide a potential treatment benefit. Other patients with SALS may want testing in order to prove that the disease is not genetic, thereby ensuring that their own family members are not at increased risk. A discussion of testing motivation in both cases would allow an opportunity for the genetic counselor to address the patient's specific concerns. For patients with SALS that do test positive for a known ALS gene mutation, genetic counseling will be vital in the test disclosure and follow-up. A patient and family with a previously low risk of hereditary disease may require additional support in dealing with the impact of a positive result.

For patients and families with genetic concerns, but no identified mutation, DNA banking and autopsy should be discussed. Once new genetic associations are discovered, DNA banking or autopsy tissue will provide a dependable source of material for testing. DNA banking may also prove beneficial if there are future improvements in genetic testing technologies, such as improved quantification of the *C9orf72* repeat.

For most positive genetic test results, the immediate major impact is on the family members, not the patient, as the genetic finding does not change a patient's treatment options. In the future, genetic test results may have greater impact on a patient's treatment options, such as providing eligibility for certain clinical trials. There are some specific gene results that could offer prognostic information to patients, such as the more rapid progression of the *SOD1* A4V mutation. Overall, however, a positive gene result will provide information regarding the risk to other family members. The majority of ALS genes are inherited in an autosomal dominant fashion meaning that the patient's own offspring will be at 50 % risk, as well as the patient's siblings. Due to the reduced penetrance of some genes and mutations, it is also possible that a positive result could reveal risk to the patient's parents.

Due to the complex genetic heterogeneity of ALS, it is advisable that predictive (presymptomatic) genetic counseling and testing only be offered when a known genetic mutation has already been identified in the family. If a mutation has not been previously identified in an affected family member, the application and interpretation of genetic testing in a healthy, at-risk individual can be difficult, if not impossible. For those with a family history consistent with autosomal dominant inheritance, but no identified family gene mutation, at-risk individuals may still benefit from counseling to address life and financial planning concerns, as well as ongoing psychosocial and educational support regarding their possible lifetime risk for ALS [49].

For an individual at 50 % risk of a known ALS gene mutation, genetic counseling should always precede any genetic testing decisions. Many neurodegenerative conditions, including ALS, follow the guidelines developed in the Huntington disease community for the provision of predictive genetic testing services [49–51]. The predictive counseling model includes two genetic counseling sessions prior to testing, as well as consultations with a neurologist, psychologist, and/or neuropsychologist, and an in-person disclosure of the result accompanied by a support person. Like other neurodegenerative conditions, there are no preventative measures and no medical interventions that can be offered to a healthy individual who tests positive for an ALS-causing mutation. Therefore, the testing should only be pursued because the individual finds a personal benefit in learning his or her own status. As in symptomatic testing, a discussion of testing motivation can provide valuable insight into the concerns and issues that are most important to an individual's predictive genetic testing decision. For individuals interested in learning their genetic status for family planning reasons, the genetic counseling session should include a detailed discussion of prenatal options such as preimplantation genetic diagnosis, prenatal testing, gamete donation, adoption, natural conception with no testing, and the decision not to pursue pregnancy. Genetic discrimination risks should be discussed with all individuals, including a discussion of the national Genetic Information Nondiscrimination Act (GINA) as well as any local state laws.

The specific mutation for which the individual is at risk can also impact the initial genetic counseling session. *C9orf72* and *TARDBP* present the challenge of not only being at risk for ALS, but also for FTD. *VCP* carries the risk of FTD, as well as inclusion body myopathy or Paget disease of bone. There is no way to predict which symptoms will eventually develop for any of these three genes and the individual needs to be counseled accordingly so that he or she can consider the wide range of potential symptoms in their testing decision. Predictions regarding age of onset are limited for most ALS genes; however, average ages of onset and ranges of onset can be provided. In addition to the spectrum of ALS and FTD phenotypes, *C9orf72* predictive testing is also complicated by the fact that this hexanucleotide expansion is not yet fully understood. As the most common genetic cause of ALS, interest in *C9orf72* predictive testing is potentially high. Clinicians and genetic counselors need to remain updated on future developments in *C9orf72* that could impact predictive genetic testing, such as the stability of the expansion and phenotypic correlations with repeat length.

13.6 Case History (Fig. 13.1)

Mr. J, a 50-year-old Caucasian male, presents in the general neurology clinic with complaints of weakness in his right leg. He indicates that the weakness has gotten progressively worse over the past 6 months and he is now struggling to complete many of his physical duties both at home and at work. Medical history is unremarkable. He is married with three children. Family history is negative for any relatives with similar symptoms or movement disorders. A neurology exam notes lower limb weakness. Further tests are ordered, including blood work, spinal tap, MRI, and electromyogram (EMG). Blood work and CSF analysis are negative; MRI is unremarkable; EMG provides evidence of lower motor neuron involvement in both his right and left leg.

The neurologist explains to Mr. J that the most likely diagnosis is ALS, a progressive neurodegenerative disease with no cure or preventative treatment. Educational materials and support resources are provided, as well as a referral to an ALS specialty clinic. Mr. and Mrs. J express concern for their children, Steve

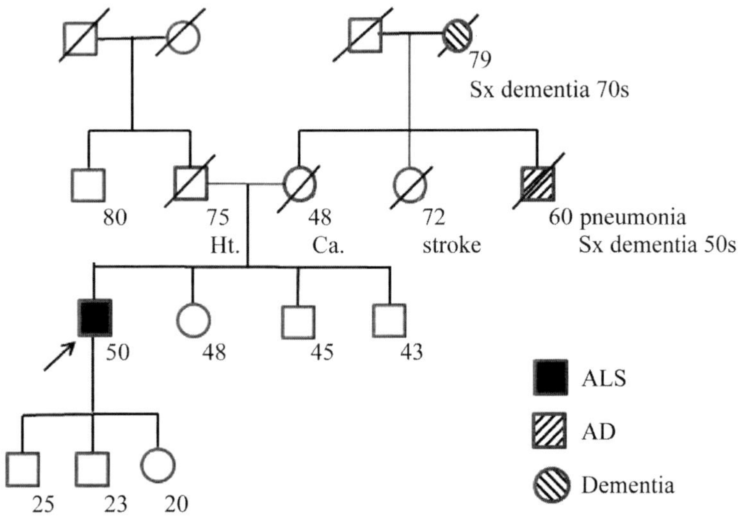

Fig. 13.1 ALS case history pedigree

aged 25, Brian aged 23, and Kelly aged 20, wondering if they will also be at risk for ALS. The doctor reassures them that without a family history of ALS the risk of a genetic cause is low, but provides them with the information for a genetic counselor that specializes in neurogenetics.

Discussion Questions

- Like many neurodegenerative diseases, a clinical diagnosis relies on ruling out other known possible causes of a patient's symptoms before making the diagnosis based on clinical criteria. Could including genetic testing as part of the routine work-up be beneficial in establishing an ALS diagnosis?
- Mr. Jones' ALS is described as being sporadic. What genes have been associated with sporadic ALS? Which, if any, are most likely based on the case report?

Mr. and Mrs. J meet with the genetic counselor and explain their interest in learning if there is an increased risk of ALS for their children. The genetic counselor explains that family history information would help to better guide their discussion, and proceeds to collect a three-generation pedigree. The family history is negative for ALS. Mr. and Mrs. J are unsure about the diagnosis, but report that Mr. J's maternal grandmother was senile in her mid-70s, dying at age 79 in a nursing home. She was unable to move or communicate for the last year of her life. There was a maternal uncle that was described as having Alzheimer disease in his 50s, presenting with personality changes and language difficulties that progressed until his death at 60 of pneumonia. His mother died at 48 of colon cancer and he has three younger siblings, ages 48, 45, and 43.

The genetic counselor explains that ALS can be associated with another neurodegenerative condition called frontotemporal degeneration (FTD), a type of dementia. She explains that, due to his positive family history of dementia, she feels that he and his family should be aware of the possible connection between these two diseases. Although the symptoms of FTD and ALS are very different, they do share certain disease proteins and can both be caused by a genetic mutation on chromosome 9. The genetic counselor provides information about this gene, *C9orf72*, as well as a brief review of other known genetic causes of ALS. Both autosomal dominant inheritance and multifactorial inheritance are discussed. The genetic counselor explains that Mr. J can choose to have genetic testing for a panel of ALS genes or just the *C9orf72* gene. Mr. J is anxious regarding any possible risk and wants to get the full panel of ALS genes offered by a commercial laboratory. The genetic counselor explains that he may have to pay for the test himself if his insurance will not cover it. Mr. J expresses that the cost is not an issue if it could be potentially helpful to his children.

Discussion Questions

- Is either testing approach, the full panel of ALS genes versus the single test for *C9orf72*, the most appropriate course of action and why?
- Patient-reported family history information can be influenced by the specific questions asked by the clinician. In the field of neurogenetics, what approaches or types of questions could help capture the most complete overview of a patient's family history?

The results of the genetic testing panel are positive for a *C9orf72* expansion. The genetic counselor meets with the patient to review the results. Mr. and Mrs. J appear to be shocked by the information. The genetic counselor prompts them, asking if this is the result they expected. Mrs. J explains that they had both hoped that the testing would be negative, allowing them to tell their children that they were not at risk for ALS. The genetic counselor asks what questions they have about the result, but Mr. and Mrs. J are both visibly upset and reluctant to speak. The genetic counselor excuses herself, saying that she wants to get a few educational materials, in order to give Mr. and Mrs. J a moment alone. Upon returning, the counselor states that she understands that the result is not what they were expecting, but she hopes to work with Mr. and Mrs. J to help them use this information in the most beneficial manner possible. Mr. J shares that, while the result is still upsetting, it was not entirely unexpected as he does feel that his uncle was likely misdiagnosed with Alzheimer disease, but really had FTD. He expresses fear that his children are at risk not only for ALS, but also for FTD. The couple shares that they have not told any of their children that Mr. J was having genetic testing; just telling them about their father's diagnosis of ALS was difficult enough. They are unsure how to proceed now that they have the results. The genetic counselor spends time exploring options for communicating the information to their adult children. Due to Mr. and Mrs. J's emotional state, she suggests that they allow themselves some time to come to terms with the result themselves, prior to approaching a discussion with any of their children. The couple agrees. The genetic counselor explains that Mr. J likely inherited the *C9orf72* mutation from his mother, which means that his three siblings are also at risk. Mr. and Mrs. J indicate that they understand, but note that they are not in regular contact with his siblings.

Discussion Questions

- Receiving a positive genetic test result can put a patient into the role of being the "messenger" of this news for the entire family. How can a genetic counselor or other clinician best prepare and help a patient in this type of situation?
- Given that there are no cures or preventative measures for ALS or FTD, is there an immediate need to tell other family members about the risk?

Three months later, Mrs. J contacts the genetic counselor by telephone. Her eldest son is newly engaged. Mr. and Mrs. J have not yet told their children about the genetic test result, nor have they told any other family members. She feels that they must tell their children, especially now that her son and his fiancée may be thinking about future family planning. She notes that her husband agrees with the decision to share the information, but that he is feeling depressed and guilty about the hereditary risk. The genetic counselor and Mrs. J discuss a plan for disclosing the information to their children and review some basic facts about the genetic result, including the 50 % inheritance risk. The genetic counselor encourages Mr. and Mrs. J to recontact her after their discussion with their children.

Two weeks later, Mrs. J calls back; they told their children about the *C9orf72* result. The genetic counselor asks Mrs. J how she feels the discussion went. Mrs. J reports that it was difficult at first, as their children had many initial questions and concerns. However, they felt that their children were very optimistic and supportive, telling their father that they loved him and that they would all work together to conquer this disease. Their children have used the Internet to research the genetic cause, and are trying to connect both their father and themselves to any research efforts to better understand this genetic form of ALS. She feels that Mr. J's mood has improved somewhat now that their children are aware and engaged in accepting this new information about the family's risk of disease. She and her children are working together to contact other family members to inform them about the genetic finding. They are also making plans for a small family reunion in the upcoming months, hoping to bring the family together before Mr. J's symptoms become progressively worse. She reports that none of their children wish to pursue predictive genetic testing at this time, but feels that they may change their minds when preventative treatment becomes an option.

Discussion Questions

- What issues would be important to discuss in terms of family and personal future planning with an individual at 50 % risk of an inherited form of ALS?
- What other support resources or referrals could be beneficial to Mr. and Mrs. J and their family members as they deal with both his recent diagnosis of ALS and a positive genetic test result?

13.7 Patient Resources

1. ALS Association
   Website: www.alsa.org
   National Headquarters: 1275 K Street NW, Suite 1050
   Washington, DC 20005
   Phone: (202) 407-8580
2. NCBI—GeneTests and GeneReviews: www.ncbi.nlm.nih.gov/sites/GeneTests/review
3. National Institute of Neurological Diseases and Stroke (NINDS)
   ALS Fact Sheet: www.ninds.nih.gov/disorders/amyotrophiclateralsclerosis/detail_ALS.htm
4. Center for Disease Control: National Amyotrophic Lateral Sclerosis (ALS) Registry
   http://wwwn.cdc.gov/als
5. International Alliance of ALS/MND Associations: http://www.alsmndalliance.org/

References

1. Wijesekera, L. C., & Leigh, P. N. (2009). Amyotrophic lateral sclerosis. *Orphanet Journal of Rare Diseases, 4*, 3.
2. Logroscino, G., Beghi, E., Zoccolella, S., Palagano, R., Fraddosio, A., Simone, I. L., et al. (2005). Incidence of amyotrophic lateral sclerosis in southern Italy: A population based study. *Journal of Neurology, Neurosurgery, and Psychiatry, 76*(8), 1094–1098.
3. Juneja, T., Pericak-Vance, M. A., Laing, N. G., Dave, S., & Siddique, T. (1997). Prognosis in familial amyotrophic lateral sclerosis: Progression and survival in patients with glu100gly and ala4val mutations in Cu, Zn superoxide dismutase. *Neurology, 48*(1), 55–57.
4. Andersen, P. M., & Al-Chalabi, A. (2011). Clinical genetics of amyotrophic lateral sclerosis: What do we really know? *Nature Reviews Neurology, 7*(11), 603–615.
5. Zoccolella, S., Beghi, E., Palagano, G., Fraddosio, A., Guerra, V., Samarelli, V., et al. (2008). Analysis of survival and prognostic factors in amyotrophic lateral sclerosis: A population based study. *Journal of Neurology, Neurosurgery, and Psychiatry, 79*(1), 33–37.
6. Neary, D., Snowden, J. S., Gustafson, L., Passant, U., Stuss, D., Black, S., et al. (1998). Frontotemporal lobar degeneration: A consensus on clinical diagnostic criteria. *Neurology, 51* (6), 1546–1554.
7. Portet, F., Cadilhac, C., Touchon, J., & Camu, W. (2001). Cognitive impairment in motor neuron disease with bulbar onset. *Amyotrophic Lateral Sclerosis and Other Motor Neuron Disorders, 2*(1), 23–29.
8. Lomen-Hoerth, C., Murphy, J., Langmore, S., Kramer, J. H., Olney, R. K., & Miller, B. (2003). Are amyotrophic lateral sclerosis patients cognitively normal? *Neurology, 60*(7), 1094–1097.
9. Traynor, B. J., Codd, M. B., Corr, B., Forde, C., Frost, E., & Hardiman, O. M. (2000). Clinical features of amyotrophic lateral sclerosis according to the El Escorial and Airlie House diagnostic criteria: A population-based study. *Archives of Neurology, 57*(8), 1171–1176.
10. Millul, A., Beghi, E., Logroscino, G., Micheli, A., Vitelli, E., & Zardi, A. (2005). Survival of patients with amyotrophic lateral sclerosis in a population-based registry. *Neuroepidemiology, 25*(3), 114–119.

11. Brooks, B. R., Miller, R. G., Swash, M., Munsat, T. L., & World Federation of Neurology Research Group on Motor Neuron Diseases. (2000). El Escorial revisited: Revised criteria for the diagnosis of amyotrophic lateral sclerosis. *Amyotrophic Lateral Sclerosis and Other Motor Neuron Disorders, 1*(5), 293–299.
12. Neumann, M., Sampathu, D. M., Kwong, L. K., Truax, A. C., Micsenyi, M. C., Chou, T. T., et al. (2006). Ubiquitinated TDP-43 in frontotemporal lobar degeneration and amyotrophic lateral sclerosis. *Science, 314*(5796), 130–133.
13. Al-Chalabi, A., Jones, A., Troakes, C., King, A., Al-Sarraj, S., & van den Berg, L. H. (2012). The genetics and neuropathology of amyotrophic lateral sclerosis. *Acta Neuropathologica, 124* (3), 339–352.
14. DeJesus-Hernandez, M., Mackenzie, I. R., Boeve, B. F., Boxer, A. L., Baker, M., Rutherford, N. J., et al. (2012). Expanded GGGGCC hexanucleotide repeat in noncoding region of C9ORF72 causes chromosome 9p-linked FTD and ALS. *Neuron, 72*(2), 245–256.
15. Renton, A. E., Majounie, E., Waite, A., Simon-Sanchez, J., Rollinson, S., Gibbs, J. R., et al. (2012). A hexanucleotide repeat expansion in C9ORF72 is the cause of chromosome 9p21-linked ALS-FTD. *Neuron, 72*(2), 257–268.
16. Andersen, P. M., Borasio, G. D., Dengler, R., Hardiman, O., Kollewe, K., Leigh, P. N., et al. (2005). EFNS task force on management of amyotrophic lateral sclerosis: Guidelines for diagnosing and clinical care of patients and relatives. *European Journal of Neurology, 12* (12), 921–938.
17. Turner, M. R., Hardiman, O., Benatar, M., Brooks, B. R., Chio, A., de Carvalho, M., et al. (2013). Controversies and priorities in amyotrophic lateral sclerosis. *Lancet Neurology, 12*(3), 310–322.
18. Radunovic, A., Mitsumoto, H., & Leigh, P. N. (2007). Clinical care of patients with amyotrophic lateral sclerosis. *Lancet Neurology, 6*(10), 913–925.
19. Byrne, S., Walsh, C., Lynch, C., Bede, P., Elamin, M., Kenna, K., et al. (2011). Rate of familial amyotrophic lateral sclerosis: A systematic review and meta-analysis. *Journal of Neurology, Neurosurgery, and Psychiatry, 82*(6), 623–627.
20. Byrne, S., Bede, P., Elamin, M., Kenna, K., Lynch, C., McLaughlin, R., et al. (2011). Proposed criteria for familial amyotrophic lateral sclerosis. *Amyotrophic Lateral Sclerosis, 12*(3), 157–159.
21. Conte, A., Lattante, S., Luigetti, M., Del Grande, A., Romano, A., Marcaccio, A., et al. (2012). Classification of familial amyotrophic lateral sclerosis by family history: Effects on frequency of genes mutation. *Journal of Neurology, Neurosurgery, and Psychiatry, 83*(12), 1201–1203.
22. Yang, Y., Hentati, A., Deng, H. X., Dabbagh, O., Sasaki, T., Hirano, M., et al. (2001). The gene encoding alsin, a protein with three guanine-nucleotide exchange factor domains, is mutated in a form of recessive amyotrophic lateral sclerosis. *Nature Genetics, 29*(2), 160–165.
23. Hadano, S., Hand, C. K., Osuga, H., Yanagisawa, Y., Otomo, A., Devon, R. S., et al. (2001). A gene encoding a putative GTPase regulator is mutated in familial amyotrophic lateral sclerosis 2. *Nature Genetics, 29*(2), 166–173.
24. Lesca, G., Eymard-Pierre, E., Santorelli, F. M., Cusmai, R., Di Capua, M., Valente, E. M., et al. (2003). Infantile ascending hereditary spastic paralysis (IAHSP): Clinical features in 11 families. *Neurology, 60*(4), 674–682.
25. Ben Hamida, M., Hentati, F., & Ben, H. C. (1990). Hereditary motor system diseases (chronic juvenile amyotrophic lateral sclerosis). Conditions combining a bilateral pyramidal syndrome with limb and bulbar amyotrophy. *Brain, 113*(Pt 2), 347–363.
26. Rabin, B. A., Griffin, J. W., Crain, B. J., Scavina, M., Chance, P. F., & Cornblath, D. R. (1999). Autosomal dominant juvenile amyotrophic lateral sclerosis. *Brain, 122*(Pt 8), 1539–1550.
27. Al-Saif, A., Al-Mohanna, F., & Bohlega, S. (2011). A mutation in sigma-1 receptor causes juvenile amyotrophic lateral sclerosis. *Annals of Neurology, 70*(6), 913–919.
28. Rosen, D. R., Siddique, T., Patterson, D., Figlewicz, D. A., Sapp, P., Hentati, A., et al. (1993). Mutations in Cu/Zn superoxide dismutase gene are associated with familial amyotrophic lateral sclerosis. *Nature, 362*(6415), 59–62. Erratum in: *Nature*, 1993, 364(6435), 362.

29. Redler, R. L., & Dokholyan, N. V. (2012). The complex molecular biology of amyotrophic lateral sclerosis (ALS). *Progress in Molecular Biology and Translational Science, 107*, 215–262.
30. Sabatelli, M., Conte, A., & Zollino, M. (2013). Clinical genetic heterogeneity of amyotrophic lateral sclerosis. *Clinical Genetics, 83*(5), 408–416.
31. Chiò, A., Borghero, G., Pugliatti, M., Ticca, A., Calvo, A., Moglia, C., et al. (2011). Large proportion of amyotrophic lateral sclerosis cases in Sardinia due to a single founder mutation of the TARDBP gene. *Archives of Neurology, 68*(5), 594–598.
32. Vance, C., Rogelj, B., Hortobagyi, T., De Vos, K. J., Nishimura, A. L., Sreedharan, J., et al. (2009). Mutations in FUS, an RNA processing protein, cause familial amyotrophic lateral sclerosis type 6. *Science, 323*(5918), 1208–1211.
33. Kwiatkowski, T. J., Jr., Bosco, D. A., Leclerc, A. L., Tamrazian, E., Vanderburg, C. R., Russ, C., et al. (2009). Mutations in the FUS/TLS gene on chromosome 16 cause familial amyotrophic lateral sclerosis. *Science, 323*(5918), 1205–1208.
34. Millecamps, S., Boillée, S., Le Ber, I., Seilhean, D., Teyssou, E., Giraudeau, M., et al. (2012). Phenotype difference between ALS patients with expanded repeats in C9ORF72 and patients with mutations in other ALS-related genes. *Journal of Medical Genetics, 49*(4), 258–263.
35. van Blitterswijk, M., DeJesus-Hernandez, M., & Rademakers, R. (2012). How do C9ORF72 repeat expansions cause amyotrophic lateral sclerosis and frontotemporal dementia: Can we learn from other noncoding repeat expansion disorders? *Current Opinion in Neurology, 25*(6), 689–700.
36. Gomez-Tortosa, E., Gallego, J., Guerrero-Lopez, R., Marcos, A., Gil-Neciga, E., Sainz, M. J., et al. (2013). C9ORF72 hexanucleotide expansions of 20-22 repeats are associated with Frontotemporal deterioration. *Neurology, 80*(4), 366–370.
37. Chio, A., Calvo, A., Mazzini, L., Cantello, R., Mora, G., Moglia, C., et al. (2012). Extensive genetics of ALS: A population-based study in Italy. *Neurology, 79*(19), 1983–1989.
38. Chio, A., Borghero, G., Restagno, G., Mora, G., Drepper, C., Traynor, B. J., et al. (2012). Clinical characteristics of patients with familial amyotrophic lateral sclerosis carrying the pathogenic GGGGCC hexanucleotide repeat expansion of C9ORF72. *Brain, 135*(Pt 3), 784–793.
39. Irwin, D. J., McMillan, C. T., Brettschneider, J., Libon, D. J., Powers, J., Rascovsky, K., et al. (2013). Cognitive decline and reduced survival in C9orf72 expansion frontotemporal degeneration and amyotrophic lateral sclerosis. *Journal of Neurology, Neurosurgery, & Psychiatry, 84*(2), 163–169.
40. Nishimura, A. L., Mitne-Neto, M., Silva, H. C., Richieri-Costa, A., Middleton, S., Cascio, D., et al. (2004). A mutation in the vesicle-trafficking protein VAPB causes late-onset spinal muscular atrophy and amyotrophic lateral sclerosis. *American Journal of Human Genetics, 75* (5), 822–831.
41. van Es, M. A., Schelhaas, H. J., van Vught, P. W., Ticozzi, N., Andersen, P. M., Groen, E. J., et al. (2011). Angiogenin variants in Parkinson disease and amyotrophic lateral sclerosis. *Annals of Neurology, 70*(6), 964–973.
42. Chow, C. Y., Landers, J. E., Bergren, S. K., Sapp, P. C., Grant, A. E., Jones, J. M., et al. (2009). Deleterious variants of FIG4, a phosphoinositide phosphatase, in patients with ALS. *American Journal of Human Genetics, 84*(1), 85–88.
43. Maruyama, H., Morino, H., Ito, H., Izumi, Y., Kato, H., Watanabe, Y., et al. (2010). Mutations of optineurin in amyotrophic lateral sclerosis. *Nature, 465*(7295), 223–226.
44. Elden, A. C., Kim, H. J., Hart, M. P., Chen-Plotkin, A. S., Johnson, B. S., Fang, X., et al. (2010). Ataxin-2 intermediate-length polyglutamine expansions are associated with increased risk for ALS. *Nature, 466*(7310), 1069–1075.
45. Johnson, J. O., Mandrioli, J., Benatar, M., Abramzon, Y., Van Deerlin, V. M., Trojanowski, J. Q., et al. (2010). Exome sequencing reveals VCP mutations as a cause of familial ALS. *Neuron*, 68(5), 857-64. Erratum in. *Neuron, 69*(2), 397.
46. Deng, H. X., Chen, W., Hong, S. T., Boycott, K. M., Gorrie, G. H., Siddique, N., et al. (2011). Mutations in UBQLN2 cause dominant X-linked juvenile and adult-onset ALS and ALS/dementia. *Nature, 477*(7363), 211–215.

47. Wu, C. H., Fallini, C., Ticozzi, N., Keagle, P. J., Sapp, P. C., Piotrowska, K., et al. (2012). Mutations in the profilin 1 gene cause familial amyotrophic lateral sclerosis. *Nature, 488* (7412), 499–503.
48. Cox, L. E., Ferraiuolo, L., Goodall, E. F., Heath, P. R., Higginbottom, A., Mortiboys, H., et al. (2010). Mutations in CHMP2B in lower motor neuron predominant amyotrophic lateral sclerosis (ALS). *PLoS ONE, 5*(3), e9872.
49. Fong, J. C., Karydas, A. M., & Goldman, J. S. (2012). Genetic counseling for FTD/ALS caused by the C9ORF72 hexanucleotide expansion. *Alzheimer's Research & Therapy, 4*(4), 27.
50. International Huntington Association (IHA) and the World Federation of Neurology (WFN) Research Group on Huntington's Chorea. (1994). Guidelines for the molecular genetics predictive test in Huntington's disease. *Neurology, 44*(8), 1533–1536.
51. Goldman, J. S., Hahn, S. E., Catania, J. W., LaRusse-Eckert, S., Butson, M. B., Rumbaugh, M., et al. (2011). Genetic counseling and testing for Alzheimer disease: Joint practice guidelines of the American College of Medical Genetics and the National Society of Genetic Counselors. *Genetics in Medicine, 13*(6), 597–605.

Chapter 14
Spinal Bulbar Muscular Atrophy: Kennedy Disease

Alison La Pean Kirschner

Spinal and bulbar muscular atrophy (SBMA), also known as Kennedy disease, is a relatively rare form of motor neuron disease. It has an estimated worldwide prevalence of 1:40,000 to 1:50,000. Like most late-onset motor neuron diseases, SBMA is generally diagnosed well into adulthood, most commonly in the fourth or fifth decade of life. Genetics may play a role in age of onset. SBMA is inherited in an X-linked recessive manner, and therefore manifestations of diagnostic clinical symptoms only affect men (however, mild symptoms have been reported in homozygous and heterozygous females). Due to its rarity, SBMA is not usually the first diagnosis considered, but can be diagnosed quite easily with a single-gene test commonly available through many testing companies. SBMA is found around the world, but most commonly in Caucasians (Northern European decent, particularly Finnish) and Japanese.

14.1 Clinical Presentation

SBMA is a slowly progressive, adult-onset motor neuron disorder. Patients typically present with proximal (greater than distal) spinal muscle weakness and bulbar muscle weakness between the ages of 20 and 66 years, most commonly in the early-to-mid-40s [1]. Patients report initial lower extremity weakness more often (50–70 %) than upper extremity weakness (31 %) [2]. Bulbar muscles are those of the tongue, pharynx, and larynx, and atrophy of these areas results in facial weakness, dysarthria (difficulty articulating words resulting in slow or slurred speech), and dysphagia (difficulty swallowing). Another common symptom is

A.L.P. Kirschner (✉)
Center for Patient Care and Outcomes Research (PCOR) & Department of Neurology, Medical College of Wisconsin, 8701 Watertown Plank Rd., Rm H3155, Milwaukee, WI 53226, USA
e-mail: alapean@mcw.edu

J.S. Goldman (ed.), *Genetic Counseling for Adult Neurogenetic Disease*,
DOI 10.1007/978-1-4899-7482-2_14

fasciculations (involuntary muscle twitching) in the tongue and around the mouth and chin. These symptoms may be preceded by muscle cramping, especially in the upper limbs and torso, and hand tremors with average age of onset in the early-to-mid-30s [2]. Patients may experience clinical or subclinical levels of sensory loss (lower motor or primary sensory neuropathy) and hyporeflexia [3]. Patients may also present with symptoms of androgen insensitivity, including gynecomastia, reduced fertility, erectile dysfunction, and testicular atrophy [2]. However, SBMA should not be ruled out based on the absence of androgen insensitivity since gynecomastia may only be present in 50 % of patients.

In general, disease progression in SBMA is slow. Patients usually experience progressive muscle weakness leading to mobility issues, first needing to use handrails for stair climbing, and then a cane or walking aid, and may become wheelchair dependent approximately 20–30 years after symptom onset, usually in their mid-50s to -60s [1]. Dysarthria and dysphagia typically occur in the early-to-mid-50s and progress as well. Patients with SBMA may suffer from bulbar palsy causing aspiration, which can lead to life-threatening respiratory tract infections (pneumonia) in later stages of disease [1, 4]. In general, patients with SBMA have a long, even normal, life span. However, it is estimated in Japanese populations that life span for men with SBMA can be 10–15 years shorter than that of the general population [4]. The most common cause of death is aspiration pneumonia.

Female heterozygous carriers of SBMA are usually asymptomatic. However, mild symptoms have been reported in female homozygous carriers and heterozygous carriers [3]. The most common symptoms are twitching and frequent muscle cramping, mild muscle weakness, hand tremor, and evidence of mild-to-chronic denervation on EMG, though more severe symptoms also have been reported [3, 5].

14.2 Diagnosis

Along with a thorough clinical neurological examination, molecular genetic testing for SBMA is considered the "gold standard" for diagnosing disease. Targeted mutation analysis is typically done using polymerase chain reaction (PCR) amplification of the trinucleotide repeat region and fragment length determination by molecular weight standards after capillary electrophoresis [1]. Given the rarity of the condition and that X-linked pedigrees can prove uninformative in many instances (particularly in small families or families with several female relatives), patients generally undergo a series of primary care and neurological evaluations prior to genetic testing. As with many slowly progressive conditions, significant delays can occur between onset of symptoms, recognition of those symptoms, initial medical evaluation (possibly including misdiagnosis), and diagnosis of SBMA. Patients with SBMA are commonly misdiagnosed. Though exact estimates are unknown, reports range from 2 to 32 % of patients who are misdiagnosed with amyotrophic lateral sclerosis (ALS) or familial ALS (FALS) due to overlapping symptoms, lack of "classic" SBMA symptoms, or subtle symptoms in early stages of disease [2]. SBMA should also be considered in the differential diagnosis of patients with essential tremor, including familiar tremor [3]. As potential therapies are developed and clinical trials continue, prompt diagnosis in order to provide early intervention is likely to become increasingly important.

The following evaluations may be done as part of a neuro-diagnostic work-up, but are not required or necessary for diagnosing SBMA:

- Electromyogram/nerve conduction studies (EMG/NCS) showing [2, 6]:
  - Progressive lower motor neuron dysfunction in arms, legs, and face
  - Low SNAP amplitude (94–100 %)
  - Low CMAP amplitude in median and perineal nerves (52 %)
  - MUNE's greater than 1 standard deviation from the mean
- Serum laboratory tests showing [1, 2]:
  - Likely decreased levels of creatinine and/or elevated levels of creatine kinase two to five times above normal (~85 % show abnormalities in both, 88–99 % will show abnormality in one)
  - Possible elevated levels of aspartate aminotransferase (AST) (72 %) and alanine aminotransferase (ALT) (60–70 %)
  - Possible elevated levels of lactate dehydrogenase (LDH) (35 %)
  - Glucose intolerance
- Muscle or nerve biopsy showing:
  - Chronic or partial denervation
  - Demyelination and remyelination on individual fibers
  - Unmyelinated fibers throughout sural nerves
- Barium pharyngeal videofluorography (a clinical measure of dysphagia) showing [1]:
  - Increased amounts of pharyngeal barium residue

Objective and quantitative assessments (not functional scales or subjective outcome measures) are more sensitive measures of early or preclinical symptoms of disease [1].

14.3 Treatment and Management

Treatment for SBMA remains primarily symptomatic, though clinical treatment trials have been done with androgen inhibitors (androgen-depleting therapies), a β_2 agonist, and exercise therapy. Some treatment trials have shown positive improvements in strength (compared to declines in the placebo group), quality of life (specific to physical activity, particularly falls), motor function (by timed 6-min walk), and less progressive dysphagia compared with controls [7–12]. Another report suggests that longer term antiandrogen therapy may inhibit the toxic accumulation of mutant androgen receptor protein in the motor neurons of the spinal cord and brainstem [10]. Though these clinical treatment trials have not shown significant results in their primary outcome measures, the results do indicate that these therapies hold some promise, particularly for those treated in the early stages of disease (<10 years from onset of symptoms). Additionally, several other therapeutic interventions that alter different molecular pathways show promise in humans, in the laboratory, or in mouse models of SBMA.

To date, no drug treatments are considered standard of care or recommended for patients with SBMA. Eating a healthy diet and incorporating regular exercise to maintain muscle mass (in order to slow disease- and age-related decline in muscle mass) and to control weight gain are generally recommended. This can potentially help patients maintain their ability to walk without the use of assistive devices; however, family and health care providers may need to encourage the use of assistive devices for safety or to preserve energy, which can improve quality of life. Patients may benefit from physical, occupational, and speech therapy referrals, as well as periodic mobility and fall assessments. Some patients with SBMA may have difficulties adjusting to their decline in physical functioning or its impact on their employment or family. Mental health assessments can be beneficial for patients with SBMA, and antidepressants and antianxiety medications may be recommended.

14.4 Genetics and Pathogenesis

SBMA is caused by a CAG trinucleotide repeat expansion in the first exon of the androgen receptor (*AR*) gene on Xq12, and thus exhibits a sex-linked recessive inheritance pattern. The nucleotides CAG, along with CAA, encode the amino acid glutamine, signified by a single-letter code, Q. Glutamine expansion diseases, therefore, are often said to have a poly-Q expansion or poly-Q tract. SBMA is part of a group of nine neurogenetic disorders caused by poly-Q expansions, the other eight of which are categorized as movement disorders (Huntington disease, dentatorubral-pallidoluysian atrophy, and six forms of spinocerebellar ataxia) [6].

Genetic testing for SBMA is widely available, though some debate exists about pathogenic and pre-mutation "borderline" repeat numbers, and lab reporting varies slightly. In general, ≤34 CAG trinucleotide repeats is within normal limits and ≥35–38 CAG trinucleotide repeats is considered pathogenic, and diagnostic of SBMA [13]. These same reference ranges apply to diagnosing carrier status in females, whereby one of the two X chromosomes carries a pathogenic CAG trinucleotide repeat expansion in the *AR* gene. The clinical significance of 35, 36, and 37 CAG trinucleotide repeats is unclear, and many genetic testing companies note that results in this range must be interpreted within the context of the proband's clinical presentation and that of other affected family members. In general, normal CAG trinucleotide repeat lengths in SBMA have been shown to be highly mitotically stable [14]. However, it has been proposed that repeats in the abnormal and "borderline" range show somatic and germline instability, likely to expand during transition to subsequent generations [15, 16]. It is also possible that repeats in the "borderline" range may represent alleles with reduced penetrance.

As with many trinucleotide repeat expansion disorders and all neurogenetic poly-Q expansion disorders, anticipation is seen during transmission and should be included in genetic counseling as appropriate. Larger poly-Q expansions inversely correlate with age of onset and clinical severity of symptoms, such as scored disability assessments, quantitative muscle strength, and activities of daily living [2]. Though there is some debate, poly-Q expansion length has not shown to be significantly correlated with disease progression [1, 2, 4]. Indeed, there is an indication that factors other than the CAG trinucleotide repeat length play a role in symptom severity and disease progression, and some studies have suggested that physical ability *before* the onset of symptoms may play an important role [1].

Unlike the other poly-Q expansion disorders, the structure and function of the mutant AR protein are well characterized. AR belongs to a family of steroid hormones, which have reduced androgen binding in patients with SBMA [17]. Studies suggest that poly-Q expansions lead to low levels of transcription of the receptor mRNA in androgen-responsive genes, thus causing some of the symptoms of androgen insensitivity seen in patients with SBMA [18]. In addition, pathogenesis for neurological symptoms is thought to be a toxic gain-of-function mechanism induced by the accumulation of aggregate mutant AR proteins in the nucleus and cytoplasm of spinal cord and brainstem motor neuron cells [19]. Accumulation of these aggregates (or nuclear inclusions) leads to neuronal dysfunction, initiating cell degeneration and loss of motor neurons [20]. Several hypotheses exist to explain the exact nature of this relationship, and most of these pathways are theoretical targets for treatment.

14.5 Genetic Counseling Issues

As with most genetic conditions, genetic testing of the proband or another affected family member will prove most informative. Establishing a genetic cause for symptoms will, in turn, provide risk information for other family members. Once a diagnosis through genetic testing has been found in one family member, other family members will be eligible for clinical assessment and genetic testing. As with all X-linked recessive disorders, all female offspring of an affected male are obligate genetic carriers, while all male offspring will be unaffected. Carrier testing for at-risk female relatives is available through the same genetic testing process. Prenatal diagnosis for carrier females is also available, though not commonly requested due to the late age of onset, relatively slow progression of symptoms, and the lack of effect on cognition or life-span. Presymptomatic testing of at-risk male family members is technically possible, but also an uncommon request for the similar reasons. If presymptomatic testing is requested by an at-risk adult, a clinical neurological assessment is recommended along with appropriate genetic counseling. Genetic testing of asymptomatic children (age <18 years) is not considered appropriate, particularly while no established effective treatment exists for the condition.

Clinicians should be aware of some of the potential psychosocial issues for patients with SBMA. In general, this patient population consists of smart, highly motivated older men, many of whom have families of their own for which they are the financial and/or caregiving patriarch. Many patients begin to show initial symptoms during significant life events, such as children leaving for college ("empty nest") or retirement. Dealing with a significant change in daily life, along with physical decline, can prove emotionally taxing. For patients who work in professions requiring a great deal of physical ability, there can be significant impact on a patient's ability to retain gainful employment. As genetic counselors, it is important to specifically ask about psychosocial issues.

Targeted family history questions

- Has anyone in the family been diagnosed with a neurological disorder?
- Has anyone in the family had a tremor?
- Has anyone in the family had muscle weakness?
- Has anyone in the family had trouble walking or used a cane or walker?
- Has anyone in the family had speech or swallowing problems?
- Has anyone in the family had sexual dysfunction or fertility issues?

14.6 Genetic Counseling for Kennedy Disease (SBMA) Case History (Fig. 14.1)

Mr. K was a 47-year-old man with a 6-year history of hand tremors, muscle cramps, and progressive muscle weakness. Upon initial evaluation at age 43 (2 years after mild symptom onset), Mr. K was initially diagnosed with "likely ALS" by his primary care physician. A referral to neurology was given, but clinic slots for new consults were booked out several weeks. In the meantime, Mr. K underwent an EMG/NCS, which showed mild lower motor neuron dysfunction. Mr. K worked as a handyman, "jack of all trades," for a local university and picked up extra weekend hours working for his friend's roofing company. Mr. K presented in neurology clinic 6 weeks later with his wife.

Genetic counseling began by asking the couple to explain the reason for referral. They understood that Mr. K had a current "likely" diagnosis of ALS, but that this consult had been recommended because his primary care physician was not a neurologist and some of his symptoms "didn't quite fit that picture," particularly his slow progression of symptoms. Mrs. K was especially anxious about the

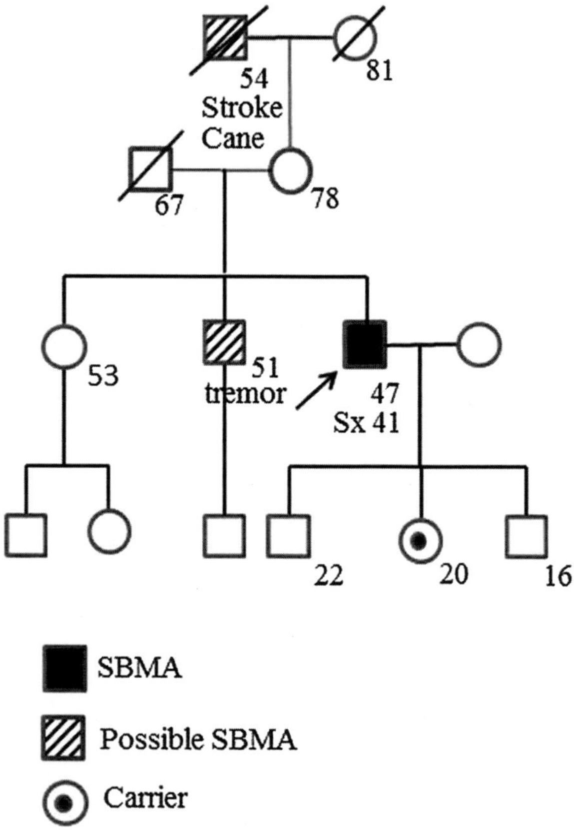

Fig. 14.1 SBMA case history pedigree

potential ALS diagnosis, since she had done quite a bit of Internet research. She was also concerned that they'd both spent years dealing with the slow progression of symptoms that were becoming more apparent and also about the recent uncertainty of not having a "firm" clinical diagnosis. The Ks both expressed frustration that no one had been able to tell them what he really had or what prognosis to expect. The genetic counselor acknowledged the feelings of fear and frustration, and assured them that the purpose of this initial appointment was to review the findings of previous studies, have a formal neurological examination, and ultimately try to find answers for the family regarding diagnosis.

A review of the family history revealed that Mr. K had an older brother and an older sister. Mr. K was on good terms with both siblings, but didn't feel particularly comfortable asking them about their medical histories. Both siblings had been quite shocked when told about Mr. K's potential diagnosis of ALS, and both denied any progressive muscle weakness, speech, or breathing issues. Mrs. K thought that Mr. K's brother had complained about a hand tremor at a recent family reunion, but no real details were discussed. The rest of the family pedigree was largely unremarkable for neurological symptoms, aside from Mr. K's maternal grandfather who used a cane to walk for a few years before an early, sudden death due to stroke. By Mr. K's mother's report, his grandfather had "knee issues" for many years, but couldn't recall a specific accident or injury that caused the problems.

Mr. K expressed concern about his employment, since it was becoming difficult to accomplish some of his usual tasks. He and Mrs. K had three children aged 16, 20, and 22, and were "nowhere near retiring" since two of the children were in college and one was still living at home in high school. They considered themselves just barely financially stable. Though Mrs. K had a part-time position as a dental receptionist, Mr. K was the family's primary financial provider. They regretted that their college-aged children had to take out student loans in order to attend university. When the genetic counselor asked what modifications or options were open to Mr. K, he became very quiet and tearful. He stated that he didn't think he had many options, and felt like he was letting his family down. Though Mrs. K disagreed and reassured him that no one in the family felt that way, Mr. K just nodded his head and quickly changed the subject.

A complete neurological evaluation was performed and findings were similar to those found by Mr. K's primary care physician. The genetic counselor and neurologist discussed with the Ks that the two most likely diagnoses were ALS and spinal and bulbar muscular atrophy (SBMA or Kennedy disease). Because of the slow disease progression, genetic testing for SBMA was ordered. The genetic counselor reviewed the genetic information for both ALS (likely sporadic) and SBMA (X-linked inheritance), including risks to the K's three children and other family members. The genetic counselor pointed out that if his genetic test results came back positive, Mr. K's daughter would be an obligate carrier for SBMA. Again, Mr. K appeared to be quite upset by this information. When asked how he felt, Mrs. K interjected that it was too soon to "play the guessing game" and that they couldn't worry about it yet. She stated that caring for Mr. K was their priority right now, and that their focus was finding out his diagnosis. They would "deal with anything else after that." When the counselor pressed the issue a bit more, asking how the Ks planned to tell their children about the testing and potential diagnoses, Mrs. K said that it was premature to involve the children in the conversation. She said that they would tell the children when they knew something definitive, particularly since both high school and college final exams were approaching. She stated that they didn't want the children to worry unnecessarily or cause a distraction for their exams. Mr. K nodded his head in agreement.

Discussion Questions

- What happens when genetic counseling turns up an ambiguous or uninformative family history? How much weight should be given to the information when deciding on genetic testing options?
- How do you help patients deal with uncertainty: short-term uncertainty or preparation for the potential of longer term uncertainty?
- Given the K's frustration over lack of information thus far, how much information should the genetic counselor provide about both ALS and SBMA including

diagnosis, disease progression, and treatment options (or lack thereof) at this initial appointment?

- How much should the genetic counselor address the family's financial and employment concerns at this initial appointment, considering that the medical team is still unclear about the diagnosis and disease course (which differs greatly between ALS and SBMA)? What, if any, resources should be discussed?
- What is the best way to deal with a family member who answers questions for the patient? Given Mr. K's emotional responses to his disease symptoms and its impact (or potential impact) on his family, how important is it to assess Mr. K's psychological state at this time in the presence of his wife? When, where, or how might be the best way to go about this?

Genetic test results for Mr. K were available a few weeks later. Because the family lived over 2 h from the clinic, the results were initially given to the Ks by phone (both were available for the call). The genetic counselor explained that the results were positive (diagnostic) for SBMA, with 42 CAG trinucleotide repeats in the AR gene. Both of the Ks seemed genuinely relieved at the news, and Mrs. K wept with joy and kept repeating, "I'm just so happy it's not ALS." Mr. K seemed to have taken the news well, but after an initial excited shout, he was fairly quiet on the phone. A follow-up appointment was scheduled a few weeks later to meet for additional genetic counseling and follow-up with the neurologist.

Mr. and Mrs. K came to clinic for the follow-up appointment with their 20-year-old daughter, Melanie, who was home on a college break. The Ks had informed all of the children about Mr. K's genetic diagnosis, but they told the counselor that it had been particularly hard on Melanie. Melanie said that she was concerned for her father, but now had concerns about herself. Since she had been out of state during the testing process, she said that she felt shocked and upset that her parents "sprang the information about carrier status on her out of the blue" when she returned home from college for the summer. It was clear from Melanie's description that she had been unprepared to hear the news, and particularly distressed that this felt like a solitary burden since her brothers did not share the same risks. She had just entered a new relationship and "didn't want to have to deal with this." When the genetic counselor asked her to say more about her feelings and worries, she stated that she was worried about what this meant for her romantic and reproductive future, and she had no idea what to tell her boyfriend. She also said that she felt embarrassed having to discuss this information in front of her parents. Mrs. K. kept repeating that she "thought her daughter should be tested."

The genetic counselor suggested that they talk briefly about X-linked inheritance and a few reproductive options with Melanie, highlighting the fact that genetic carrier testing for SBMA was certainly possible, but not medically necessary at this time (since Melanie would be an obligate carrier). The genetic counselor also highlighted that medical research is advancing rapidly for SBMA treatment options (should she have an at-risk child in the future). A brief description of ART, PGD, sex selection, and prenatal testing were also discussed. After that, the genetic counselor suggested that Melanie could make her own follow-up appointment to discuss these issues and options in further detail. Melanie chose to leave the room, but said that the information provided was enough to "calm her down" because it gave her alternative options to think about.

Once the attention for the appointment was turned back to Mr. K and his new diagnosis, the genetic counselor asked how the Ks had been processing the information. Mrs. K said that she was thrilled with the information and thanked the genetic counselor. Mr. K said that he was also happy with the diagnosis of SBMA, given the alternative. Mrs. K mentioned that Mr. K had been depressed over the past few months, and, since the telephone call, had seen his primary care provider and a psychologist. They were monitoring him for depression, and had started him on a low dose of antidepressant medication. Mr. K said that he didn't notice any improvement, but acknowledged that he had only been taking the medication for 1 week. He repeated his initial concern about being able to provide for his family. He acknowledged that his wife was very supportive, but that sometimes it was difficult to talk to her about those issues. The genetic counselor suggested that Mr. K get in touch with the KDA support network, so that he might share his experiences and concerns with other men who had his diagnosis. Both of the Ks seemed to appreciate this idea.

Discussion Questions

- What do you do when a support person or family member unexpectedly takes over an appointment, particularly when it is at the patient's request?
- How appropriate are large family discussions during genetic counseling? If you feel like the discussion is becoming too personal for one of the participants, when do you draw the line? How do you mitigate or steer the conversation?

14.7 Resource for Patients

Kennedy Disease Association website: www.kennedysdisease.org/

Kennedy Disease Association Facebook page: www.facebook.com/pages/Kennedys-Disease-Association/325990476576/

References

1. Hashizume, A., Katsuno, M., Banno, H., Suzuki, K., Suga, N., Mano, T., et al. (2012). Longitudinal changes of outcome measures in spinal and bulbar muscular atrophy. *Brain, 135*(9), 2838–2848.
2. Rhodes, L. E., Freeman, B. K., Auh, S., Kokkinis, A. D., La Pean, A., Chen, C., et al. (2009). Clinical features of spinal and bulbar muscular atrophy. *Brain, 132*(12), 3242–3251.

3. Schmidt, B. J., Greenberg, C. R., Allingham-Hawkins, D. J., & Spriggs, E. L. (2002). Expression of X-linked bulbospinal muscular atrophy (Kennedy disease) in two homozygous women. *Neurology, 59*(5), 770–772.
4. Atsuta, N., Watanabe, H., Ito, M., Banno, H., Suzuki, K., Katsuno, M., et al. (2006). Natural history of spinal and bulbar muscular atrophy (SBMA): A study of 223 Japanese patients. *Brain, 129*(6), 1446–1455.
5. Greenland, K. J., Beilin, J., Castro, J., Varghese, P. N., & Zajac, J. D. (2004). Polymorphic CAG repeat length in the androgen receptor gene and association with neurodegeneration in a heterozygous female carrier of Kennedy's disease. *Journal of Neurology, 251*(1), 35–41.
6. Sambataro, F., & Pennuto, M. (2012). Cell-autonomous and non-cell-autonomous toxicity in polyglutamine diseases. *Progress in Neurobiology, 97*(2), 152–172.
7. Fernández-Rhodes, L. E., Kokkinis, A. D., White, M. J., Watts, C. A., Auh, S., Jeffries, N. O., et al. (2011). Efficacy and safety of dutasteride in patients with spinal and bulbar muscular atrophy: A randomised placebo-controlled trial. *Lancet Neurology, 10*(2), 140–147.
8. Katsuno, M., Banno, H., Suzuki, K., Adachi, H., Tanaka, F., & Sobue, G. (2010). Clinical features and molecular mechanisms of spinal and bulbar muscular atrophy (SBMA). *Advances in Experimental Medicine and Biology, 685*, 64–74.
9. Suzuki, K., Banno, H., Katsuno, M., Adachi, H., Tanaka, F., & Sobue, G. (2012). Disease-modifying therapy for spinal and bulbar muscular atrophy (SBMA). *Brain and Nerve, 64*(3), 237–244.
10. Banno, H., Katsuno, M., Suzuki, K., Takeuchi, Y., Kawashima, M., Suga, N., et al. (2009). Phase 2 trial of leuprorelin in patients with spinal and bulbar muscular atrophy. *Annals of Neurology, 65*(2), 140–150.
11. Banno, H., Katsuno, M., Suzuki, K., & Sobue, G. (2011). Dutasteride for spinal and bulbar muscular atrophy. Comment on: Efficacy and safety of dutasteride in patients with spinal and bulbar muscular atrophy: A randomised placebo-controlled trial. *Lancet Neurology, 10*(2), 113–115.
12. Querin, G., D'Ascenzo, C., Peterle, E., Ermani, M., Bello, L., Melacini, P., et al. (2013). Pilot trial of clenbuterol in spinal and bulbar muscular atrophy. *Neurology, 80*(23), 2095–2098.
13. La Spada, A. (1999). Spinal and bulbar muscular atrophy. [Updated 2011 Oct 13]. In: R. A. Pagon, M. P. Adam, T. D. Bird, et al. (Eds.), *GeneReviews™* [Internet]. Seattle, WA: University of Washington, Seattle; 1993–2013. Available from: http://www.ncbi.nlm.nih.gov/books/NBK1333/ar Dystrophy Association: www.mda.org
14. Finsterer, J. (2010). Perspectives of Kennedy's disease. *Journal of Neurological Sciences, 298* (1–2), 1–10.
15. Katsuno, M., Banno, H., Suzuki, K., Takeuchi, Y., Kawashima, M., Tanaka, F., et al. (2008). Molecular genetics and biomarkers of polyglutamine diseases. *Current Molecular Medicine, 8* (3), 221–234.
16. Rosales-Reynoso, M. A., Ochoa-Hernández, A. B., & Barros-Núñez, P. (2009). Diseases caused by triplet expansion. *Revista de Neurologia, 49*, 79–87.
17. Warner, C. L., Griffin, J. E., Wilson, J. D., Jacobs, L. D., Murray, K. R., Fischbeck, K. H., et al. (1992). X-linked spinomuscular atrophy: A kindred with associated abnormal androgen receptor binding. *Neurology, 42*(11), 2181–2184.
18. Choong, C. S., Kemppainen, J. A., Zhou, Z. X., & Wilson, E. M. (1996). Reduced androgen receptor gene expression with first exon CAG repeat expansion. *Molecular Endocrinology, 10* (12), 1527–1535.
19. Piccioni, F., Simeoni, S., Andriola, I., Armatura, E., Bassanini, S., Pozzi, P., et al. (2001). Polyglutamine tract expansion of the androgen receptor in a motoneuronal model of spinal and bulbar muscular atrophy. *Brain Research Bulletin, 56*(3–4), 215–220.
20. Adachi, H., Katsuno, M., Minamiyama, M., Waza, M., Sang, C., Nakagomi, Y., et al. (2005). Widespread nuclear and cytoplasmic accumulation of mutant androgen receptor in SBMA patients. *Brain, 128*, 659–670.

Chapter 15
Hereditary Spastic Paraplegia

Alice B. Schindler

Hereditary spastic paraplegia (HSP), also called familial spastic paraparesis (FSP), refers to a group of inherited disorders that are characterized by length-dependent distal axonopathy of the corticospinal tracts (upper motor neurons), resulting in progressive, lower limb spasticity (stiffness), and weakness. The cell bodies of these neurons are located in the motor cortex area of the brain. The axons travel to the brainstem and down the spinal cord and relay instructions to lower motor neurons located along the brainstem and spinal cord. Lower motor neurons then carry the message out to the muscles. When upper motor neurons degenerate, the correct messages cannot reach the lower motor neurons, and the lower motor neurons cannot transmit the correct messages to the muscles. As the degeneration continues, spasticity, and weakness increase. The legs are affected because degeneration occurs primarily at the ends of the longest nerves in the spinal cord, which control the legs. In some cases, the upper body can be minimally affected as well, leading to problems with the arms or speech and swallowing muscles [1, 2].

Electronic supplementary material Supplementary material is available in the online version of this chapter at 10.1007/978-1-4899-7482-2_15. Videos can also be accessed at http://www.springerimages.com/videos/978-1-4899-7481-5.

A.B. Schindler (✉)
Neurogenetics Branch, NINDS/NIH, 10 Center Drive, Building 10 Room 5S-219, Bethesda, MD 20892-1671, USA
e-mail: schindlerab@mail.nih.gov

J.S. Goldman (ed.), *Genetic Counseling for Adult Neurogenetic Disease*,
DOI 10.1007/978-1-4899-7482-2_15

Discussion Questions

- How might childlike behavior and parental dependency influence genetic counseling?
- How might family dynamics make discussing suspected depression in one family member difficult? Where are the counseling boundaries? How much should the counselor intercede?
- How could variable expressivity affect individuals psychosocially?

While the results of the SPG11 testing were negative, sequencing of SPG15 revealed that both Jane and John were compound heterozygotes for mutations in SPG15, confirming the diagnosis of SPG15. The results were communicated to the family by phone and they returned for a follow-up visit to discuss results and undergo parental testing. Mrs. X indicated that her oldest daughter would be attending clinic and was desperate to learn her status, so the entire family presented for the second visit. The family dynamics were unchanged from the previous visit. Both the neurologist and genetic counselor were present to discuss the results with the family. Mrs. X indicated that she was relieved to finally have a diagnosis for her children, and was excited by the prospect of beginning drug therapy and possibly stem cell therapy. Since her last visit, she had been doing a lot of research on the Internet. She explained that her children were prepared to try anything to find a cure. She believed that since the neurologist worked on HSPs in his lab, he would begin studying her children and would subsequently develop a cure. The neurologist and genetic counselor discussed the results of the testing in detail, clarifying that the SPG15 mutations explained Jane's and John's symptoms. The genetic counselor discussed the inheritance pattern of SPG15, describing how Mr. and Mrs. X were most likely both unaffected carriers who, unknowingly, had each passed on an SPG15 mutation to their children. Mrs. X was flabbergasted and indicated that she and her husband were in no way related and did not understand how this could have happened to them. The counselor explained the nuances of the compound heterozygous results again and agreed that families are often puzzled and stunned by these types of results, given parental health status and lack of family history. Even in conditions that are extremely rare and have a low carrier frequency, it was still possible for parents to be carriers and have affected children; parental testing would help to clarify this. In these cases, the families have no prior knowledge, so it can be quite upsetting and may take time and further discussion to accept. When asked, both Jane and John indicated that it was important for them to have a diagnosis, but that they did not anticipate that the diagnosis would change anything. Mr. X agreed. Mrs. X added that she was extremely fearful for her oldest daughter who might be a carrier; she was successful and was engaged, and she did not want her carrier status to affect her life. The genetic counselor asked the older sister how she felt, and she admitted that she was terrified of being a carrier and did not want to have children who were affected like her siblings. The counselor tried to engage the family in exploring how HSP had impacted their lives and affected their relationships with one another. Both Jane and John responded that they had grown up with this progressive condition and had learned to deal with it. Mrs. X indicated that she preferred to focus on the future and on curing her children by participating in research. Mr. X said that he would continue to support his children in their endeavors. The oldest sister stated that she left home for college when she was 18 years old and later had traveled for work, only returning home for holidays. She did not take an active role in her siblings' lives, and this was her first time attending a clinic appointment. She came to the visit in the hopes of learning her status and helping her siblings by being part of the research.

The neurologist and counselor revisited the goals of their research and discussed that, while there were currently no treatments or cures for HSPs, through continued research, therapies might be identified. The counselor acknowledged that participating in research on rare conditions can be frustrating for both families and researchers because the science does not always move as quickly as everyone would like. She reiterated the importance of remaining hopeful and of continuing physical and occupational therapy. She encouraged them to join the SPF, a group she felt was helpful for emotional as well as medical support. The counselor also invited all family members to contact her or the neurologist on a regular basis with questions about new therapies, as navigating the information available on the Internet, especially with regard to stem cells and gene therapies, could be difficult and, in some cases, misleading.

The parents and the oldest daughter elected to proceed with carrier testing and had their blood drawn. The results were returned 2 months later with the following results: Mr. and Mrs. X were heterozygotes and the oldest daughter was negative for both mutations. The tetrad (Mr. and Mrs. X, Jane, and John) returned to clinic annually for follow-up and natural history studies.

Discussion Questions

- What are some challenges when counseling several family members in a group setting?
- How could the counselor address the older sister's anxiety without detracting from the experience of the affected patients?
- How can managing patient and family expectations influence counseling? How does the absence of specific therapies or medical management change this?
- How can managing expectations in a research setting be different from a clinical setting?

15.7 Patient Resources

Spastic Paraplegia Foundation, Inc.
PO Box 1208
Fortson GA 31808-1208
Phone: 877-773-4483 (toll-free)
Email: information@sp-foundation.org
sp-foundation.org

National Institute of Neurological Disorders and Stroke (NINDS)
PO Box 5801
Bethesda MD 20824
Phone: 800-352-9424 (toll-free); 301-496-5751; 301-468-5981 (TTY)
Hereditary Spastic Paraplegia Information Page
www.clinicaltrials.gov

References

1. Harding, A. E. (1983). Classification of the hereditary ataxias and paraplegias. *Lancet, 1*(8334), 1151–1155.
2. Blackstone, C. (2012). Cellular pathways of hereditary spastic paraplegia. *Annual Review of Neuroscience, 35*, 25–47.
3. McMonagle, P., Webb, S., & Hutchinson, M. (2002). The prevalence of "pure" autosomal dominant hereditary spastic paraparesis in the island of Ireland. *Journal of Neurology, Neurosurgery, and Psychiatry, 72*(1), 43–46.
4. Orlacchio, A., Kawarai, T., Totaro, A., Errico, A., St George-Hyslop, P. H., Rugarli, E. I., et al. (2004). Hereditary spastic paraplegia: Clinical genetic study of 15 families. *Archives of Neurology, 61*(6), 849–855.
5. Schüle, R., & Schöls, L. (2011). Genetics of hereditary spastic paraplegias. *Seminars in Neurology, 31*(5), 484–493.
6. Fink, J. K., & Hedera, P. (1999). Hereditary spastic paraplegia: Genetic heterogeneity and genotype-phenotype correlation. *Seminars in Neurology, 19*(3), 301–309.
7. Ngudi, D. D., Kuo, Y. H., Van Montagu, M., & Lambein, F. (2012). Research on motor neuron diseases konzo and neurolathyrism: Trends from 1990 to 2010. *PLoS Neglected Tropical Diseases, 6*(7), e1759.
8. Kenwrick, S., Ionasescu, V., Ionasescu, G., Searby, C., King, A., Dubowitz, M., et al. (1986). Linkage studies of X-linked recessive spastic paraplegia using DNA probes. *Human Genetics, 73*(3), 264–266.
9. Fonknechten, N., Mavel, D., Byrne, P., Davoine, C. S., Cruaud, C., Bönsch, D., et al. (2000). Spectrum of SPG4 mutations in autosomal dominant spastic paraplegia. *Human Molecular Genetics, 9*(4), 637–644.
10. Sauter, S., Miterski, B., Klimpe, S., Bönsch, D., Schöls, L., Visbeck, A., et al. (2002). Mutation analysis of the spastin gene (SPG4) in patients in Germany with autosomal dominant hereditary spastic paraplegia. *Human Mutation, 20*(2), 127–132.
11. Depienne, C., Tallaksen, C., Lephay, J. Y., Bricka, B., Poea-Guyon, S., Fontaine, B., et al. (2006). Spastin mutations are frequent in sporadic spastic paraparesis and their spectrum is different from that observed in familial cases. *Journal of Medical Genetics, 43*(3), 259–265.
12. Alvarez, V., Sánchez-Ferrero, E., Beetz, C., Díaz, M., Alonso, B., Corao, A. I., et al. (2010). Mutational spectrum of the SPG4 (SPAST) and SPG3A (ATL1) genes in Spanish patients with hereditary spastic paraplegia. *BMC Neurology, 10*, 89.
13. Magariello, A., Muglia, M., Patitucci, A., Ungaro, C., Mazzei, R., Gabriele, A. L., et al. (2010). Mutation analysis of the SPG4 gene in Italian patients with pure and complicated forms of spastic paraplegia. *Journal of Neurological Sciences, 288*(1–2), 96–100.
14. Dürr, A., Camuzat, A., Colin, E., Tallaksen, C., Hannequin, D., Coutinho, P., et al. (2004). Atlastin1 mutations are frequent in young-onset autosomal dominant spastic paraplegia. *Archives of Neurology, 61*(12), 1867–1872.

15. Hehr, U., Bauer, P., Winner, B., Schule, R., Olmez, A., Koehler, W., et al. (2007). Long-term course and mutational spectrum of spatacsin-linked spastic paraplegia. *Annals of Neurology, 62*(6), 656–665.
16. Stevanin, G., Azzedine, H., Denora, P., Boukhris, A., Tazir, M., Lossos, A., et al. (2008). Mutations in SPG11 are frequent in autosomal recessive spastic paraplegia with thin corpus callosum, cognitive decline and lower motor neuron degeneration. *Brain, 131*(Pt 3), 772–784.
17. Goizet, C., Boukhris, A., Maltete, D., Guyant-Maréchal, L., Truchetto, J., Mundwiller, E., et al. (2009). SPG15 is the second most common cause of hereditary spastic paraplegia with thin corpus callosum. *Neurology, 73*(14), 1111–1119.
18. Schüle, R., Brandt, E., Karle, K. N., Tsaousidou, M., Klebe, S., Klimpe, S., et al. (2009). Analysis of CYP7B1 in non-consanguineous cases of hereditary spastic paraplegia. *Neurogenetics, 10*(2), 97–104.
19. Schüle, R., & Schöls, L. (2011). Genetics of hereditary spastic paraplegias. *Seminars in Neurology, 31*(5), 484–493.
20. Goizet, C., Boukhris, A., Durr, A., Beetz, C., Truchetto, J., Tesson, C., et al. (2009). CYP7B1 mutations in pure and complex forms of hereditary spastic paraplegia type 5. *Brain, 132*(Pt 6), 1589–1600.
21. Schlipf, N. A., Schüle, R., Klimpe, S., Karle, K. N., Synofzik, M., Schicks, J., et al. (2011). Amplicon-based high-throughput pooled sequencing identifies mutations in CYP7B1 and SPG7 in sporadic spastic paraplegia patients. *Clinical Genetics, 80*(2), 148–160.
22. Arnoldi, A., Crimella, C., Tenderini, E., Martinuzzi, A., D'Angelo, M. G., Musumeci, O., et al. (2012). Clinical phenotype variability in patients with hereditary spastic paraplegia type 5 associated with CYP7B1 mutations. *Clinical Genetics, 81*(2), 150–157.

Part V
The Neuropathies and Channelopathies

options, she would need to have genetic testing to confirm her status, even if she shows no evidence of CMT.

In addition to discussing natural history, management issues should also be raised. While patients may want to know what to do about the condition, they may also be frustrated by the lack of available medications. A common concern for patients and families is the progressive loss of ambulation. Patients may need psychological help transitioning to the next level of ambulation aid, such as shoe inserts, AFOs, or walkers/wheelchairs/scooters. Each stage of ambulation progression requires the patient to come to terms with their diagnosis and true needs. A helpful website is bareyourbrace.com, which highlights people who have embraced their disability and AFOs.

Although there is no published data addressing the length of time between symptom development and diagnosis of CMT, anecdotal evidence suggests that many people with CMT may be misdiagnosed. Additionally, some affected people may feel that medical treatment is unavailable. Yet, there are treatments to help symptoms: AFOs for ambulation and medication for neuropathic pain. Research opportunities are available and often make patients feel that they are being proactive in dealing with their disease [14].

16.6 Case History (Fig. 16.1)

A woman presented at a neurology clinic with her 3-year-old daughter. The child had been referred to the clinic by an orthopedic surgeon because of tight heel cords. Her pediatrician had originally referred her to the orthopedic surgeon because she was walking on her toes. The orthopedic surgeon took a thorough family history (Fig. 16.1) and found it suggestive of neuropathy. Examining the mother, the surgeon found that she had moderately high arches and fatigue. A motor and sensory exam on the mother found reduced strength in foot dorsiflexion (raising the foot) and foot eversion, as well as some atrophy of the intrinsic hand muscles. A nerve conduction study was ordered for both mother and daughter, and both velocities were found to be slowed—22 m/s in the ulnar nerve for the mother (normal >50 m/s), and 12 m/s for the daughter (normal >22 m/s for a 3-year-old). Genetic testing was ordered on the mother, and she was found to have a duplication of the *PMP22* gene, confirming a diagnosis of CMT1A. The mother returned to receive her results from the genetic counselor.

The genetic counselor (GC) met with the patient (P) for genetic counseling about CMT. She asked P if she knew the reason for the referral, and P understood that she was diagnosed with CMT. P told GC that she had done some reading on the Internet and wondered if other people in her family were affected, like her brother who had "funny-looking" feet. Examining P's pedigree, GC noted this possibility, but suggested that they discuss CMT and P's specific type of CMT based on the genetic testing results, before discussing the potential risk to other family members.

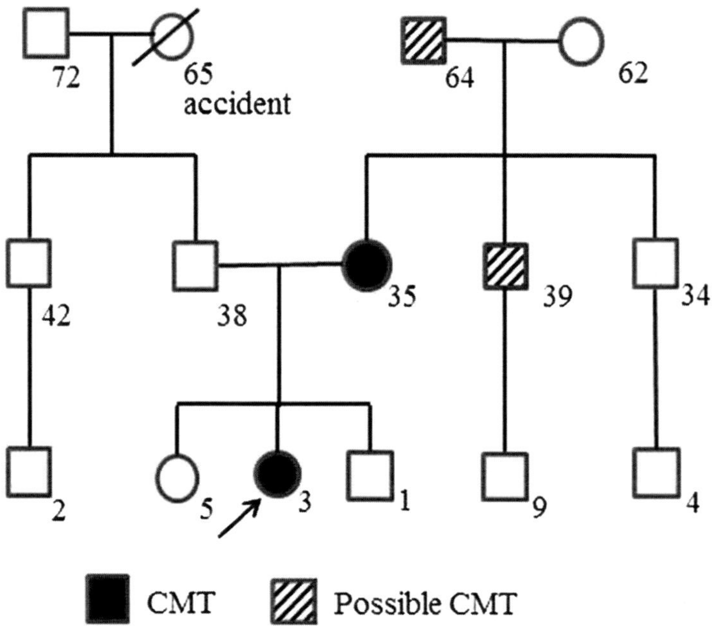

Fig. 16.1 CMT case history pedigree

GC and P then discussed the nature of CMT. During this discussion, P was surprised to learn that some of the symptoms she had were part of CMT. GC mentioned difficulty with proprioception and the feelings of imbalance that may occur when closing the eyes or in dark or crowded areas. P noted that she needed to place her elbow against the shower wall when washing her hair. GC then discussed the mechanism by which an elbow can keep the whole body steady.

GC also talked to P about bracing. Since she was having difficulty with balance and proprioception, a reasonable next step was AFOs. Although her physician had already recommended AFOs, she was initially resistant to trying them. She believed that her walking was fine, just a little slower than others. GC agreed that thinking about using AFOs was a big step, and acknowledged that this must be quite a shock. P had just received this new diagnosis of CMT, and she had to think about various recommendations for changes in her daily life. P agreed, but noted that she was getting used to the diagnosis, as it explained a lot about her and the way she grew up. She knew that she was slow and clumsy, but she thought it was just she. Now she had a condition that she could cite as the reason for her problems. That being said, she still did not think that AFOs would be of use to her.

GC asked if she could talk to P more about her walking. She asked questions aimed at determining whether P had a noticeable foot drop: "Do people know it is you coming down the hall before they see you?" "Would you say that your feet slap when you walk?" "Do you get tired when walking a long distance?" "When standing still, do you feel like you are steady or do you need to step backward or bob up and down to maintain balance?" P answered that people always knew that she was coming down the hall, her feet slapped, she got tired when walking (and occasionally used walking aids such as a grocery cart to help with distances), and she could stand still, but in a crouch. Based on these answers, GC told her that she was experiencing foot drop because of the CMT. She discussed the mechanism behind the foot drop and the tiring steppage gait that results. She told P that, though she was not going to want to hear it, proper bracing could help all of these things. P understood this, but still did not have interest in pursuing braces. Probing more, GC was finally able to discover that P was actually worried about other people noticing that she was wearing braces. GC was frank—she told P that braces would make her impairments less noticeable, not more. People would not know it was she walking down the hall because they would not hear her coming. Furthermore, by wearing pants and socks, the brace would not be visible. Additionally, braces would help keep the Achilles tendon stretched, preventing the arches from getting high. They also would align the feet properly to reduce the stress on her ankles, knees, hips, and back, making arthritis less likely in the future. P was surprised. GC then challenged her to try one on and just see how it felt. P reluctantly agreed.

Discussion Questions

- The genetic counselor spent a lot of time on disease management. Do you see this as part of the role of a genetic counselor?
- The patient offered some reasons why she was resistant to AFOs. Do you think there are other reasons why she did not want to get a pair? What would these be? How could the genetic counselor have addressed these other unspoken issues?

Having discussed management issues, GC redirected the conversation back to the type of CMT that was in the family and the inheritance pattern. P knew from her doctor that she had CMT1A. GC asked P what she knew about CMT1A, and discussed information about the extra copy of *PMP22* that causes the condition. GC raised the possibility that P's father, who had high arches and walked with a walker, could also be affected with CMT1A. P appeared prepared for this possibility; however, she made a sarcastic comment thanking her dad for her CMT. P asked again about her brother, whom she had brought up previously in the conversation. She had read on the Internet that men cannot pass down the condition to their sons, but her brother seemed to have some symptoms similar to herself. GC then explained autosomal dominant inheritance versus X-linked inheritance. She discussed how CMT1A is inherited in an autosomal dominant manner, so there is a 50/50 chance of passing down the condition in each pregnancy of a person affected with the condition. P's reading about the lack of male-to-male transmission applied only to people with X-linked forms of CMT. GC then informed P that her brother could be tested either genetically or through an NCS to see if he was affected with CMT1A. In this case, if he were found to have slowed nerve conductions, he would be given a genetic diagnosis of CMT1A, even without a genetic test. It would be his decision, and GC and P discussed the pros and cons of testing. GC told P that she would be happy to speak with her brother about these issues if he had questions or concerns.

P suddenly looked tearful. When GC asked what was upsetting her, P answered that she was responsible for passing the condition on to her daughter. Even though she had not known about the condition and couldn't have kept her daughter from getting it, she clearly felt very guilty. GC expressed empathy for P and asked her if she was also upset at her father, who may have passed the condition on to her. She said no, she couldn't be mad at her father for doing something he didn't know he was doing and had no control over. GC then asked P why she would feel guilty for doing the same thing. She, too, had no control over which chromosome was passed to her children.

P wondered whether all of her children could be affected, since each had the chance of inheriting the extra copy of the gene. GC again discussed the 50/50 chance in each pregnancy for a child to inherit the extra copy of *PMP22*. P asked if she should have her other children tested. GC stated that, in general, asymptomatic children were not tested, and only if difficulties developed that required a diagnosis for proper management would testing be discussed. Otherwise it was better not to label the children. P responded that they were good kids. P sighed, indicating that she had learned more information than she had expected. GC acknowledged that these meetings could be overwhelming. GC told P that she would be happy to go over any of this information again in the future and would send her a summary letter. P was grateful for both of these and left feeling more empowered about her condition.

Discussion Questions

- What does the genetic counselor mean by "non-genetic genetic testing" and do you feel that this is a good option for some patients?
- What do you think about the genetic counselor not testing the other children of the patient, but offering to discuss it again in the future?

16.7 Patient Resources

Charcot Marie Tooth Association (CMTA)—www.cmtausa.org

- Support and Action Groups

  Muscular Dystrophy Association (MDA)—http://www.mda.org

- Support groups (may be in conjunction with CMTA)
- Funding of CMT research
- Provide $500 per year in repairs to AFOs or other aids
- Can provide items from loan closet if needed (some wheelchairs, bath seats, etc.)

  Hereditary Neuropathies Foundation (HNF)—http://www.hnf-cure.org

References

1. Skre, H. (1974). Genetic and clinical aspects of Charcot-Marie-Tooth's disease. *Clinical Genetics, 6*(2), 98–118.
2. Saporta, A. S., Sottile, S. L., Miller, L. J., Feely, S. M., Siskind, C. E., & Shy, M. E. (2011). Charcot-Marie-Tooth disease subtypes and genetic testing strategies. *Annals of Neurology, 69* (1), 22–33.
3. Sheth, S., Francies, K., Siskind, C. E., Feely, S. M., Lewis, R. A., & Shy, M. E. (2008). Diabetes mellitus exacerbates motor and sensory impairment in CMT1A. *Journal of the Peripheral Nervous System, 13*(4), 299–304.
4. Feely, S. M. E., Laura, M., Siskind, C. E., Sottile, S., Davis, M., Gibbons, V. S., et al. (2011). MFN2 mutations cause severe phenotypes in most patients with CMT2A. *Neurology, 76*(20), 1690–1696.
5. Pitceathly, R. D., Murphy, S. M., Cottenie, E., Chalasani, A., Sweeney, M. G., Woodward, C., et al. (2012). Genetic dysfunction of MT-ATP6 causes axonal Charcot-Marie-Tooth disease. *Neurology, 79*(11), 1145–1154.
6. Blair, I. P., Nash, J., Gordon, M. J., & Nicholson, G. A. (1996). Prevalence and origin of de novo duplications in Charcot-Marie-Tooth disease type 1A: First report of a de novo duplication with a maternal origin. *American Journal of Human Genetics, 58*(3), 472–476.
7. Lewis, R. A., McDermott, M. P., Herrmann, D., Hoke, A., Clawson, L. L., Siskind, C., et al. (2013). High dose ascorbic acid treatment in CMT-1A: Results of a randomized double masked controlled trial. *JAMA Neurology, 70*(8), 981–987.
8. Micallef, J., Attarian, S., Dubourg, O., Gonnaud, P. M., Hogrel, J. Y., Stojkovic, T., et al. (2009). Effect of ascorbic acid in patients with Charcot-Marie-Tooth disease type 1A: A multicentre, randomised, double-blind, placebo-controlled trial. *Lancet Neurology, 8*(12), 1103–1110.
9. Pareyson, D., Reilly, M. M., Schenone, A., Fabrizi, G. M., Cavallaro, T., Santoro, L., et al. (2011). Ascorbic acid in Charcot-Marie-Tooth disease type 1A (CMT-TRIAAL and CMT-TRAUK): A double blind randomised trial. *Lancet Neurology, 10*(4), 320–328.
10. Shy, M. E., Siskind, C., Swan, E. R., Krajewski, K. M., Doherty, T., Fuerst, D. R., et al. (2007). CMT1X phenotypes represent loss of *GJB1* gene function. *Neurology, 68*(11), 849–855.
11. Shy, M. E., Chen, L., Swan, E. R., Taube, R., Krajewski, K. M., Herrmann, D., et al. (2008). Neuropathy progression in Charcot-Marie-Tooth disease type 1A. *Neurology, 70*(5), 378–383.
12. Siskind, C. E., Murphy, S. M., Ovens, R., Polke, J., Reilly, M. M., & Shy, M. E. (2011). Phenotype expression in women with CMT1X. *Journal of the Peripheral Nervous System, 16* (2), 102–107.
13. Siskind, C. E., & Shy, M. E. (2011). Genetics of neuropathies. *Seminars in Neurology, 31*(5), 494–505.
14. Siskind, C. E., Panchal, S., Smith, C. O., Feely, S. M. E., Dalton, J. C., Schindler, A. B., et al. (2013). Genetic counseling for Charcot Marie Tooth disease (CMT). *Journal of Genetic Counseling, 22*(4), 422–436.

Chapter 17
Channelopathies

Carly E. Siskind

The periodic paralyses are a group of autosomal dominant disorders characterized by episodes of paralysis with corresponding fluctuations in serum potassium levels. The periodic paralyses, caused by defects in the calcium or sodium ion channels, are collectively known as channelopathies. The periodic paralyses caused by reduced serum potassium are called hypokalemic periodic paralyses (HypoKPP). Hyperkalemic periodic paralysis (HyperKPP) is a condition caused by increased serum potassium, though some people with HyperKPP have a normal serum potassium level during an attack.

17.1 Clinical Presentation

HypoKPP is the most common of the periodic paralyses, affecting about 1:100,000 people, with reduced penetrance in women [1]. During an attack, the characteristic findings are by episodic flaccid paralysis of the limbs (but not the breathing or facial muscles) and corresponding decreased serum potassium levels. Between attacks, the serum potassium levels are normal. Patients often wake up with paralysis after a day of vigorous exercise and/or a salty, carbohydrate-rich dinner, both of which are common precipitants [2, 3]. Usual onset of symptoms occurs during the first two decades of life, with an average age of onset at 15 years [3]. The attacks usually last for hours to days with gradual resolution. The frequency of the attacks can vary and tend to decrease after 40 years of age. The day prior to an attack, some patients may have a slight prodrome, including parasthesias, fatigue, or cognitive changes [4].

C.E. Siskind (✉)
Stanford Hospital and Clinics Neuroscience Center, Stanford University, 300 Pasteur Dr., Suite A342D, M/C 5235, Stanford, CA 94305, USA
e-mail: csiskind@stanfordmed.org

J.S. Goldman (ed.), *Genetic Counseling for Adult Neurogenetic Disease*,
DOI 10.1007/978-1-4899-7482-2_17

period. Dietary changes include eating frequent small meals and avoiding high carbohydrate loads. In addition, people with HyperKPP should avoid fasting.

Supplemental potassium administered at the beginning of a HypoKPP attack can decrease the length and/or intensity of paralysis. The usual recommended dose is 20–30 mEq/l orally every 15–30 min until serum potassium is normalized [4].

Randomized clinical trials have been performed using acetazolamide and dichlorphenamide. Acetazolamide is a carbonic anhydrase inhibitor that causes potassium to be excreted in urine. This medication was found to improve muscle strength in patients with HypoKPP, particularly in the limb-girdle muscles, and to decrease the number of attacks [5, 7]. Acetazolamide appears to be effective in people with specific mutations, but some patients are nonresponders, and some patients have worsened on the medication [3]. In some patients with HyperKPP and myotonia, acetazolamide was found to be effective for episodic weakness [8]. This benefit may be mutation specific [3].

A randomized double-blind placebo-controlled crossover trial of dichlorphenamide for both HypoKPP and potassium sensitive periodic paralysis (which included HyperKPP and paramyotonia congenita with periodic paralysis) demonstrated a significantly lower rate of attack using the medication than during the placebo phase [9]. Patients may benefit from one or both medications.

Since people with HypoKPP are at increased risk for pre- and post-anesthetic weakness and malignant hyperthermia, medical providers should be notified of the condition whenever anesthesia is to be given.

17.4 Genetics

The periodic paralyses are autosomal dominant conditions. Incomplete penetrance is seen in HypoKPP, with males being affected more than females in a ratio of 2:1 [3]. In particular, the R528H *CACNA1S* mutation seems to have lower penetrance than other mutations [10–12]. Penetrance for the R528H mutation is 45 % in females versus 90 % in males, and for the R1239H mutation is 71 % in females and 91 % in males [12]. Males and females are affected equally in HyperKPP.

HypoKPP is caused by mutations in two genes: *CACNA1S* and *SCN4A*. The first, causing HypoKPP1, is a calcium ion channel gene and the second, causing HypoKPP2, encodes a sodium ion channel. Sixty-four percent of people with HypoKPP have a mutation in one of these two genes [3]. About 1/3 of HypoKPP mutations are the result of *de novo* mutations. HyperKPP is also caused by mutations in *SCN4A*, making it allelic to HypoKPP2. Common mutations in the *SCN4A* gene causing HyperKPP are T704M and M1592V [8] (Table 17.1).

HypoKPP and HyperKPP exhibit some genotype-phenotype correlations. In one study on HypoKPP patients with mutations in *CACNA1S* or *SCN4A*, the mean age of onset was found to be 10 years versus 22 years for those without a known mutation [3]. Those with the *CACNA1S* R1239H mutation presented at an average age of 7 years versus 14 years with an R528H mutation. HypoKPP attacks were

Table 17.1 Features of HypoKPP and HyperKPP (based on [3, 13])

	HypoKPP1	HypoKPP2	HyperKPP
Gene	*CACNA1S*	*SCN4A*	*SCN4A*
Age of onset	First/second decade	Later onset	First decade
Potassium features	K levels decreased during attack	K levels decreased during attack	K provokes attack K levels may or may not be increased at the beginning of attack
Attack length	Hours to days	Hours	1–4 h
Attack triggers	Carbohydrate load, rest after exercise, salty foods, stress	Rest after exercise, sweets/high carbs, salt, cold, stress	K loading, rest after exercise, cold, hunger, stress, illness
Fixed proximal weakness	Present	Less likely to develop	Possible
Myotonia	–	Rare	55–90 %

most common during the teenage years, regardless of mutation. Exercise was found to be the most common trigger, regardless of specific mutation. Residual weakness after an attack occurred in 72 % of patients with mutations in these genes and only 20 % in those without [3].

The same study looked at characteristics of people with HyperKPP. Of the 99 people with HyperKPP, 82 had mutations in *SCN4A*. Two mutations in *SNC4A* account for the majority of mutations—T704M (61 %) and M1592V (16 %). The average age of onset was younger for those with mutations (2 years of age) than those without mutations (14 years of age). All patients with a T704M mutation presented with symptoms before 1 year of age. The average number of attacks per month was 16 in mutation carriers and 6 in non-carriers. Those with T704M mutation averaged 1 attack per day lasting for 8 h; those with the M1592V mutation had 3 attacks per month lasting for 89 h. However, for all patients with mutations in *SCN4A*, attacks averaged 16 per month with 24 h per attack. The triggers for HyperKPP were also analyzed. The most common trigger was rest after exercise, causing attacks in 80 % of *SCN4A* mutation carriers and 69 % of those without mutations. The second most common trigger was cold temperature, causing an attack in 54 % with a mutation and 38 % without. Clinical myotonia (with corresponding electrical myotonia) was present in 74 % of those with mutations and 55 % of those without. Fixed proximal weakness was found in 60 % with mutations and 89 % without [3].

17.5 Genetic Counseling Issues

The periodic paralyses have a unique set of issues affecting patients. Because they are autosomal dominant conditions, usually a parent has been affected with the condition and is able to note symptoms in the children. However, if there is a new mutation in the family, getting a diagnosis of periodic paralysis can be both medically and psychologically challenging. Often the first issue that arises is the fear that accompanies waking up paralyzed, as the person believes that he/she is dying. Then, because of the intermittent symptoms, as well as the normal exams and laboratory studies between attacks, the medical community may question patients' reports, and patients may be suspected of faking symptoms or of having psychosomatic symptoms. These issues can cause some patients to refrain from seeking medical attention or to be distrustful of the medical profession. Fear of disbelief may also cause them to avoid sharing symptoms with friends or relatives. Providers should be careful about the terms they use with these patients.

A lack of family history may be due to *de novo* mutations, incomplete penetrance, misattributed-paternity, or undisclosed adoption. When family history is not present, the genetic counselor must address the utility of testing the parents in order to predict the risk for other family members. Although the neurologist should handle medical management, the genetic counselor may wish to reinforce lifestyle management and anesthesia dangers.

17.6 Case History (Fig. 17.1)

A 17-year-old male presented to neurogenetics clinic after a very disconcerting episode at home in which he awoke unable to move. Although able to breathe, he could not move any of his extremities. He was terrified and thought that he was dying. His mother found him and called 911. By the time he was transported to the hospital and seen by a doctor, he had started to recover from his paralysis. The ED (emergency department) doctor pulled his mother aside and told her that the patient was faking or was having a psychosomatic episode of weakness, and suggested that she take him to a psychiatrist. The mother called her ex-husband from the ED. He reported having had similar episodes when younger and had seen a neurologist about the condition. At his suggestion, the family made an appointment with the neurogenetics clinic.

The genetic counselor (GC) welcomed the patient (P) and his mother (M). The three of them discussed the reasons for presenting to neurogenetics. P was very withdrawn, but M said that they had come at the suggestion of her ex-husband because of his history of similar symptoms. The GC began by addressing P and asking him about his attack. P mumbled a bit and seemed hesitant, but eventually told the GC about waking up paralyzed. The GC acknowledged that the attack must have been very scary, and asked about his experience in the Emergency

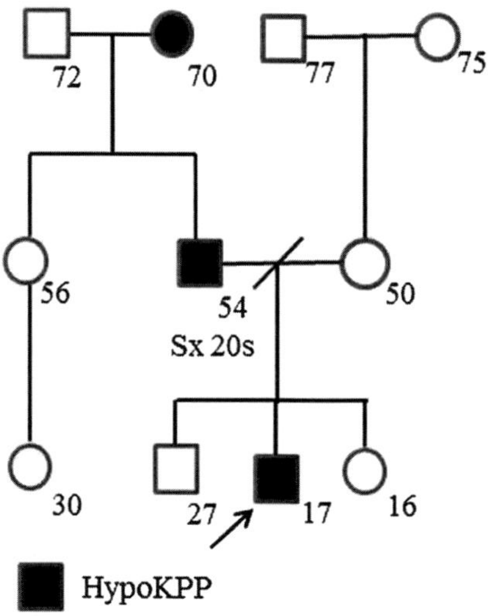

Fig. 17.1 HypoKPP case history pedigree

Department. P turned red, seemed angry, and shook his head. The GC asked P if he was upset about his time in the ED. P nodded.

The GC asked P if he knew the name of his condition. P shook his head no. The GC told him that it was called periodic paralysis, which causes sudden episodes of weakness, often when people are sleeping, and then goes away. Between attacks, lab tests and clinical exams are normal. It is common for people with periodic paralysis to be told that they are faking their reported symptoms. During this discussion, P's demeanor changed. His eyes got wider, and he leaned forward in his chair. When asked whether this sounded similar to his situation, he responded yes—that he had woken up paralyzed and terrified, only to go to see the doctors (who are supposed to help!) and be told that he was making it up. This was frustrating and embarrassing. His mother didn't know what to do.

GC turned to the mother, asking whether this experience was frustrating and embarrassing for her as well. M nodded her head. She was flabbergasted—how could nothing be wrong when just an hour before, her son was unable to move? She had called his father from the ED, and that was when she was told that he had had similar symptoms when he was a child. GC asked if this made her feel better. M said no, but at least it was a lead in the right direction. GC asked P if knowing his father had the same trouble helped with adjusting to the diagnosis. P seemed to consider this point and eventually said yes, but he wished he had known about it before the episode. M, though, was clearly angry.

GC took a detailed family history, and found that the paternal grandmother had been in a wheelchair since 60 years of age. She asked M if the grandmother had experienced any paralytic episodes when she was younger. M did not know of any such episodes. GC talked to M and P about incomplete penetrance in females who have periodic paralysis, explaining that a person can have the gene mutation without paralytic attacks. It is possible, then, that P's paternal aunt also carried the gene mutation with no symptoms. Her daughter could also be a carrier. As some mutations have lower penetrance than others, genetic testing on P could clarify the risks to his aunt and cousin. As GC discussed this reason for genetic testing, P appeared to be getting angry. GC asked P what he was thinking about. He wondered why he would find out information to help his dad's side of the family when they had never done anything to help him. GC explored P's feelings of abandonment, and also discussed the benefits and risks of testing.

Discussion Questions

- The genetic counselor spent a lot of time discussing non-genetic issues. Why did she do this and was it a good use of time?
- How does this case demonstrate the importance of "being present" for patients?

GC, M, and P discussed the diagnosis of periodic paralysis. Based on the disease prevalence and P's age of onset, HypoKPP type 1 was the likely diagnosis. GC discussed other features of HypoKPP that can occur over time, including muscle weakness, as might have been the case for P's paternal grandmother. Management issues, such as lifestyle changes, were discussed. Additionally, GC explained the genetics of the disease and that genetic testing was possible. M asked about her other children and grandchild. GC addressed the possibility that they could be tested if a mutation was found in P. At the end of the session, the family elected to pursue genetic testing for HypoKPP. He was found to carry a mutation in *CACNA1S*.

Discussion Questions:

- Should P's brother or sister be worried about HypoKPP, given that they have not had any symptoms?
- What other issues could be discussed in a counseling session with a family such as this one when a parent has an unrevealed disease and the parents are divorced?
- How does the genetic counselor's knowledge of the condition assist with anticipatory guidance?

17.7 Patient Resources

The Periodic Paralysis Association: http://www.periodicparalysis.org/
The Muscular Dystrophy Association: www.mda.org

References

1. Fontaine, B., Vale-Santos, J., Jurkat-Rott, K., Reboul, J., Plassart, E., Rime, C. S., et al. (1994). Mapping of the hypokalaemic periodic paralysis (HypoPP) locus to chromosome 1q31-32 in three European families. *Nature Genetics, 6*(3), 267–272.
2. Fontaine, B. (2008). Periodic paralysis. *Advances in Genetics, 63*, 3–23.
3. Miller, T. M., Dias da Silva, M. R., Miller, H. A., Kwiecinski, H., Mendell, J. R., Tawil, R., et al. (2004). Correlating phenotype and genotype in the periodic paralyses. *Neurology, 63*(9), 1647–1655.
4. Venance, S. L., Cannon, S. C., Fialho, D., Fontaine, B., Hanna, M. G., Ptacek, L. J., et al. (2006). The primary periodic paralysis: Diagnosis, pathogenesis and treatment. *Brain, 129*(Part 1), 8–17.
5. Links, T. P., Zwarts, M. J., & Oosterhuis, H. J. G. H. (1988). Improvement of muscle strength in familial hypokalaemic periodic paralysis with acetazolamide. *Journal of Neurology, Neurosurgery, and Psychiatry, 51*(9), 1142–1145.
6. Fournier, E., Arzel, M., Sternberg, D., Vicart, S., Laforet, P., Eymard, B., et al. (2004). Electromyography guides toward subgroups of mutation in muscle channelopathies. *Annals of Neurology, 56*(5), 650–661.
7. Griggs, R. C., Engel, W. K., & Resnick, J. S. (1970). Acetazolamide treatment of hypokalemic periodic paralysis. *Annals of Internal Medicine, 73*(1), 39–48.
8. Ptacek, L. J., Tawil, R., Griggs, R. C., Meola, G., McManis, P., Barohn, R. J., et al. (1994). Sodium channel mutations in acetazolamide-responsive myotonia congenital, paramyotonia congenital, and hyperkalemic periodic paralysis. *Neurology, 44*(8), 1500–1503.
9. Tawil, R., McDermott, M. P., Brown, R., Shapiro, B. C., Ptacek, L. J., McManis, P. G., et al. (2000). Randomized trials of dichlorphenamide in the periodic paralyses. *Annals of Neurology, 47*(1), 46–53.
10. Elbaz, A., Vale-Santos, J., Jurkat-Rott, K., Lapie, P., Ophoff, R. A., Bady, B., et al. (1995). Hypokalemic periodic paralysis and the dihydropyridine receptor (CACNL1A3): Genotype/phenotype correlations for two predominant mutations and evidence for the absence of a founder effect in 16 Caucasian families. *American Journal of Human Genetics, 56*(2), 374–380.
11. Kawamura, S., Ikeda, Y., Tomita, K., Watanabe, N., & Seki, K. (2004). A family of hypokalemic periodic paralysis with CACNA1S gene mutation showing incomplete penetrance in women. *Internal Medicine, 43*(3), 218–222.
12. Sternberg, D., Maisonobe, T., Jurkat-Rott, K., Nicole, S., Launay, E., Chauveau, D., et al. (2001). Hypokalaemic periodic paralysis type 2 caused by mutations at codon 672 in the muscle sodium channel gene SCN4A. *Brain, 124*(Part 6), 1091–1099.
13. Raja Rayan, D. L., & Hanna, M. G. (2010). Skeletal muscle channelopathies: Nondystrophic myotonias and periodic paralysis. *Current Opinion in Neurology, 23*(5), 466–476.

Part VI
The Adult Muscular Dystrophies

Chapter 18
Overview of Adult Muscular Dystrophies

Joline Dalton and Jacinda B. Sampson

Muscular dystrophy (MD) is defined as a deterioration of normal muscle structure, with a resultant increase in connective and adipose tissue around muscle fibers. It is genetically determined and genetically diverse. Although MD is characterized by its principal effect on skeletal muscles, some forms of MD also affect the heart, smooth muscle, brain, eye, gastrointestinal tract, and reproductive and endocrine systems. Consequently, disease-related symptoms during the course of the illness can be surprisingly diverse, ranging from muscle weakness, stiffness, and pain to syncope, swallowing difficulties, mental deficits, vision problems, and infertility.

The prognosis for patients varies markedly according to the type of MD. The onset of MD may vary significantly between subtypes, ranging from the neonatal period to late adulthood. Many classic childhood-onset forms of MD can present in adulthood with a different clinical course. Regardless of age of onset, MD may also vary significantly in its progression.

This chapter focuses on genetic counseling for adults affected with several forms of muscular dystrophy. The heterogeneity between and within different subtypes presents genetic counselors with challenges in genetic diagnosis and explanation of the clinical course of the conditions.

J. Dalton (✉)
Paul and Sheila Wellstone Muscular Dystrophy Center, University of Minnesota, 2101 6th St. SE MC, Minneapolis, MN 55455, USA
e-mail: jcdalton@umn.edu

J.B. Sampson
Department of Neurology, Columbia University Medical Center, 630 W. 168th St., Box 16, New York, NY 10032, USA
e-mail: js4171@cumc.columbia.edu

J.S. Goldman (ed.), *Genetic Counseling for Adult Neurogenetic Disease*,
DOI 10.1007/978-1-4899-7482-2_18

18.1 Genetic Counseling Issues for All Muscular Dystrophies

Over 500 genes are associated with neuromuscular disease. These genes play a role in different pathways involved with muscle development, structure, and function. Genetic phenomena, such as anticipation, germline mosaicism, and pleiotropy, are demonstrated by certain muscular dystrophies, and impact diagnosis and genetic counseling.

- *Purpose of genetic testing*: Genetic testing for muscular dystrophy can provide several benefits for the patient and their family. For many forms of muscular dystrophy, genetic testing is the first line of testing for confirmation of the diagnosis. Genetic confirmation can shorten the diagnostic odyssey and avoid invasive testing. Genetic confirmation can also allow for inclusion in clinical trials, which may be specific to the mutation type as well as the gene mutated. Some of the current treatment strategies are gene specific, so a definitive diagnosis can aid management of the conditions. In addition, genetic confirmation is often essential to provide accurate information about inheritance and allow carrier and presymptomatic testing of family members.
- *Presymptomatic and carrier genetic testing*: Once a causal mutation has been identified in an affected family member, presymptomatic or carrier testing is possible. However, because testing formerly was not as available and had lower sensitivity, identification of the affected family member might not have been possible. In these cases, medical records, including past electromyography (EMG), nerve conduction velocities (NCVs), and muscle biopsy reports, can be essential to establish the diagnosis in the affected individual and allow for testing of the family.
- *Pregnancy and neuromuscular disease*: Family planning for people with muscular dystrophy family histories raises significant genetic counseling issues. Not only do couples need to consider the risk of mutant gene transmission, but also women affected with a neuromuscular condition may be at a higher risk for pregnancy complications. Complications can sometimes include decreased fertility, miscarriage, preterm labor and the need for intervention during delivery (including cesarean delivery), and increased anesthesia risks. Additionally, pregnancy can worsen symptoms, which may or may not return to baseline after delivery. Though many women affected with neuromuscular disease have uneventful pregnancies, pregnancy management and risks warrant discussion during genetic counseling.
- *Genetic testing for muscular dystrophy*: The muscular dystrophies are a heterogeneous group of conditions. The number of genes associated with any subtype of muscular dystrophy ranges from 2 to 30 [1]. The heterogeneity has led to the clinical availability of testing panels, which allow for testing several genes simultaneously. Determination of the best approach for testing is based on several factors including clinical presentation, management questions, patient's

insurance, and the patient's motivation for testing. The increasing clinical utility of whole-exome or -genome sequencing may change testing strategies and diagnostic approaches.

- *Pleiotropic presentation of muscular dystrophy*: Some genes associated with muscular dystrophy have several different phenotypes associated with them. Currently almost 700 described neuromuscular conditions are associated with mutations in over 300 genes [1]. Thus, some genes causing neuromuscular disease cause a myriad of clinical presentations. The laminopathies provide one such example. Laminopathies, a group of inherited conditions caused by mutations in the *LMNA* gene, exhibit a wide variety of clinical symptoms and syndromes, including Emery-Dreifuss muscular dystrophy, limb-girdle muscular dystrophy type 1B, dilated cardiomyopathy with conduction system disease (DCM-CSD), familial partial lipodystrophy, Charcot-Marie-Tooth type 2, and progeria [2]. Given the rarity of the conditions and the complexity of clinical presentations, patients often struggle with the "name" of their condition and the best way to describe it to others. Likewise, patient literature on these conditions may be limited. Genetic counselors play an important role in translating the diagnosis to the patient, helping the patient describe it to others, and guiding patients toward appropriate information on the Internet.
- *Transition services for muscular dystrophy*: Improvements in clinical care have increased the life-span from the teens to the third and fourth decades for several childhood-onset muscular dystrophies. Genetic counselors can play an important role not only in helping young adults understand the genetics of their condition, but also helping to provide support and access services.
- *Genetically unconfirmed diagnosis of muscular dystrophy*: Despite the growing number of identified genes causing muscular dystrophies, 30–50 % of affected individuals do not have genetic confirmation of their diagnosis, even after comprehensive genetic testing. The lack of diagnosis makes patients uneasy about their prognosis. The progressive nature of muscular dystrophies implies that patients will lose skills and independence. However, if patients do not know their diagnosis and prognosis, decisions about education, housing, career planning, and family planning are difficult.
- *Implications for the patient and their family*: A genetic diagnosis of muscular dystrophy has a potential impact on the patient and their family members. These diseases can affect the ability to work, type of housing, participation in hobbies and activities, and reproductive options. Families struggle with the intricacies of going on disability collecting social security, and health insurance. In addition, these conditions can often change the roles of family members, forcing a spouse, sibling, or child to become a caregiver and/or breadwinner. Some patients will need personal care attendants (PCAs) or nursing to assist with activities of daily living, including dressing, personal cares, and household needs. While home modification and arranging PCA service are certainly outside the scope of genetic counseling, this information is important when talking about prognosis and what it means to have a form of muscular dystrophy.

18.2 Family History Questions Pertinent to Muscular Dystrophy

The clinical descriptions and names of muscular dystrophies often focus on muscle involvement and loss of muscle function; however, many are multi-system conditions. In addition, many muscular dystrophies are variable within families, presenting with different ages of onset, progression, and clinical manifestations. A detailed family history can be instrumental in establishing the diagnosis. The following questions can help determine the presence or absence of muscle diseases in the family:

- Is there any family history of diabetes? If so, was it type 1 or 2?
- Is there any family history of cataracts? If so, at what age did they present?
- Does anyone use assistance walking devices like a wheelchair, cane, or brace? If so, at what age did they start using them?
- Did anyone have polio or post-polio symptoms?
- Is there a family history of heart issues, cardiomyopathy, ICD placement, pacemaker, transplant, etc.? If so, at what age?
- Is there any family history of muscle disease or consistent muscle aches?
- Is there any family history of intellectual disabilities or behavioral issues (i.e., autism, ADHD)?

18.3 Treatment of Myopathies, Muscular Dystrophy, and Myotonic Disorders

No cures exist for genetic myopathy, muscular dystrophy, or myotonic disorders, and treatment remains supportive. However, a growing number of novel therapeutic approaches are being developed. Notifying patients, families, and other health professionals about new treatment trials can provide hope and optimism. Practice guidelines and/or care standards are available for some forms of neuromuscular disease and should be used as guides for care and management. Some medications are available to help treat symptoms associated with these conditions. Prednisone has been shown to prolong ambulation in Duchenne muscular dystrophy (DMD) [3]. Physical and occupational therapy can help patients find adaptive means to perform activities of daily living and conserve energy, and maintain independence. Orthotics can help maintain ambulation and prevent falls. Power mobility is often necessary to maintain independence; however, it can require significant home modification and the need for new transportation [4]. Preventing fractures and maintaining bone health can help preserve function and independence [5]. Cardiac and respiratory screening should be performed on all affected individuals or presumed affected individuals regardless of the subtype of neuromuscular disease [6, 7]. Often cardiac and respiratory deficiencies can be present long before an individual reports symptoms. Keeping up to date on vaccination for influenza, pneumococcus, and pertussis may be beneficial in preventing morbidity [7]. Detecting respiratory decline can prompt important discussions of advance directives and choices regarding tracheostomy/mechanical ventilation. Noninvasive ventilation (NIV) if respiratory decline is detected can provide symptomatic relief, as well as prolong survival.

Anesthesia can pose a risk for malignant hyperthermia in certain types of neuromuscular disease [8, 9]. Likewise patients with or at risk for respiratory deficiencies may need additional monitoring of cardiac and respiratory function during and after a procedure [8, 9]. Some forms of neuromuscular disease, including the dystrophinopathies and myotonic dystrophy, have significant CNS involvement including cognitive impairment and behavior issues; thus, neuropsychological assessment can help identify potential issues to assist educators and family members in helping the patient reach their potential [10]. Education of community medical providers about management and diagnosis of neuromuscular disease is an important role for neuromuscular care centers. This field has exploded with new care standards, genetic tests, and clinical trials. The improvement in care has changed many of these conditions from childhood killers to chronic diseases. Genetic counselors in these clinics can help educate the community about these advances.

References

1. Kaplan, J. C. (2009). Gene table of monogenic neuromuscular disorders (nuclear genome only) 19(1), January 2009. *Neuromuscular Disorders, 19*(1), 77–98.
2. Carboni, N., Politano, L., Floris, M., Mateddu, A., Solla, E., Olla, S., et al. (2013). Overlapping syndromes in laminopathies: A meta-analysis of the reported literature. *Acta Myologica, 32*(1), 7–17.
3. Moxley, R. T., Pandya, S., Ciafaloni, E., Fox, D. J., & Campbell, K. (2010). Change in natural history of Duchenne muscular dystrophy with long-term corticosteroid treatment: Implications for management. *Journal of Child Neurology, 25*(9), 1116–1129.
4. Abresch, R. T., Carter, G. T., Han, J. J., & McDonald, C. M. (2012). Exercise in neuromuscular diseases. *Physical Medicine and Rehabilitation Clinics of North America, 23*(3), 653–673.
5. Joyce, N. C., Hache, L. P., & Clemens, P. R. (2012). Bone health and associated metabolic complications in neuromuscular diseases. *Physical Medicine and Rehabilitation Clinics of North America, 23*(4), 773–799.
6. Benditt, J. O., & Boitano, L. J. (2013). Pulmonary issues in patients with chronic neuromuscular disease. *American Journal of Respiratory and Critical Care Medicine, 187*(10), 1046–1055.
7. Kostareva, A., Sejersen, T., & Sjoberg, G. (2013). Genetic spectrum of cardiomyopathies with neuromuscular phenotype. *Frontiers in Bioscience (Scholar Edition), 5*, 325–340.
8. Romero, A., & Joshi, G. P. (2013). Neuromuscular disease and anesthesia. *Muscle and Nerve, 48*(3), 451–460.
9. Loughnan, T., & Loughnan, A. J. (2013). Overview of the introduction of neuromuscular monitoring to clinical anaesthesia. *Anaesthesia and Intensive Care, 41*(Suppl 1), 19–24.
10. Perumal, A. R., Rajeswaran, J., & Nalini, A. (2013). Neuropsychological Profile of Duchenne Muscular Dystrophy. *Appl Neuropsychol Child*, 1–9, 2014.

19.1.1 Clinical Presentation of Myofibrillar Myopathy

Myofibrillar myopathy is characterized by slowly progressive weakness. Distal muscle weakness is present in about 80 % of individuals and is more pronounced than proximal weakness in about a quarter of cases [2]. A minority of individuals also experience sensory symptoms and muscle stiffness, aching, or cramps. Peripheral neuropathy is present in about 20 % of affected individuals, and overt cardiomyopathy occurs in 15–30 % of cases. Currently myofibrillar myopathy includes eight genetically distinct subtypes, which are relatively homogenous [2].

19.1.2 Diagnosis of Myofibrillar Myopathy

The gold standard for diagnosis of myofibrillar myopathies is muscle biopsy. Muscle biopsy histology shows variable fiber sizes with grouping of small fibers and trichrome staining demonstrates amorphous, granular, or hyaline deposits. In addition, rimmed vacuoles and congophila can be seen. Although muscle biopsy remains the gold standard, the characteristic findings are dependent on obtaining the biopsy from the correct muscle and on the pathological interpretation [3].

19.1.3 Genetics of Myofibrillar Myopathy

The myofibrillar myopathies are primarily inherited in an autosomal dominant pattern. However, isolated autosomal recessive cases and an X-linked dominant form have been described. Sporadic cases resulting from *de novo* mutations have been reported, and the absence of a family history does not exclude the diagnosis (Table 19.1).

19.1.4 Genetics Testing for Myofibrillar Myopathy

Genetic testing is available for myofibrillar myopathy; however, clinically available genetic testing only provides genetic confirmation in 50 % of cases [4]. Research exome testing has led to the identification of novel forms of myofibrillar myopathy [5]. While genetic confirmation is often the most desirable endpoint for diagnosis, most mutations are private, and interpretation of variants of unknown significance is complicated by limited family history and/or limited or lack of a muscle biopsy sample. Alternatively, muscle magnetic resonance imaging (MRI) and ultrasound can help in determining the pattern of involved muscles and

Table 19.1 MFM subtypes (adapted from [1])

MFM subtype	Gene/ protein	Age of onset	Clinical features	Inheritance
Alpha-B crystallinopathy	*CYRAB*	11–62	Distal and proximal weakness; respiratory involvement; cataracts; hypertrophic cardiomyopathy	AD, AR (rare)
BAG3-related myofibrillar myopathy	*BAG3*	Childhood	Rigid spine; cardiomyopathy; respiratory insufficiency; elevated CK	AD
Desminopathy	*DES*	11–62	Distal, proximal, scapuloperoneal and facial muscle weakness; respiratory insufficiency; dilated cardiomyopathy; arrhythmia	AD, AR
DNAJB6-related myofibrillar myopathy	*DNAJB6*	Adulthood	Distal weakness	AD
FHL1-related myofibrillar myopathy	*FHL1*	Childhood	Manifesting carriers; rapidly progressing; scapuloperoneal involvement	X-linked
Filaminopathy	*FLNAC*	38–57	Distal weakness; elevated CK; respiratory insufficiency; peripheral neuropathy	AD
Myotilinopathy	*TTID*	Adulthood	Distal weakness; cardiomyopathy; peripheral neuropathy	AD
Zaspopathy	*LDB3*	Adulthood	Distal weakness; cardiac disease; peripheral neuropathy	AD

aid in diagnosis or selection of muscle to biopsy [6–8]. Genetic counseling is essential for patients to understand the benefits and limitations of testing and the implications of a positive, negative, or indeterminate genetic test result.

19.2 Distal Myopathies

The distal myopathies refer to a heterogeneous group of disorders that predominantly affect the distal muscles. This rare group of disorders can be misdiagnosed as a neuropathy because of the pattern of weakness.

19.2.1 Clinical Presentation of the Distal Myopathies

The distal myopathies present with atrophy and/or weakness of the muscle in the hands, feet, forearm, and lower leg. Distal myopathies can have creatine kinase (CK) elevations ranging from slightly increased to greater than ten times normal. Over 20 subtypes have been described that vary in age of onset, primary muscle affected, and multi-systemic features. Most forms of distal myopathies only cause muscle weakness and present in adulthood, even after the fifth or sixth decade of life. However, myotonic dystrophy (discussed in Chap. 20) can occur at any age.

19.2.2 Diagnosis of Distal Myopathy

Diagnosis of the distal myopathies is typically established by creatine kinase (CK) level, electromyogram (EMG), nerve conduction velocities (NCV), and muscle biopsies. The pattern of muscle weakness involved in distal myopathy is clinically similar to that of Charcot-Marie-Tooth (CMT), a form of hereditary peripheral neuropathy; however, distal myopathy is not associated with sensory changes. An EMG is essential to exclude neuropathy. Muscle biopsy changes can range from mildly myopathic to dystrophic, and may or may not contain rimmed vacuoles. Some features in muscle biopsy may be more common in certain subtypes of distal myopathy and may aid in diagnosis [10]. The patchy muscle involvement of the distal myopathies makes muscle MRI and ultrasound extremely beneficial to diagnosis and clarification of variants of unknown significance obtained through genetic testing [6].

19.2.3 Genetics of Distal Myopathy

The genes associated with the distal myopathies encode proteins that play a role in muscle structure, development, and regulation of contraction. Some proteins have isoforms that play a role in all three. The location and type of mutations within the gene may account for the multiple disease phenotypes [9]. Most distal myopathies are autosomal dominant, but can appear to be sporadic because of *de novo* mutations. The early onset forms may typically have an autosomal recessive inheritance pattern (Table 19.2).

Table 19.2 Hereditary distal myopathies (adapted from [10])

Condition	Gene/protein	Decade affected
Autosomal dominant forms		
Welander distal myopathy	*TIA1*/T-cell intracellular antigen-1	5th–6th
Tibial muscular dystrophy (TMD, Udd myopathy)	*TTN/Titin*	4th–5th
Distal myotilinopathy	*TTID/Myotilin*	6th–7th
Zaspopathy (Markesbery–Griggs)	*LDB*/Z-disk alternatively spliced PDZ-domain-containing protein (ZASP)	5th–6th
Matrin3 distal myopathy (VCPDM, MPD2)	*MATR3*/Matrin3	4th–5th
VCP-mutated distal myopathy	*VCP/Valosin-containing protein*	4th–5th
Alpha-B crystallin-mutated distal myopathy	*CRYAB*/αB-crystallin	2nd–3rd
Desminopathy	*DES*/Desmin	2nd–3rd
Distal ABD-filaminopathy	*FLNC/Filamin-C*	2nd–3rd
Laing distal myopathy (MPD1)	*MYH7*/Beta-MyHHC	1st
KLHL9-mutated distal myopathy	*KLHL9*/Kelch-like homologue protein 9	1st
Myotonic dystrophy type 1	*DMPK trinucleotide expansion*	Any age
Autosomal recessive forms		
Distal nebulin myopathy	*NEB/Nebulin*	1st
Miyoshi myopathy (MM)	*DYSF/Dysferlin*	2nd–3rd
Distal anoctaminopathy	*ANO5/Anoctamin-5*	3rd–4th
Distal myopathy with rimmed vacuoles (DMRV)	*GNE*/bifunctional UDP-*N*-acetylglucosamine 2-epimerase/*N*-acetylmannosamine kinase	2nd–3rd

19.2.4 Genetic Testing for the Distal Myopathies

The distal myopathies can be clinically indistinguishable, and additionally some mutations in the same gene can present with different muscle involvement. Thus, testing with genetic panels is often the most cost-effective option [11]. Due to the rarity of the distal myopathies, sensitivity of genetic testing is unknown. At least six clinically described phenotypes still lack identified genetic causes. Families without a genetically confirmed diagnosis may be ideal candidates for whole exome sequencing or research testing. Variants of unknown significance are found frequently. Myotonic dystrophy, a polynucleotide repeat disorder, is one of the most common distal myopathies, and should be considered on the differential, since patients may not complain of myotonia—it will be discussed separately. Several of the known genes have been well described, and review of genetic literature, as well as consultation with experts, may help in clarifying the pathogenicity of the variants of uncertain significance. Given the late onset of several of these conditions, most individuals have already made many of their life choices by the time they are diagnosed.

19.2.5 *Genetic Counseling for Distal Myopathy Case History (Fig. 19.1)*

Mr. T was a 65-year-old male with a 20-year history of a progressive distal myopathy. He now required braces for ambulation. He contacted the genetic counselor to make an appointment to discuss genetic testing for the distal myopathies. During this phone conversation, it became apparent that Mr. T had no ongoing neurological care for his myopathy and, in fact, had not seen a neurologist since he was diagnosed. The genetic counselor said that in order to better diagnose his condition, he could be seen in the Muscular Dystrophy Association clinic with which the genetic counselor was associated. Mr. T agreed, and an appointment was made in the multidisciplinary clinic.

Mr. and Mrs. T came to the appointment and Mr. T was evaluated by the neurologist and physical therapist, and was registered with the Muscular Dystrophy Association (MDA). The neurological exam revealed distal muscle weakness and a modestly elevated creatine kinase of 800 U/L. An electromyogram (EMG) was performed and demonstrated a myopathic process. The neurologist provided the clinical diagnosis of a distal myopathy. Mr. T was referred back to the genetic counselor to discuss genetic confirmation. Mr. T revealed that for the past two

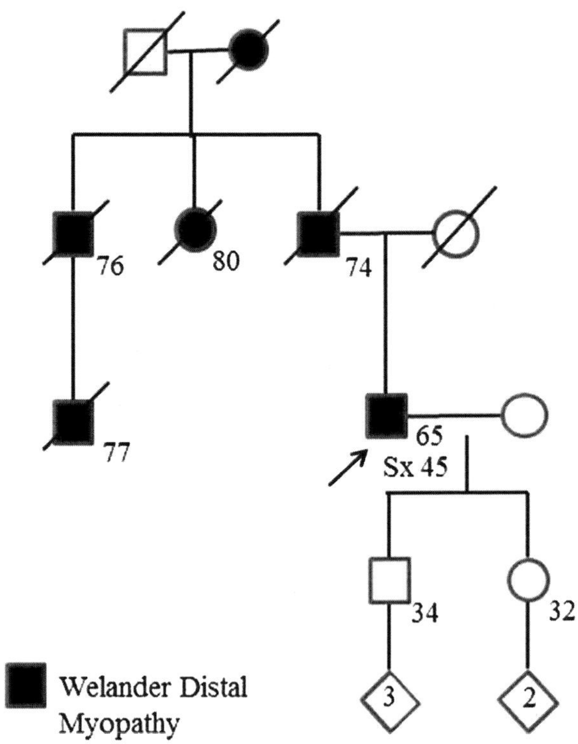

Fig. 19.1 Welander distal myopathy case history pedigree

decades he had chosen not to tell his adult children of his diagnosis. However, the recent death of a family member due to complications of familial distal myopathy prompted the disclosure of his diagnosis to his children. Mr. T's two adult children were in their 30s and had completed their families. The revelation resulted in such tension in the immediate family that his children refused to speak to him. Mr. T decided to pursue genetic testing in hopes of family peace. His children wished to have presymptomatic testing in order to know their risk and the risk to their children. Mr. T was aware that the first step for their presymptomatic testing was providing genetic confirmation of his diagnosis.

The genetic counselor then obtained a five generation pedigree, which revealed that Mr. T's father, paternal grandmother, paternal aunt, paternal uncle, and paternal first cousin were clinically diagnosed with Welander distal myopathy. The family was of German decent. After reviewing the family history, the genetic counselor described autosomal dominant inheritance and the risk to his children and grandchildren. The genetic counselor reviewed the genetic tests available for distal myopathy, and told them that the gene for Welander distal myopathy, *TIA1*, was not yet available as a single gene test. Given the clinical overlap between the distal myopathies, testing for known forms, including sequencing *CAV3*, *TTN*, and *VCP*, was a reasonable option. If these were negative, they would pursue testing for the myofibrillar myopathies, given the respiratory involvement note in Mr. T's father's medical record. The genetic counselor also discussed the potential benefits of genetic confirmation, explaining that it might provide more prognostic information about his condition and could potentially help direct care and management. Likewise knowing the diagnosis could help establish services for needed care. Mr. T and his wife were very motivated to establish a genetic diagnosis to allow for presymptomatic testing and begin mending the broken family relationships. The genetic counselor had a frank discussion about the limitations of genetic testing, and that it was likely that these tests might not provide genetic confirmation. Additionally, the genetic counselor discussed how they would move forward with the family if the results were negative. Mr. and Mrs. T remained very hopeful and said that they would "cross that bridge when they came to it." Observing that Mrs. T took copious notes throughout the session, the genetic counselor asked if it would be helpful to have a detailed clinic note about the session. They were enthusiastic about providing evidence for their children that they were obtaining additional information. The genetic counselor also provided them with contact cards so that the family could call the genetic counselor directly.

Discussion Questions

- Are decisions to obtain genetic confirmation ever without external influence? To what extent does the genetic counselor need to assure that the patient is acting autonomously?
- What is the value of providing patients with copies of their medical records including genetic counseling clinic notes?

- What role should genetic counselors play in care coordination? Is there a conflict of interest in referring the patients to the genetic counselor's clinic?
- How could the diagnosing clinic have helped Mr. T to be more honest with his children?

Despite extensive testing, Mr. T's diagnosis remained genetically unconfirmed. Mr. T established clinical care in the MDA clinic and started attending clinic regularly. The genetic counselor became part of his ongoing care team and helped coordinate newly available genetic tests for distal myopathy. Mrs. T and the counselor had a long conversation about his decision not to tell his children. She had hoped for years that Mr. T would say something every time a grandchild asked about his braces. She had felt very conflicted about her relationship with her husband, children, and grandchildren. She was very loyal to her husband, as he now needed more and more of her help with activities of daily living. At the end of the conversation she stated that it was good to talk to someone who could understand.

Mr. and Mrs. T became involved in the MDA, and participated in annual education and social events. Mr. T provided his family with notes from clinic visits. Eventually his sons came to an understanding, and the family dynamic continued to improve. Mr. T's condition progressed considerably. He could not ambulate long distances and required a scooter. Mr. and Mrs. T purchased an accessible home. The genetic counselor stayed involved in the case, and called to tell the couple that testing was now available for a newly identified Welandar distal myopathy gene, *TIA1* [12]. Once again, the genetic results were negative.

Discussion Questions

- How does a genetic counselor establish an ongoing relationship with patients and families?
- What role should patient advocacy groups play in clinic? What benefit do you think they had on this family and others?
- How does a genetic counselor display understanding and empathy? How do you gain skills of empathy for conditions for which you have no personal experience?
- For how long is a genetic counselor responsible for updating patients on new genetic testing?

19.3 Metabolic Myopathies

The metabolic myopathies refer to inherited forms of exercise intolerance and rhabdomyolysis that lead to progressive muscle weakness, chronic pain, and fatigue.

19.3.1 Clinical Presentation of the Metabolic Myopathies

The metabolic myopathies are a rare group of inherited conditions caused by inefficient or ineffective energy production within the muscle [13]. The three primary metabolic myopathies are mitochondrial myopathies, lipid metabolism myopathies, and glycogen metabolism myopathies [14].

The mitochondrial myopathies may present with multi-systemic features [15]. The age of onset can range from childhood to adulthood. The associated muscle fatigue is generalized and not necessarily correlated with strenuous or aerobic exercise. Proximal and ocular muscles, resulting in ptosis, are sometimes involved. Mitochondrial disorders are often suspected if two or more organ systems are involved and/or there is a persistently elevated lactic acid level.

Disorders of glycogen storage associated with myopathy typically result in exercise-induced muscle pain and fatigue and progressive muscle weakness [16]. Elevated CK can occur with exercise; when severe, extensive muscle breakdown, or rhabdomyolysis, can occur, manifesting as muscle pain, weakness, myoglobinuria (dark urine), hyperkalemia, and kidney failure. Onset varies from childhood to adulthood. The subtype of glycogen storage disease may determine the extent to which the first few minutes of aerobic exercise are tolerated [17].

In some cases, after about 7 or 8 min of exercise the muscle can start to use alternative sources of energy from fats and sugars supplied from the liver and so the symptoms ease. This phenomenon is called the "second wind" and is most common in glycogen storage disease type V or McArdle disease [18]. A subset of individuals affected with a glycogen storage disease can have progressive muscle weakness. For example, acid maltase deficiency can mimic limb-girdle muscular dystrophy in muscle pattern involvement and progression [19, 20].

Disorders of fatty acid oxidation or lipid metabolism that present with myopathy include CPT2 deficiency. The myopathic forms of these conditions are rare and can present any time from childhood to adulthood. Fatty acid oxidation disorders are variable both within and between subtypes, ranging from isolated trigger-induced attacks of muscle weakness to progressive muscle weakness and frequent muscle pain with moderate exercise. In fatty acid oxidation disorders, exercise is the most common trigger, but infections, fasting, cold, anesthesia, and sleep deprivation can also trigger attacks [21].

19.3.2 Diagnosis of Metabolic Myopathy

Since most events of rhabdomyolysis are situation based, a metabolic myopathy is not considered unless there are several reported episodes. Diagnosis of metabolic myopathies can be a long process. Due to nonspecific symptoms of muscle cramps, general pain, fatigue, and inability to exercise or stay active, affected individuals may appear to be lazy or malingering. The gold standard of diagnosis for metabolic myopathies is muscle biopsy. The sample can be evaluated by histological and biochemical analysis to look for reduction or absence of enzyme activity [22]. Some forms of mitochondrial myopathies have histological features such as ragged blue or red fibers that provide insight for diagnosis as well as a direction for genetic testing [15].

19.3.3 Genetics of Metabolic Myopathy

The metabolic myopathies are a heterogeneous group of conditions that can be inherited in most known inheritance patterns: matrilineal, autosomal dominant, or autosomal recessive. The disorders of glycogen storage and fatty acid oxidation are typically autosomal recessive; however, some are X-linked forms.

19.3.4 Genetic Testing for the Metabolic Myopathies

Genetic confirmation may be pursued after diagnosis is established by muscle biopsy. If a muscle sample is not available or if patients do not want invasive procedures, a skin biopsy can be utilized or genetic testing can be performed. Genetic testing for the mitochondrial disorders can be complicated by the heteroplasmy of mitochondrial mutations in different tissues. Additionally a number of nuclear genes are associated with these conditions, e.g., *POLG*-related mitochondrial disorders, which is one of the more common mitochondrial myopathies [23]. Although a variety of algorithms can be used to guide testing, a neuromuscular expert best establishes diagnosis. Establishing a diagnosis either by biopsy, genetic testing, or other means can be an important part of the coping process for patients with these conditions. If acid maltase deficiency is identified, enzyme replacement therapy can improve symptoms. For other metabolic myopathies, definitive diagnosis can give validation to their symptoms that may have been dismissed for much of their lives.

References

1. Selcen, D. (2011). Myofibrillar myopathies. *Neuromuscular Disorders, 21*(3), 161–171.
2. Selcen, D., Ohno, K., & Engel, A. G. (2004). Myofibrillar myopathy: Clinical, morphological and genetic studies in 63 patients. *Brain, 127*(Pt 2), 439–451.
3. Vattemi, G., Neri, M., Piffer, S., Vicart, P., Gualandi, F., Marini, M., et al. (2011). Clinical, morphological and genetic studies in a cohort of 21 patients with myofibrillar myopathy. *Acta Myologica, 30*(2), 121–126.

4. Selcen, D., & Engel, A. G. (2012). Myofibrillar myopathy. In: R. A. Pagon, M. P. Adam, T. D. Bird, C. R. Dolan, C. T. Fong, K. Stephens (Eds.) *GeneReviews*™ [Internet]. Seattle, WA: University of Washington, Seattle; 1993–2013. 2005 January 28 [updated 2012 October 29]
5. Griggs, R., Vihola, A., Hackman, P., Talvinen, K., Haravuori, H., Faulkner, G., et al. (2007). Zaspopathy in a large classic late-onset distal myopathy family. *Brain, 130*(Pt 6), 1477–1484.
6. Joshi, P. R., Glaser, D., Dreßel, C., Kress, W., Weis, J., & Deschauer, M. (2014). Anoctamin 5 muscular dystrophy associated with a silent p.Leu115Leu mutation resulting in exon skipping. *Neuromuscular Disorders, 24*(1), 43–47.
7. Peterle, E., Fanin, M., Semplicini, C., Padilla, J. J., Nigro, V., & Angelini, C. (2013). Clinical phenotype, muscle MRI and muscle pathology of LGMD1F. *Journal of Neurology, 260*(8), 2033–2041.
8. Sarkozy, A., Deschauer, M., Carlier, R. Y., Schrank, B., Seeger, J., Walter, M. C., et al. (2012). Muscle MRI findings in limb girdle muscular dystrophy type 2L. *Neuromuscular Disorders, 22*(Suppl 2), S122–S129.
9. Laing, N. G. (2012). Genetics of neuromuscular disorders. *Critical Reviews in Clinical Laboratory Sciences, 49*(2), 33–48.
10. Udd, B. (2012). Distal myopathies—new genetic entities expand diagnostic challenge. *Neuromuscular Disorders, 22*(1), 5–12.
11. Kraya, T., & Zierz, S. (2013). Distal myopathies: From clinical classification to molecular understanding. *Journal of Neural Transmission, 120*(Suppl 1), S3–S7.
12. Hackman, P., Sarparanta, J., Lehtinen, S., Vihola, A., Evila, A., Jonson, P. H., et al. (2013). Welander distal myopathy is caused by a mutation in the RNA-binding protein TIA1. *Annals of Neurology, 73*, 500–509.
13. D'Amico, A., & Bertini, E. (2013). Metabolic neuropathies and myopathies. *Handbook of Clinical Neurology, 113*, 1437–1455.
14. Das, A. M., Steuerwald, U., & Illsinger, S. (2010). Inborn errors of energy metabolism associated with myopathies. *Journal of Biomedicine and Biotechnology, 2010*, 340849.
15. Selcen, D., & Engel, A. G. (2011). Myofibrillar myopathies. *Handb Clin Neurol, 101*, 143–154.
16. Gargiulo, M., Herson, A., Michon, C. C., Hogrel, J. Y., Doppler, V., Laloui, K., et al. (2013). Attitudes and expectations of patients with neuromuscular diseases about their participation in a clinical trial. *Revue Neurologique (Paris), 169*(8–9), 670–676.
17. DiMauro, S., & Spiegel, R. (2011). Progress and problems in muscle glycogenoses. *Acta Myologica, 30*(2), 96–102.
18. Miteff, F., Potter, H. C., Allen, J., Teoh, H., Roxburgh, R., & Hutchinson, D. O. (2011). Clinical and laboratory features of patients with myophosphorylase deficiency (McArdle disease). *Journal of Clinical Neuroscience, 18*(8), 1055–1058.
19. Teener, J. W. (2012). Late-onset Pompe's disease. *Seminars in Neurology, 32*(5), 506–551.
20. Pascual, J. M., & Roe, C. R. (2013). Systemic metabolic abnormalities in adult-onset acid maltase deficiency: Beyond muscle glycogen accumulation. *JAMA Neurology, 70*(6), 756–763.
21. Bennett, M. J. (2010). Pathophysiology of fatty acid oxidation disorders. *Journal of Inherited Metabolic Disease, 33*(5), 533–537.
22. Kurt, B., Gulcan Kurt, Y., & Akgul, E. O. (2013). Importance of muscle biopsy in diagnosis of muscle diseases. *Biochemical and Biophysical Research Communications, 435*(4), 513.
23. Stumpf, J. D., Saneto, R. P., & Copeland, W. C. (2013). Clinical and molecular features of POLG-related mitochondrial disease. *Cold Spring Harbor Perspectives in Biology, 5*(4), a011395.

Chapter 20
The Muscular Dystrophies

Joline Dalton, Jill S. Goldman, and Jacinda B. Sampson

The muscular dystrophies are a heterogeneous group of conditions that cause progressive muscle weakness, characterized on muscle biopsy by degenerating/regenerating muscle fibers, fibrosis, and fatty replacement.

20.1 Dystrophinopathies

The dystrophinopathies include a spectrum of muscle diseases caused by mutations in the dystrophin gene, *DMD*, including Duchenne muscular dystrophy, Becker muscular dystrophy, and isolated dilated cardiomyopathy.

Electronic supplementary material Supplementary material is available in the online version of this chapter at 10.1007/978-1-4899-7482-2_20. Videos can also be accessed at http://www.springerimages.com/videos/978-1-4899-7481-5.

J. Dalton (✉)
Paul and Sheila Wellstone Muscular Dystrophy Center, University of Minnesota, 2101 6th St. SE MC, Minneapolis, MN 55455, USA
e-mail: jcdalton@umn.edu

J.S. Goldman
Taub Institute, Columbia University Medical Center, 630 W. 168th St., Box 16, New York, NY 10032, USA
e-mail: jg2673@cumc.columbia.edu

J.B. Sampson
Department of Neurology, Columbia University Medical Center, 630 W. 168th St., Box 16, New York, NY 10032, USA
e-mail: js4171@cumc.columbia.edu

J.S. Goldman (ed.), *Genetic Counseling for Adult Neurogenetic Disease*,
DOI 10.1007/978-1-4899-7482-2_20

20.1.1 Clinical Presentation of the Dystrophinopathies

Duchenne muscular dystrophy affects 1 in 3,500 males. Onset is typically at age 3 and results in progressive muscle weakness, cardiomyopathy, respiratory insufficiency, and loss of ambulation at or before age 12, though this can be delayed with corticosteroid treatment [1]. DMD can be associated with specific learning disabilities, autism spectrum disorder, and/or attention-deficit/hyperactivity disorder (ADD/ADHD) [2, 3]. In the last decade, the life expectancy of DMD has increased from the teens to the 30s or 40s [4, 5]. Families should be informed that living into adulthood is now the norm instead of the exception.

Becker muscular dystrophy (BMD) is a less severe form of dystrophinopathy. The age of onset can range from childhood to late adulthood; BMD is defined as loss of ambulation after age 13; however, due to the blurring of boundaries caused by DMD corticosteroid use, a classification of an intermediate form with loss of ambulation between age 13 and 16 is being used. Late-onset BMD may be mutation specific, with some mutations consistently showing a milder clinical presentation, with ambulation being retained much longer [6–10].

Female carriers of DMD can manifest any or all of the symptoms [11], though typically less severely than in males with DMD. For example, only a small percentage of female carriers are at risk to develop cardiomyopathy (10–30 %) or progressive weakness (7–10 %). However, being a manifesting DMD carrier is now recognized as an underdiagnosed form of muscular dystrophy, and can be seen without a family history of an affected male [12, 13].

20.1.2 Diagnosis of Dystrophinopathies

(DMD video clip Part 1)

Dystrophinopathy is generally suspected if a male or female has a highly elevated creatine kinase (CK) (often greater than 10,000 U/L), proximal muscle weakness, and hypertrophic calves. A reduction or absence of dystrophin on muscle biopsy demonstrated either by immunohistochemistry or western blot analysis remains the gold standard in the absence of genetic confirmation. Genetic testing is often the first line of diagnosis due to high sensitivity and specificity of current methodologies.

20.1.3 Genetics of Dystrophinopathies

The *DMD* gene is located on the X chromosome and is the largest known gene in the genome. The large size is thought to play a role in the high *de novo* mutation rate [14]. The dystrophinopathies are hallmark examples of genetic phenomena such as germ line mosaicism and skewed X-inactivation in manifesting carriers [15–17]. Since the dystrophin protein is involved in maintaining muscle cell membrane integrity, insufficient production or defective dystrophin can cause muscle cell breakdown. When cell breakdown is greater than cell replacement, progressive muscle weakness occurs. Over 5,000 identified dystrophin mutations have been identified, the majority of which (60–70 %) are deletions. The location and type of mutation (reading frame rule) can provide some insight for prognosis [18]. Additionally several genetic modifiers are thought to play a role in disease variability [19, 20].

20.1.4 Genetic Testing for the Dystrophinopathies

(DMD video clip Part 2)

Several methodologies are employed to identify genetic mutations within the dystrophin gene. Since therapeutic approaches may be mutation dependent, genetic confirmation is essential for inclusion in clinical trials [21]. Most laboratories employ a stepwise approach, first searching for the more common mutations—deletions and duplications, and then, if no mutations are identified, sequencing the gene. This process is typically more cost effective. Patient advocacy groups recognize the importance of genetic confirmation, and, when cost is prohibitive, have initiated programs to cover genetic testing. Carrier testing is generally recommended after the identification of a family mutation. However, if an affected individual is unavailable, genetic testing for dystrophin mutations can be performed and is becoming highly sensitive. Due to the high *de novo* mutation rate and germ line mosaicism, genetic counselors can help families understand carrier risk.

20.2 Limb-Girdle Muscular Dystrophy

Limb-girdle muscular dystrophy (LGMD) is characterized by progressive proximal muscle weakness, an elevated creatine kinase level, and muscle degeneration/regeneration pattern on muscle biopsy [22].

20.2.1 Clinical Presentation of the LGMD

LGMD refers to a group of inherited muscular dystrophies that are characterized by muscle weakness and wasting of shoulder and pelvic girdle muscles. Depending on the specific subtype, LGMD affects 1/123,000 to 1/14,500 people. LGMD is a progressive condition with onset from childhood to adulthood. Proximal (close to the trunk) skeletal muscles are affected first, but with disease progression, more distal muscles can become weak. LGMD can also present like a metabolic myopathy; however, in these conditions unlike the metabolic myopathies, CK seldom returns to normal after a rhabdomyolysis event [23].

20.2.2 Diagnosis of LGMD

Generally, the diagnosis of LGMD is made if an individual has predominantly shoulder and hip muscle weakness, elevated creatine kinase (CK) levels, and dystrophic changes on muscle biopsy [24–26]. A muscle biopsy can help reveal the type of LGMD. Special stains can be used to determine the absence or presence of proteins. Finding an absent or reduced protein narrows the causal gene candidates [27]. Because dystrophin is an important part of the dystrophin-sarcoglycan complex, it is important to rule out mutations in dystrophin as the cause of the muscular dystrophy. Finally, muscle imaging is becoming a helpful and noninvasive tool in the diagnosis of LGMD [27].

20.2.3 Genetics of LGMD

The dystrophin-sarcoglycan complex (DSC) is located on the membrane of the muscle cell and helps the muscle withstand everyday wear and tear. Improperly formed DSC can cause a rapid breakdown of muscle, which results in the loss of muscle cells and muscle weakness. Over 20 forms of LGMD are known, and can be divided into two types based on inheritance pattern: autosomal dominant LGMD1 and autosomal recessive LGMD2. LGMD1 and LGMD2 are further divided into subtypes based on the causative mutation. The subgroups are designated by letters (Table 20.1).

20.2.4 Genetic Testing for the LGMD

Because the different forms of LGMD can be clinically indistinguishable, testing with gene panels is the most efficient way to provide genetic confirmation [28]. Families without a genetically confirmed diagnosis may be ideal candidates for whole exome sequencing. As with all muscle diseases, private mutations and variants of unknown significance can complicate results.

Table 20.1 The LGMDs (adapted from [26])

Disease name (synonym)	Populations with founder mutations	Gene symbol	Inheritance
Myotilinopathy (LGMD1A)	None	*MYOT*	AD
LGMD1B	None	*LMNA*	AD
Caveolinopathy (LGMD1C)	None	*CAV3*	AD
LGMD1D	None	*DES*	AD
LGMD1E	None	*DNAJB6*	AD
Alpha-sarcoglycanopathy (LGMD2D)	None	*SGCA*	AR
Beta-sarcoglycanopathy (LGMD2E)	Amish	*SGCB*	AR
Gamma-sarcoglycanopathy (formerly SCARMD) (LGMD2C)	North Africans; Gypsies	*SGCG*	AR
Delta-sarcoglycanopathy (LGMD2F)	Brazilian	*SGCD*	AR
Calpainopathy (LGMD2A)	Amish, La Reunion Island, Basque (Spain), Turkish	*CAPN3*	AR
Dysferlinopathy (LGMD2B)	Libyan Jewish	*DYSF*	AR
LGMD2G	Italian	*TCAP*	AR
LGMD2H	Manitoba Hutterites only	*TRIM32*	AR
LGMD2I	Unknown	*FKRP*	AR
LGMD2J	Finland	*TTN*	AR
LGMD2K	Turkish	*POMT1*	AR
LGMD2L	Northern European	*ANO5*	AR
LGMD2M	Unknown	*FKTN*	AR
LGMD2N	Unknown	*POMT2*	AR
LGMD2O	Unknown	*POMGNT1*	AR
LGMD2Q	Turkish	*PLEC*	AR

20.3 Emery-Dreifuss Muscular Dystrophy (EDMD)

Emery-Dreifuss muscular dystrophy (EDMD) is a rare form of MD affecting an estimated 1/100,000 individual [29]. EDMD is characterized by joint contractures that precede muscle weakness and progressive, often severe cardiac involvement with cardiac conduction defects [30].

20.3.1 Clinical Presentation of the EDMD

EDMD is suspected in the presence of contractures prior to weakness. EDMD is considered a slowly progressive muscular dystrophy. It is often associated with cardiac problems including both cardiomyopathy and cardiac conduction defects [31].

20.3.2 Diagnosis of EDMD

Diagnosis is typically made clinically by the presence of contractures, especially at the elbows.

20.3.3 Genetics of EDMD

EDMD is caused by a mutation in any of the three genes that encode proteins associated with the nuclear envelope, *LMNA*, *EMD*, and *FHL1* [29]. Both *EMD* and *FHL1* are X-linked, with *FLH1* being X-linked dominant and female are affected. *LMNA* mutations typically cause an autosomal dominant form of EMD but can be recessive, and is often the result of a *de novo* mutation.

20.3.4 Genetic Testing for EDMD

Genetic testing for EDMD is usually done in a stepwise manner beginning with the most common genes, *LMNA* and *EMD* [29]. Other rare causes, including *FHL1* and other contracture disorder such as the collagen-VI-related disorders, are investigated if the first tier of testing is negative.

20.4 Facioscapulohumeral Muscular Dystrophy (FSHD)

Facioscapulohumeral muscular dystrophy (FSHD) causes slowly progressive muscle weakness and is characterized by scapular winging [32].

20.4.1 Clinical Presentation of the FSHD

FSHD is characterized by muscle weakness in the face, shoulders, upper arms, and lower legs. The weakness may be asymmetric [33]. Typical onset is in the teens or twenties. However, FSHD shows significant inter- and intra-familial variability both in age of onset and presenting symptoms, which can lead to difficulties in diagnosis. Infantile-onset FSHD with hearing loss and retinal changes is considered a rare form of FSHD [33, 34]. Hearing loss and retinal changes (Coats' disease) are also complications sometimes seen in the adult-onset form. The infantile form may be underdiagnosed and symptoms of FSHD may be unrecognized during childhood.

20.4.2 Diagnosis of FSHD

Diagnosis of FSHD is typically made clinically, with genetic testing as the gold standard. Muscle biopsy shows no specific changes [35], but may have an inflammatory infiltrate, which may be misleading, and result in misdiagnosis of myositis.

20.4.3 Genetics of FSHD

FSHD is an autosomal dominant condition primarily caused by a deletion on chromosome 4. The deletion within the D4Z4 repeat region results in changes in methylation [36–38]. A second FSHD gene, *SMCHD1*, has been identified and can be either a genetic cause of FSHD (in the presence of the permissive haplotype) or act as a disease modifier [39].

20.4.4 Genetic Testing of FSHD

A deletion of the D4Z4 repeat region on chromosome 4 is present in 95 % of individuals affected with FSHD. Detection of the deletion is complicated by the large size of the region and a genetically similar region located on chromosome 10. The deletion of D4Z4 repeats on chromosome 10 does not cause FSHD. A translocation between the chromosome 10 region and the D4Z4 region on chromosome 4 occurs frequently, occurring in 20 % of the general population without causing disease [36]. The D4Z4 deletion alone is not sufficient to cause FSHD1; a permissive allele, 4qA161, which allows polyadenylation and stabilization of DUX4 transcripts, is required to manifest FSHD1. Genetic strategies have been developed to detect both copies of D4Z4. In general the normal size of the FSHD region is greater than 40 kbs (or 40,000 base pairs). In individuals with FSHD, the size of the region is less than 35 kbs (or 35,000 base pairs). A grey zone of 35–40 kbs exists where some individuals will be symptomatic and others will not. In the event that genetic testing for the common mutation is negative and clinical suspicion is high, follow-up testing with alternate probes can be helpful. Additionally, testing of *SCHMD1* can be performed for the second less common cause of FSHD, now clinically called FSHD2 [40].

20.5 Oculopharyngeal Muscular Dystrophy (OPMD)

Oculopharyngeal muscular dystrophy (OPMD) is characterized by late-onset ptosis, dysphagia, and lower extremity weakness.

20.5.1 Clinical Presentation of the OPMD

OPMD is a condition that typically affects the muscles necessary for swallowing and eyelid movement. The muscles of the upper arms and legs can also be affected. Typically symptoms start appearing in the 50s and progress slowly; however a great deal of variability exists, even within families. OPMD is more common in the French Canadian population, but may be under-recognized in other populations [41].

20.5.2 Diagnosis of OPMD

OPMD is generally a clinical diagnosis, which is confirmed by genetic testing. EMG or muscle biopsy can be useful in excluding mitochondrial disorders or bulbar onset ALS early in the disease.

20.5.3 Genetics of OPMD

OPMD is an autosomal dominant condition caused by a polyalanine repeat within polyadenylate binding protein nuclear 1 encoded by the *PABPN1* gene located on chromosome 14 [42]. When homozygous, a modifier allele of seven GCG repeats can cause autosomal recessive OPMD, and also increase severity. The size of the polyalanine repeat appears to correlate with the severity of the condition and the age of onset.

20.5.4 Genetic Testing for the OPMD

Genetic test for OPMD involves determining the size of the GCN repeat within the *PABPN1* gene (abbreviated GCN because all four codons, GCA, GCT, GCC, and GCG, encode alanine). The normal size of the GCN repeat is ten repeats. At least one copy of 12 or more GCN repeats confirms the diagnosis of OPMD. When homozygous the GCN repeat size of 11 can cause autosomal recessive OPMD.

20.6 Congenital Muscular Dystrophy (CMD)

Congenital muscular dystrophy (CMD) is a clinically and genetically heterogeneous group of disease that presents from infancy through childhood, but will not be discussed in this chapter. Many of the genes associated with CMD can cause an LGMD phenotype [43].

20.7 Genetic Counseling Case History of a Transitional Age Patient

Mr. R, a 23-year-old male patient affected with Duchenne muscular dystrophy, requested a genetic counseling appointment for genetic testing and discussion of research participation. Mr. R was a long-standing patient in the Muscular Dystrophy Association (MDA) clinic. He had genetic testing during childhood, which did not identify a genetic mutation.

Mr. R, accompanied by his mother, arrived for the genetic counseling session. The genetic counselor began by asking Mr. R if he had any specific questions. Mr. R told her how his online research regarding possible treatment strategies had caused him to wonder about his mutation and research participation. The genetic counselor then inquired about his current life. He was enrolled in a part-time master's program in computer science and living independently.

The genetic counselor then reviewed family history and learned that Mr. R was an only child, and that there was no family history of any neuromuscular disorder. She discussed the inheritance of the dystrophinopathies and the fact that one-third of cases are due to a new mutation. She stated that if he wanted to have children, none of his sons would be affected or at risk of passing on the dystrophin mutation; however, all of his daughters would be carriers. Mr. R's mother remained quiet during the session, and denied having any questions or concerns. However, when the genetic counselor discussed the risk to DMD carriers for cardiomyopathy, and that cardiac screening was recommended for DMD carriers, she said that she was not interested in carrier testing and was already undergoing cardiac care for an arrhythmia. The genetic counselor discussed how other women in the family might be at risk, and could be offered carrier testing.

The counselor then explained the changes in technologies that allowed for better analysis of the dystrophin gene, and that most (>90 %) mutations were now identifiable. She discussed different mutation types and the research study for dystrophin nonsense mutations at their clinic. Mr. R elected to have genetic testing, and the genetic counselor and Mr. R made arrangements to discuss the results by phone.

The results revealed a deletion of exons 8–17 within the dystrophin gene. The genetic counselor explained how this meant that he was not eligible for the nonsense mutation clinical trial. The genetic counselor also discussed that the current exon skipping antisense polymers under development were not directed at this region. Mr. R asked about participation in other clinical studies. The clinical research team was currently enrolling for a natural history study for non-ambulatory DMD patients. The genetic counselor described the study, and facilitated Mr. R's enrollment.

Several years later, the genetic counselor met Mrs. R at an MDA function. Mrs. R remarked about the hope that was generated by her son's genetic counseling, testing, and research participation, and thanked her for arranging them.

Discussion Questions

- In this scenario the genetic counselor was both a genetic counselor and research coordinator. How do genetic counselors balance wearing many hats without creating a conflict of interest?
- How do you tailor a genetic counseling session if the primary information sought is not inheritance and risk to future generations? What is the genetic counselor's responsibility to raise awareness in family members of carrier-associated risks?
- How often should return patients be offered genetic counseling? Is the need for genetic testing or reviewing results the only reason for a follow-up consult?
- Working closely with a patient advocacy group, like the Muscular Dystrophy Association (MDA), often requires attendance at social functions and support groups. What positive and negative impact can this have on the providers' clinical practice?

References

1. Morrison, L. A. (2011). Dystrophinopathies. *Handbook of Clinical Neurology, 101*, 11–39.
2. Perumal, A. R., Rajeswaran, J., et al. (2013). Neuropsychological profile of Duchenne muscular dystrophy. *Applied Neuropsychology. Child.* 0: 1–9, 2014.
3. Pane, M. L., Lombardo, M. E., Alfieri, P., D'Amico, A., Bianco, F., Vasco, G., et al. (2012). Attention deficit hyperactivity disorder and cognitive function in Duchenne muscular dystrophy: Phenotype-genotype correlation. *Journal of Pediatrics, 161*(4), 705–709.e1.
4. Eagle, M., Baudouin, S. V., Chandler, C., Giddings, D. R., Bullock, R., & Bushby, K. (2002). Survival in Duchenne muscular dystrophy: Improvements in life expectancy since 1967 and the impact of home nocturnal ventilation. *Neuromuscular Disorders, 12*(10), 926–929.
5. Kieny, P., Chollet, S., Delalande, P., Le Fort, M., Magot, A., Pereon, Y., et al. (2013). Evolution of life expectancy of patients with Duchenne muscular dystrophy at AFM Yolaine de Kepper centre between 1981 and 2011. *Annals of Physical and Rehabilitation Medicine, 56* (6), 443–454.
6. Flanigan, K. M., Dunn, D. M., von Niederhausern, A., Howard, M. T., Mendell, J., Connolly, A., et al. (2009). DMD Trp3X nonsense mutation associated with a founder effect in North American families with mild Becker muscular dystrophy. *Neuromuscular Disorders, 19*(11), 743–748.
7. Gentil, C., Leturcq, F., Ben Yaou, R., Kaplan, J. C., Laforet, P., Pénisson-Besnier, I., et al. (2012). Variable phenotype of del45-55 Becker patients correlated with nNOSmu mislocalization and RYR1 hypernitrosylation. *Human Molecular Genetics, 21*(15), 3449–3460.

8. Flanigan, K. M., Dunn, D. M., von Niederhausern, A., Soltanzadeh, P., Howard, M. T., Sampson, J. B., et al. (2011). Nonsense mutation-associated Becker muscular dystrophy: Interplay between exon definition and splicing regulatory elements within the DMD gene. *Human Mutation, 32*(3), 299–308.
9. Witting, N., Duno, M., & Vissing, J. (2013). Becker muscular dystrophy with widespread muscle hypertrophy and a non-sense mutation of exon 2. *Neuromuscular Disorders, 23*(1), 25–28.
10. Acsadi, G., Moore, S. A., Chéron, A., Delalande, O., Bennett, L., Kupsky, W., et al. (2012). Novel mutation in spectrin-like repeat 1 of dystrophin central domain causes protein misfolding and mild Becker muscular dystrophy. *Journal of Biological Chemistry, 287*(22), 18153–18162.
11. Soltanzadeh, P., Friez, M. J., Dunn, D., von Niederhausern, A., Gurvich, O. L., Swoboda, K. J., et al. (2010). Clinical and genetic characterization of manifesting carriers of DMD mutations. *Neuromuscular Disorders, 20*(8), 499–504.
12. Mercier, S., Toutain, A., Toussaint, A., Raynaud, M., de Barace, C., Marcorelles, P., et al. (2013). Genetic and clinical specificity of 26 symptomatic carriers for dystrophinopathies at pediatric age. *European Journal of Human Genetics, 21*(8), 855–863.
13. Brioschi, S., Gualandi, F., Scotton, C., Armaroli, A., Bovolenta, M., Falzarano, M. S., et al. (2012). Genetic characterization in symptomatic female DMD carriers: Lack of relationship between X-inactivation, transcriptional DMD allele balancing and phenotype. *BMC Medical Genetics, 13*, 73.
14. Mukherjee, M., Chaturvedi, L. S., Srivastava, S., Mittal, R. D., Mittal, B., et al. (2003). De novo mutations in sporadic deletional Duchenne muscular dystrophy (DMD) cases. *Experimental and Molecular Medicine, 35*(2), 113–117.
15. Yoshioka, M., Yorifuji, T., & Mituyoshi, I. (1998). Skewed X inactivation in manifesting carriers of Duchenne muscular dystrophy. *Clinical Genetics, 53*(2), 102–107.
16. Ferreiro, V., Szijan, I., & Giliberto, F. (2004). Detection of germline mosaicism in two Duchenne muscular dystrophy families using polymorphic dinucleotide (CA)n repeat loci within the dystrophin gene. *Molecular Diagnosis, 8*(2), 115–121.
17. van Essen, A. J., Mulder, I. M., van der Vlies, P., van der Hout, A. H., Buys, C. H., Hofstra, R. M., et al. (2003). Detection of point mutation in dystrophin gene reveals somatic and germline mosaicism in the mother of a patient with Duchenne muscular dystrophy. *American Journal of Medical Genetics. Part A, 118A*(3), 296–298.
18. Muntoni, F., Torelli, S., & Ferlini, A. (2003). Dystrophin and mutations: One gene, several proteins, multiple phenotypes. *Lancet Neurology, 2*(12), 731–740.
19. Pegoraro, E., Hoffman, E. P., Piva, L., Gavassini, B. F., Cagnin, S., Ermani, M., et al. (2011). SPP1 genotype is a determinant of disease severity in Duchenne muscular dystrophy. *Neurology, 76*(3), 219–226.
20. Swaggart, K. A., & McNally, E. M. (2013). Modifiers of heart and muscle function: Where genetics meets physiology. *Experimental Physiology, 99*(4), 621–626.
21. Ferlini, A., Neri, M., Gualandi, F., et al. (2013). The medical genetics of dystrophinopathies: Molecular genetic diagnosis and its impact on clinical practice. *Neuromuscular Disorders, 23* (1), 4–14.
22. Guglieri, M., Straub, V., Bushby, K., & Lochmüller, H. (2008). Limb-girdle muscular dystrophies. *Current Opinion in Neurology, 21*(5), 576–584.
23. Pena, L., Kim, K., & Charrow, J. (2010). Episodic myoglobinuria in a primary gamma-sarcoglycanopathy. *Neuromuscular Disorders, 20*(5), 337–339.
24. Pegoraro, E., & Hoffman, E. P. (2012). Limb-Girdle muscular dystrophy overview. In: R. A. Pagon, M. P. Adam, T. D. Bird, C. R. Dolan, C. T. Fong, R. J. H. Smith, & K. Stephens (Eds.), *GeneReviews*™ [Internet]. Seattle, WA, University of Washington, Seattle; 1993–2013. 2000 June 08 [updated 2012 August 30].
25. Eymard, B., & Levy, N. (2012). Diagnostic strategy for limb-girdle muscular dystrophies. *Revue Neurologique (Paris), 168*(12), 919–926.

26. Mitsuhashi, S., & Kang, P. B. (2012). Update on the genetics of limb girdle muscular dystrophy. *Seminars in Pediatric Neurology, 19*(4), 211–218.
27. Sarkozy, A., Deschauer, M., Carlier, R. Y., Schrank, B., Seeger, J., Walter, M. C., et al. (2012). Muscle MRI findings in limb girdle muscular dystrophy type 2L. *Neuromuscular Disorders, 22*(Suppl 2), S122–S129.
28. Ghosh, P. S., & Zhou, L. (2012). The diagnostic utility of a commercial limb-girdle muscular dystrophy gene test panel. *Journal of Clinical Neuromuscular Disease, 14*(2), 86–87.
29. Puckelwartz, M., & McNally, E. M. (2011). Emery-Dreifuss muscular dystrophy. *Handbook of Clinical Neurology, 101*, 155–166.
30. Bonne, G., Leturcq, F., & Ben Yaou, R. (2013). Emery-Dreifuss muscular dystrophy. In: R. A. Pagon, M. P. Adam, T. D. Bird, C. R. Dolan, C. T. Fong, R. J. H. Smith, & K. Stephens (Eds.), *GeneReviews*™ [Internet]. Seattle, WA, University of Washington, Seattle; 1993–2013. 2004 September 29 [updated 2013 January 17].
31. Parmar, M. S., & Parmar, K. S. (2012). Emery-Dreifuss humeroperoneal muscular dystrophy: Cardiac manifestations. *The Canadian Journal of Cardiology, 28*(4), 516. e511–513.
32. van der Maarel, S. M., Miller, D. G., Tawil, R., Filippova, G. N., & Tapscott, S. J. (2012). Facioscapulohumeral muscular dystrophy: Consequences of chromatin relaxation. *Current Opinion in Neurology, 25*(5), 614–620.
33. Lamperti, C., Fabbri, G., Vercelli, L., D'Amico, R., Frusciante, R., Bonifazi, E., et al. (2010). A standardized clinical evaluation of patients affected by facioscapulohumeral muscular dystrophy: The FSHD clinical score. *Muscle and Nerve, 42*(2), 213–217.
34. Lutz, K. L., Holte, L., Kliethermes, S. A., Stephan, C., & Mathews, K. D. (2013). Clinical and genetic features of hearing loss in facioscapulohumeral muscular dystrophy. *Neurology, 81* (16), 1374–1377.
35. Wood-Allum, C., Brennan, P., Hewitt, M., Lowe, J., Tyfield, L., & Wills, A. (2004). Clinical and histopathological heterogeneity in patients with 4q35 facioscapulohumeral muscular dystrophy (FSHD). *Neuropathology and Applied Neurobiology, 30*(2), 188–191.
36. van der Maarel, S. M., Deidda, G., Lemmers, R. J., Bakker, E., van der Wielen, M. J., Sandkuijl, L., et al. (1999). A new dosage test for subtelomeric 4;10 translocations improves conventional diagnosis of facioscapulohumeral muscular dystrophy (FSHD). *Journal of Medical Genetics, 36*(11), 823–828.
37. Tassin, A., Laoudj-Chenivesse, D., Vanderplanck, C., Barro, M., Charron, S., Ansseau, E., et al. (2013). DUX4 expression in FSHD muscle cells: How could such a rare protein cause a myopathy? *Journal of Cellular and Molecular Medicine, 17*(1), 76–89.
38. Richards, M., Coppee, F., Thomas, N., Belayew, A., & Upadhyaya, M. (2012). Facioscapulohumeral muscular dystrophy (FSHD): An enigma unravelled? *Human Genetics, 131*(3), 325–340.
39. Sacconi, S., Lemmers, R. J., Balog, J., van der Vliet, P. J., Lahaut, P., van Nieuwenhuizen, M. P., et al. (2013). The FSHD2 gene SMCHD1 is a modifier of disease severity in families affected by FSHD1. *The American Journal of Human Genetics, 93*(4), 744–751.
40. Mitsuhashi, S., Boyden, S. E., Estrella, E. A., Jones, T. I., Rahimov, F., Yu, T. W., et al. (2013). Exome sequencing identifies a novel SMCHD1 mutation in facioscapulohumeral muscular dystrophy 2. *Neuromuscular Disorders, 23*(12), 975–980.
41. Ruegg, S., Lehky Hagen, M., Hohl, U., Kappos, L., Fuhr, P., Plasilov, M., et al. (2005). Oculopharyngeal muscular dystrophy—An under-diagnosed disorder? *Swiss Medical Weekly, 135*(39–40), 574–586.
42. Banerjee, A., Apponi, L. H., Apponi, L. H., Pavlath, G. K., Corbett, A. H., et al. (2013). PABPN1: Molecular function and muscle disease. *FEBS Journal, 280*(17), 4230–4250.
43. Cirak, S., Foley, A. R., Herrmann, R., Willer, T., Yau, S., Stevens, E., et al. (2013). ISPD gene mutations are a common cause of congenital and limb-girdle muscular dystrophies. *Brain, 136* (Pt 1), 269–281.

Chapter 21
The Myotonic Dystrophies

Joline Dalton, Jill S. Goldman, and Jacinda B. Sampson

The clinical definition of myotonia is delayed relaxation of muscles. Myotonia can be caused by various factors, including genetic mutations. The conditions that cause myotonia are subdivided by their associated clinical symptoms as either myotonic dystrophy or non-dystrophic myotonia.

21.1 Myotonic Dystrophy: DM Type 1

(*DM Type 1 video clip Part 1 and 2*)

Electronic supplementary material Supplementary material is available in the online version of this chapter at 10.1007/978-1-4899-7482-2_21. Videos can also be accessed at http://www.springerimages.com/videos/978-1-4899-7481-5.

J. Dalton (✉)
Paul and Sheila Wellstone Muscular Dystrophy Center, University of Minnesota, 2101 6th St. SE MC, Minneapolis, MN 55455, USA
e-mail: jcdalton@umn.edu

J.S. Goldman
Taub Institute, Columbia University Medical Center, 630 W. 168th St., Box 16, New York, NY 10032, USA
e-mail: jg2673@cumc.columbia.edu

J.B. Sampson
Department of Neurology, Columbia University Medical Center, 630 W. 168th St., Box 16, New York, NY 10032, USA
e-mail: js4171@cumc.columbia.edu

J.S. Goldman (ed.), *Genetic Counseling for Adult Neurogenetic Disease*,
DOI 10.1007/978-1-4899-7482-2_21

21.1.1 Clinical Presentation

Myotonic dystrophy is a progressive, multi-systemic condition that causes muscle weakness and myotonia (the inability of muscles to relax after use). Individuals with myotonic dystrophy can have cataracts, intestinal pseudo-obstruction and other gastrointestinal abnormalities, male infertility, insulin insensitivity and diabetes, and cardiac conduction defects [1]. Fatigue is common and can neither be completely controlled by medication nor explained by respiratory insufficiency [2]. Both myotonia and weakness can lead to decreased hand dexterity, which can interfere with activities of daily living and work. Muscle weakness is typically more pronounced in distal and facial muscles, and swallowing can be affected. Myotonia and muscle weakness associated with myotonic dystrophy can become more pronounced during pregnancy [3–5].

Two types of myotonic dystrophy, type 1 (DM1) and type 2 (DM2), have been described. They are genetically heterogeneous, but the adult-onset forms have overlap of clinical symptoms. Myotonic dystrophy type 2 (DM2), previously described as proximal myotonia and muscle weakness (PROMM), can present with either proximal or distal weakness. In general, although musculoskeletal pain is more problematic in DM2, it is generally milder than DM1 and includes respiratory insufficiency less often [6, 11] (Table 21.1).

A more severe form of myotonic dystrophy type 1, called congenital myotonic dystrophy type 1, is characterized by neonatal hypotonia and failure to thrive due to respiratory and feeding difficulties. Sometimes polyhydramnios, club feet, and other signs of decreased fetal movements are detectable by ultrasound during pregnancy [8]. Infants that survive past the first few years of life have delayed developmental milestones, often have some degree of learning difficulties and/or behavioral problems, and often later develop progressive muscle weakness. Additionally, a juvenile form of myotonic dystrophy type 1 causes progressive weakness, and intellectual, psychiatric, and behavioral problems [9, 10]. The congenital form has not been described in myotonic dystrophy type 2.

Adult myotonic dystrophy type 1 can include facial weakness (with ptosis, temporal muscle wasting, and "fish-mouth"), male-pattern baldness, hypophonic speech, "Christmas tree" cataracts, grip myotonia, distal greater than proximal

Table 21.1 Clinical symptoms of DM1 and DM2 (adapted from [7])

Symptom	DM1	DM2
Myotonia	+	+
Iridescent cataracts	+	+
Weakness	+	+
Cardiac arrhythmia	+	+
Testicular failure	+	+
Hyperinsulinemia	+	+
Hypo IgG	+	+
Cognitive difficulties	+	–
Congenital/juvenile onset	+	–
CNS effects	+	+/–

weakness, and increased risk of cardiac arrhythmias and cardiomyopathy. The risk of sudden death due to cardiac conduction abnormalities and arrhythmias requires cardiac monitoring [11].

21.1.2 Diagnosis of Myotonic Dystrophy

The diagnosis of myotonic dystrophy can be established by identification of clinical or electrical myotonia and presence of other multi-systemic features. However, EMG sometimes may not reveal myotonia in DM2 [11]. Muscle biopsy may sometimes show ringbindin, a swirling pattern of cytoskeletal elements, but is more often abnormal but non-diagnostic. With its high sensitivity and specificity, genetic testing is often pursued instead of invasive testing. Due to the multi-systemic features of myotonic dystrophy, patients should be followed for symptoms for other conditions. Since the constellation of DM features is not recognized, a diagnostic odyssey may occur [12].

21.1.3 Genetics of Myotonic Dystrophy

Myotonic dystrophy type 1 is caused by a CTG expansion in the 3′UTR of the *DMPK* gene located on chromosome 19. An expansion of 100 or more CTG repeats typically causes symptoms of the condition. Some degree of correlation between age of onset and repeat number exists; however, because of the overlap in symptoms, the size of expansion cannot predict the prognosis [13]. There is also variability in repeat size among tissues and over time. Because the expansion can increase in each generation, anticipation is seen in DM1. Thus, in subsequent generations, age of onset may decrease and severity increase [14, 15]. The size of the repeat tends to expand more when maternally transmitted. Therefore, a greater risk of congenital myotonic dystrophy type 1 exists with maternal transmission, though cases have been reported with paternal transmission [16]. Most infants with congenital myotonic dystrophy have greater than 1,000 repeats, with a range of 500–2,000 [17]. The repeat range of 4–37 is considered normal and 38–50 is considered a premutation range, which may expand in the next generation. People with repeats of 51–100 not only have a risk of next generation expansion, but also may develop mild symptoms such as cataracts late in life [11].

Myotonic dystrophy type 2 (DM2) is caused by a CCTG repeat expansion in the *ZNF9* gene. The expansion ranges from approximately 75 to greater than 11,000 CCTG repeats. The CCTG repeat tract is very unstable and tends to increase as a person ages (somatic expansion). However, the size of the repeat cannot predict age of onset or severity [11].

Genetic testing for myotonic dystrophy is greater than 90 % accurate [18]. Genetic confirmation helps to explain many symptoms and clinical issues they may have experienced, and allows for better treatment of present symptoms, and appropriate surveillance for cardiac complications.

21.2 Non-dystrophic Myotonia

21.2.1 Clinical Presentation of the Non-dystrophic Myotonia

Non-dystrophic myotonic disorders are conditions that produce myotonia without associated with muscle weakness or symptoms other than cramping or pain [19].

21.2.2 Diagnosis of Non-dystrophic Myotonia

The non-dystrophic myotonias are typically diagnosed by the presence of clinical myotonia and/or electromyogram (EMG) evidence. Depending on patient's desire and the clinical suspicion, genetic confirmation may be warranted.

21.2.3 Genetics of Non-dystrophic Myotonia

As many as one-third of cases of non-dystrophic myotonia are caused by mutations in the ion channel genes, specifically the chloride channel gene, *CLCN1*, and the sodium channel gene, *SCN4A* [20, 21]. Myotonia congenita is associated with *CLCN1*; it is referred to as Thomsen myotonia if dominant, and Becker myotonia if recessive. Paramyotonia, which is myotonia worsening with exercise, is mostly associated with *SCN4A*, and rarely *CLCN1* [22–24]. The role of the chloride channel is to keep skeletal muscle electrically stable. It works to maintain voluntary use of muscles by regulating the flow of chloride ions. Ions act as cell signals, and too much or too little of an ion produces a reaction, such as a muscle contraction. If the chloride channel is not working properly, the muscle cannot repolarize or relax efficiently after contraction, leading to stiffening of the muscle. Sometimes cold can make this process even slower, and people with myotonia often have a "warm-up effect" in which their muscle responds "normally" when warmed up. Mutations in the chloride channel gene can also be a modifier gene in myotonic dystrophy type 2 [25].

SCN4A encodes a voltage-gated sodium channel, which can be associated with paramyotonia or hyperkalemic periodic paralysis. The disruption of the sodium levels results in changes in potassium levels, which causes weakness or myotonias depending on the *SCN4A* mutation. *SCN4A*-related myotonia is significantly worse when muscles are cold. The *SCN4A*-related conditions are inherited in an autosomal dominant pattern [26].

21.3 Myotonic Dystrophy Case History

Mr. A was a 37-year-old man with progressive muscle weakness and fatigue. He presented to his family physician because he felt sluggish and depressed. The physician ran some routine lab tests that revealed that Mr. A had borderline diabetes and hypothyroidism. However, the doctor also noted a myotonic grip and hypophonic voice, and referred him to a neurologist. The neurological exam and medical history led to a diagnosis of myotonic dystrophy, and he was referred to cardiology and ophthalmology for evaluations and to genetic counseling for genetic confirmation of his diagnosis.

The genetic counselor (GC) greeted Mr. A and asked if he understood why he had been referred. Mr. A replied that he was supposed to have a test to prove that he had DM. The counselor then explained that there were two different forms of DM, and that the test was important to differentiate between them in order to guide prognosis and management. She also explained that it was important information for Mr. and Mrs. A if they wished to have children, as well as for other family members. He replied that they wanted children but could not get pregnant. The counselor told him that male infertility was a possible but not universal symptom of DM1, and that he might still father a child. The counselor then explained the genetics of DM1 and 2, and the difference in symptoms between the two. Mr. A remarked that he had no family history of DM. The counselor said that she would like to take a more detailed family history. The family history revealed that Mr. A was an only child. Mr. A's father was a 65-year-old melanoma survivor and was generally in good health, as were the extended members of the paternal side. The paternal grandparents had lived into their 80s and died of liver failure and stroke. His mother was 63, had no neurological problems, but had a heart condition of some kind. Mr. A did not know the details. His maternal grandmother had died of breast cancer in her 60s and the maternal grandfather had died of a heart condition in his 70s. His maternal aunt also had a heart problem and one of her sons had died suddenly at age 46 of a heart attack. Mr. A remarked that he felt that his greatest risk was heart disease, not a neurological disease. The genetic counselor explained that cardiac conditions could be a part of DM, and asked if his mother had ever been evaluated by a neurologist. He did not know the answer to this question. The GC suggested that he ask her and ask if she would be willing to have a neurological evaluation. He said that he would do so. Mr. A completed the paperwork, informed consent for genetic testing, and set up an appointment to come back with his wife for results.

A month later Mr. and Mrs. A came for the result session. Mr. A was found to have an expansion of 234 CTG repeats in the *DMPK* gene. The genetic counselor told the couple that this confirmed that Mr. A had DM1. They then talked about his symptoms, including the infertility, and his prognosis for the future. She reminded him of the importance of being followed by an ophthalmologist and cardiologist. She also discussed the couple's plans for reproduction and the risk to children. Mrs. A said that they were thinking about the possibility of sperm donation, but had not yet decided. They wanted to wait until Mr. A was fully evaluated to better understand his prognosis. Contraceptive use until his evaluation by a fertility specialist was recommended.

The GC then returned to his family history, pointing to the cardiac history and sudden death of his cousin. Mr. A became very concerned about his mother, but then the concern turned to anger. He asked how she could have had this family history and never pursued a full work-up. The GC reminded him that without the neurological symptoms, it was unlikely that a cardiologist would think about DM1. She acknowledged that he must be feeling some anger that he inherited the gene, but said that his mother clearly had no way of knowing that she carried it. The GC explained anticipation and how his mother probably carried a much lower repeat number. To be balanced, she discussed that it is also possible his father has a low repeat number—an increased incidence of certain cancers, including melanoma, has been reported in DM1 [27]. She asked him if he planned to share the information with his mother. He said that he probably would. The GC said that it was actually important information for her and her doctor. Mr. A agreed to discuss it with her. The GC gave him her card to pass onto his mother.

Later that week, the GC received a call from Mr. A's mother. She was very concerned both about her son's health and about her own genetic status. She was horrified that she might have "caused his disease." The GC validated her feelings and explained that she had no way of knowing that she carried the gene and could not be held responsible. She asked if the senior Mrs. A would like to make an appointment for herself to learn more about DM1 and genetic testing. She said that she would.

Mr. A's mother attended a genetic counseling session and decided to move forward with her own testing. She said that she would schedule a neurological evaluation and have testing at that time. The neurological evaluation revealed very mild weakness, with mild myotonia on EMG. The genetic testing revealed a CTG expansion of 142. The genetic counselor encouraged Mrs. A to pass this information on to her cardiologist and to schedule an ophthalmology exam for cataracts. They also discussed informing the extended family about the diagnosis. Mrs. A said that she would do so.

Discussion Questions

- In what ways do disorders with anticipation affect patients and families differently than disorders without anticipation?
- How does counseling about multi-systemic diseases differ from single system disorders?
- In the above case history, the genetic counselor accepted several family members as her patients. How do you prevent conflict of interest and confidentiality breaches when you see different family members?
- How much reproductive counseling would you do for Mr. and Mrs. A at the result session?

References

1. Turner, C., & Hilton-Jones, D. (2010). The myotonic dystrophies: Diagnosis and management. *Journal of Neurology, Neurosurgery, and Psychiatry, 81*(4), 358–367.
2. Laberge, L., Gagnon, C., & Dauvilliers, Y. (2013). Daytime sleepiness and myotonic dystrophy. *Current Neurology and Neuroscience Reports, 13*(4), 340.
3. Dufour, P., Berard, J., et al. (1997). Myotonic dystrophy and pregnancy. A report of two cases and a review of the literature. *European Journal of Obstetrics, Gynecology, and Reproductive Biology, 72*(2), 159–164.
4. Khan, Z. A., & Khan, S. A. (2009). Myotonic dystrophy and pregnancy. *The Journal of the Pakistan Medical Association, 59*(10), 717–719.
5. Rudnik-Schoneborn, S., Schneider-Gold, C., Raabe, U., Kress, W., Zerres, K., & Schoser, B. G. (2006). Outcome and effect of pregnancy in myotonic dystrophy type 2. *Neurology, 66* (4), 579–580.
6. George, A., Schneider-Gold, C., Zier, S., Reiners, K., & Sommer, C. (2004). Musculoskeletal pain in patients with myotonic dystrophy type 2. *Archives of Neurology, 61*(12), 1938–1942.
7. Ranum, L. P., & Day, J. W. (2002). Myotonic dystrophy: Clinical and molecular parallels between myotonic dystrophy type 1 and type 2. *Current Neurology and Neuroscience Reports, 2*(5), 465–470.
8. Erikson, A., Forsberg, H., Drugge, U., & Holmgren, G. (1995). Outcome of pregnancy in women with myotonic dystrophy and analysis of CTG gene expansion. *Acta Paediatrica, 84* (4), 416–418.
9. Steyaert, J., Umans, S., Willekens, D., Legius, E., Pijkels, E., de Die-Smulders, C., et al. (1997). A study of the cognitive and psychological profile in 16 children with congenital or juvenile myotonic dystrophy. *Clinical Genetics, 52*(3), 135–141.
10. Douniol, M., Jacquette, A., Cohen, D., Bodeau, N., Rachidi, L., Angeard, N., et al. (2012). Psychiatric and cognitive phenotype of childhood myotonic dystrophy type 1. *Developmental Medicine and Child Neurology, 54*(10), 905–911.
11. Wicklund, M. P. (2013). The muscular dystrophies. *Continuum (Minneapolis Minnesota), 19* (6 Muscle Disease), 1535–1570.
12. Hilbert, J. E., Ashizawa, T., Day, J. W., Luebbe, E. A., Martens, W. B., McDermott, M. P., et al. (2013). Diagnostic odyssey of patients with myotonic dystrophy. *Journal of Neurology, 260*(10), 2497–2504.
13. Hamshere, M. G., Harley, H., et al. (1999). Myotonic dystrophy: The correlation of (CTG) repeat length in leucocytes with age at onset is significant only for patients with small expansions. *Journal of Medical Genetics, 36*(1), 59–61.
14. Martorell, L., Monckton, D. G., Gamez, J., & Baiget, M. (2000). Complex patterns of male germline instability and somatic mosaicism in myotonic dystrophy type 1. *European Journal of Human Genetics, 8*(6), 423–430.
15. Martorell, L., Monckton, D. G., Sanchez, A., Lopez De Munain, A., & Baiget, M. (2001). Frequency and stability of the myotonic dystrophy type 1 premutation. *Neurology, 56*(3), 328–335.
16. Zeesman, S., Carson, N., & Whelan, D. T. (2002). Paternal transmission of the congenital form of myotonic dystrophy type 1: A new case and review of the literature. *American Journal of Medical Genetics, 107*(3), 222–226.
17. Tsilfidis, C., MacKenzie, A. E., Mettler, G., Barceló, J., & Korneluk, R. G. (1992). Correlation between CTG trinucleotide repeat length and frequency of severe congenital myotonic dystrophy. *Nature Genetics, 1*(3), 192–195.
18. Kamsteeg, E. J., Kress, W., Catalli, C., Hertz, J. M., Witsch-Baumgartner, M., Buckley, M. F., et al. (2012). Best practice guidelines and recommendations on the molecular diagnosis of myotonic dystrophy types 1 and 2. *European Journal of Human Genetics, 20*(12), 1203–1208.
19. Matthews, E., Fialho, D., Tan, S. V., Venance, S. L., Cannon, S. C., Sternberg, D., et al. (2010). The non-dystrophic myotonias: Molecular pathogenesis, diagnosis and treatment. *Brain, 133* (Pt 1), 9–22.

20. Trip, J., Drost, G., Ginjaar, H. B., Nieman, F. H., van der Kooi, A. J., de Visser, M., et al. (2009). Redefining the clinical phenotypes of non-dystrophic myotonic syndromes. *Journal of Neurology, Neurosurgery, and Psychiatry, 80*(6), 647–652.
21. Jurkat-Rott, K., & Lehmann-Horn, F. (2010). State of the art in hereditary muscle channelopathies. *Acta Myologica: Myopathies and Cardiomyopathies, 29*(2), 343–350.
22. Dunø, M., Colding-Jørgensen, E., Grunnet, M., Jespersen, T., Vissing, J., & Schwartz, M. (2004). Difference in allelic expression of the CLCN1 gene and the possible influence on the myotonia congenita phenotype. *European Journal of Human Genetics, 12*(9), 738–743.
23. Gurgel-Giannetti, J., Senkevics, A. S., Zilbersztajn-Gotlieb, D., Yamamoto, L. U., Muniz, V. P., Pavanello, R. C., et al. (2012). Thomsen or Becker myotonia? A novel autosomal recessive nonsense mutation in the CLCN1 gene associated with a mild phenotype. *Muscle and Nerve, 45*(2), 279–283.
24. Cardani, R., Giagnacovo, M., Botta, A., Rinaldi, F., Morgante, A., Udd, B., et al. (2012). Co-segregation of DM2 with a recessive CLCN1 mutation in juvenile onset of myotonic dystrophy type 2. *Journal of Neurology, 259*(10), 2090–2099.
25. Ursu, S. F., Alekov, A., Mao, N. H., & Jurkat-Rott, K. (2012). ClC1 chloride channel in myotonic dystrophy type 2 and ClC1 splicing in vitro. *Acta Myologica: Myopathies and Cardiomyopathies, 31*(2), 144–153.
26. Saleem, R., Setty, G., Khan, A., Farrell, D., & Hussain, N. (2013). Phenotypic heterogeneity in skeletal muscle sodium channelopathies: A case report and literature review. *Journal of Pediatric Neurosciences, 8*(2), 138–140.
27. Win, A. K., Perattur, P. G., Pulido, J. S., Pulido, C. M., & Lindor, N. M. (2012). Increased cancer risks in myotonic dystrophy. *Mayo Clinical Proceedings, 87*(2), 130–135.

Part VII
Neurocutaneous Syndromes

Chapter 22
Overview of Neurocutaneous Syndromes

Amanda Bergner

The neurocutaneous syndromes are a diverse group of over 100 described disorders that are unified by involvement of the nervous system and the skin. Other organ systems, such as the eyes, kidneys, and heart, are often involved. Outside of the nervous system, common findings include hypo- or hyper-pigmentation of the skin, cutaneous and/or internal vascular dysplasias, neoplasms (primarily benign, but sometimes malignant) and overgrowth. Primary neurocutaneous syndromes are developmental conditions that involve genetic dysregulation. Secondary neurocutaneous disorders are not developmental in nature, but rather result as a complication of another condition, often metabolic. The distinction between primary and secondary neurocutaneous syndromes is important, as both pathogenesis and prognosis differ.

Diagnosis of primary neurocutaneous syndromes is typically made using a combination of clinical exam and diagnostic testing. Most primary neurocutaneous syndromes can be diagnosed based on established clinical criteria and do not require genetic testing, though genetic testing can sometimes assist with the diagnostic process and is often used to inform management of the family. The most frequent clinical evaluations include neurology, dermatology, and ophthalmology to obtain the clinical history and examine the most commonly affected body systems for the presence of characteristic features of each condition. Diagnostic testing that can assist evaluation includes X-ray, MRI, CT scan, EEG, and blood and/or urine tests.

Although the majority appear to be sporadic, many primary neurocutaneous syndromes exhibit Mendelian inheritance patterns. All types of Mendelian

A. Bergner (✉)
Department of Neurology, Johns Hopkins University School of Medicine, 600 North Wolfe Street, Phipps 117, Baltimore, MD 21287, USA

McKusick-Nathans Institute of Genetic Medicine, Johns Hopkins University School of Medicine, 600 North Wolfe Street, Phipps 117, Baltimore, MD 21287, USA
e-mail: abergne1@jhmi.edu

J.S. Goldman (ed.), *Genetic Counseling for Adult Neurogenetic Disease*,
DOI 10.1007/978-1-4899-7482-2_22

inheritance patterns have been described among the primary neurocutaneous syndromes, including autosomal dominant (as in neurofibromatosis and tuberous sclerosis), autosomal recessive (as in ataxia telangiectasia), and X-linked (as in incontinentia pigmenti) [1]. The most common syndromes based on known incidence are neurofibromatosis (including neurofibromatosis 1, neurofibromatosis 2, and schwannomatosis) and tuberous sclerosis, which will be discussed in this chapter. As with other conditions addressed in this book, the counseling issues presented in the context of the conditions reviewed in detail here may be relevant to many other primary neurocutaneous syndromes.

22.1 Genetic Counseling Issues for Neurocutaneous Syndromes

Primary neurocutaneous syndromes are developmental, and therefore, present at birth. However, many symptoms may not appear until later in life. As such, patients can experience lifelong issues and concerns. When considering the genetic counseling issues for adults with primary neurocutaneous syndromes, several common themes recur.

22.1.1 Accuracy of Diagnosis

In many primary neurocutaneous syndromes, features present at birth or in childhood may recede, fade, be corrected, or be removed by adulthood, potentially making a physical exam less than fully informative when assessing for specific diagnostic criteria. Additionally, medical records from childhood may not be readily available for review, and adults may not remember the details of their medical care from childhood. Another concern is that a diagnosis made in childhood may no longer be accurate given changes in medical understanding during the intervening years. Prior to offering genetic counseling for an adult with a primary neurocutaneous syndrome, it is imperative to confirm the diagnosis by current standards. A thorough physical exam coupled with a detailed medical history and review of medical records is often necessary to determine the accuracy of a diagnosis. In cases in which the current diagnostic criteria cannot be met, but a particular diagnosis is suspected, genetic counseling should be undertaken with the caveat that the information provided only applies if the diagnosis is in fact accurate. In these situations, genetic testing can often assist in confirming a specific diagnosis.

22.1.2 Inheritance Pattern and De Novo Mutations

In order to provide accurate genetic counseling, the inheritance pattern of the condition in question must be known, as primary neurocutaneous syndromes can be inherited in a variety of ways. Additionally, in the setting of autosomal dominant conditions, not every affected adult has an affected parent. Each autosomal dominant primary neurocutaneous syndrome has its own rate of *de novo* mutation. For instance, while 50 % of adults with neurofibromatosis have an affected parent, only about a third of adults with tuberous sclerosis do [1, 2].

22.1.3 Mosaicism

Adults with an autosomal dominant primary neurocutaneous syndrome due to a *de novo* mutation may have a mosaic form of the condition in question. The original putative mutation could have been somatic and occurred during the cascade of cell divisions during pregnancy rather than in the germ cells. Mosaicism can impact the calculation of reproductive risk for an adult with a primary neurocutaneous syndrome who is interested in having children, as the mutation may not be present in every cell of their body, including their germ cells. The possibility of mosaicism can also impact the ability to locate a mutation, depending on the tissue type that is used for testing [3].

22.1.4 Availability of Comprehensive Genetic Testing

The availability of comprehensive genetic testing for primary neurocutaneous syndromes varies. Many conditions are single-gene disorders for which genetic testing is available and comprehensive. For example, one gene, *Nf1*, causes neurofibromatosis 1 (NF1), and approximately 97 % of people meeting clinical criteria for this condition are found to have a mutation in this gene [3]. Some conditions are associated with multiple genes, though still have a fairly high rate of mutation detection when combined. Thus, tuberous sclerosis, which is associated with *TSC1* and *TSC2*, has a combined sensitivity of approximately 85 % for people meeting clinical criteria for this condition [4]. However, other primary neurocutaneous syndromes have not yet been fully characterized, such as schwannomatosis for which the known genes only account for approximately 40–50 % of affected individuals.

Without the availability of comprehensive genetic testing, many aspects of genetic counseling can be complicated, such as confirming a diagnosis, offering reproductive options, and interpreting negative test results. Additionally, it is important to know the conditions for which one gene test is appropriate versus a panel of gene tests. One must also know which tissue to send for testing to allow for the greatest likelihood of mutation detection. Thus, prior to offering genetic testing to an adult with a primary neurocutaneous syndrome, a complete understanding of the genes involved, the tests available, the sensitivity of each test, and the appropriate tissue to send for testing must be obtained.

22.1.5 Reproductive Decision-Making

Adults with primary neurocutaneous syndromes are often diagnosed prior to having children themselves, though this is not always the case. Symptoms may be subclinical and diagnosed only when an affected child is born. When working with an adult with a primary neurocutaneous syndrome, it is important to assess whether they already have children and whether they are desirous of having children in the future. Genetic testing and counseling regarding recurrence risk and options for prenatal testing and interventions are appropriate for this population and frequently requested. Some adult patients indicate that they have already decided not to have children of their own, either to prevent passing a syndrome to their children or because of the uncertainty about their own health and capacities as they age. It is important to assess the patient's understanding about the inheritance pattern and likelihood of passing a syndrome to a child to be certain that the information upon which these decisions are based is correct and complete.

22.1.6 Stigma and Discrimination

Many adults with primary neurocutaneous syndromes will have symptoms that are evident to others, including both physical and functional differences. It is common for people with these disorders to report experiences of stigmatization and discrimination throughout their life, particularly if symptoms occur in routinely exposed parts of the body, such as the face or hands [5]. In order to provide appropriate support to maximize current psycho-emotional functioning, it is important to assess whether stigma or discrimination has been a large part of a patient's life. It is also common for these experiences to impact reproduction and medical care decision-making. Providers with an understanding of this aspect of their patients' experience are often better able to form positive partnerships around management choices.

22.1.7 Recurrent Loss/Progression of Symptoms

Primary neurocutaneous syndromes are often progressive, with symptoms increasing in number and/or severity across the life span. Additionally, medical interventions can themselves introduce further morbidity, as in the loss of hearing upon surgical removal of a vestibular schwannoma that was impinging on the brain stem of a patient with neurofibromatosis 2 (NF2). By adulthood, many people with primary neurocutaneous syndromes have already experienced multiple functional losses and may have many ahead of them. It is important for providers working with this population to appreciate the chronicity of loss that might exist for their patients and to address this directly as part of the management plan. Depression and anxiety are frequently reported comorbidities with primary neurocutaneous disorders, and can be related to the current or expected progression of symptoms.

22.1.8 Uncertainty

Uncertainty about possible future symptoms is a reality with these conditions. It is not possible to predict which symptoms will occur, when they will arise, or how much of an impact they will have. This uncertainty can challenge both emotional and psychological well-being. Directly addressing the uncertainty can be beneficial to the patient by identifying ways in which they may manage this aspect of their condition most successfully.

22.2 Family History Questions Pertinent to Primary Neurocutaneous Syndromes

Targeted questions about family history can help determine if a condition is hereditary and assist with diagnosis. A three generation pedigree should always be obtained and include documentation of any medical condition, particularly those impacting the neurologic, dermatologic, and ophthalmologic systems. When taking a pedigree, questions that are relevant to the specific diagnosis under consideration should be asked. Some examples are listed below:

- Does anyone have spots on their skin that are either darker or lighter than the rest of their body?
- Does anyone have cancer or tumors?
- Has anyone had a growth/mass removed?
- Does anyone have lumps or bumps under their skin that do not go away?
- Does anyone have trouble hearing or have ringing in their ears?
- Does anyone have trouble seeing or any other eye problems?

- Does anyone have seizures?
- Does anyone have a heart defect or an arrhythmia?
- Did anyone have bone problems at birth or as a young child?
- Does anyone have kidney problems, including diabetes?
- Does anyone have trouble walking?
- Does anyone have hypertension, stroke, or other vascular problems?

References

1. Jenterra, G., Synder, S. L., & Narayanan, V. (2006). Genetic aspects of neurocutaneous disorders. *Seminars in Pediatric Neurology, 3*(1), 43–47.
2. DeBella, K., Szudek, J., & Friedman, J. M. (2000). Use of the National Institutes of Health criteria for diagnosis of neurofibromatosis 1 in children. *Pediatrics, 105*(3), 608–615.
3. Boyd, K. P., Korf, B. R., & Theos, A. (2009). Neurofibromatosis type 1. *Journal of the American Academy of Dermatology, 61*(1), 1–14.
4. Sancak, O., Nellist, M., Goedbloed, M., Elfferich, P., Wouters, C., Maat-Kievit, A., et al. (2005). Mutational analysis of the TSC1 and TSC2 genes in a diagnostic setting: Genotype–phenotype correlations and comparison of diagnostic DNA techniques in Tuberous Sclerosis Complex. *European Journal of Human Genetics, 13*(6), 731–741.
5. Vranceanu, A. M., Merker, V. L., Park, E., & Plotkin, S. R. (2013). Quality of life among adult with neurofibromatosis 1, neurofibromatosis 2 and schwannomatosis: A systematic review of the literature. *Journal of Neuro-Oncology, 114*(3), 257–262.

Chapter 23
Neurofibromatosis

Amanda Bergner

Neurofibromatosis 1 (NF1) is the most common inherited neurologic disease, with an estimated incidence of 1/3,300 and approximately 100,000 affected individuals in the USA [1]. NF1 is an autosomal dominant genetic condition that results from mutations in the *Nf1* gene. Mutations in this gene appear to be fully penetrant, such that any person with an underlying *Nf1* mutation will exhibit symptoms of NF1. About 50 % of people with NF1 have inherited an *Nf1* mutation from one of their parents; the other 50 % have a *de novo Nf1* mutation. Symptoms of NF1 can vary widely within and between families, indicating the likely role of modifier genes in this disease process, though none have yet been identified [2]. NF1 is thought to be pan-ethnic without gender bias. Highly specific and sensitive clinical criteria exist which are the basis for the majority of diagnoses, though genetic testing is available and can be of assistance in cases involving individuals who do not yet meet clinical criteria.

23.1 Clinical Presentation

(*NF video clip Part 1*)

Electronic supplementary material Supplementary material is available in the online version of this chapter at 10.1007/978-1-4899-7482-2_23. Videos can also be accessed at http://www.springerimages.com/videos/978-1-4899-7481-5.

A. Bergner (✉)
Department of Neurology, Johns Hopkins University School of Medicine, 600 North Wolfe Street, Phipps 117, Baltimore, MD 21287, USA

McKusick-Nathans Institute of Genetic Medicine, Johns Hopkins University School of Medicine, 600 North Wolfe Street, Phipps 117, Baltimore, MD 21287, USA
e-mail: abergne1@jhmi.edu

J.S. Goldman (ed.), *Genetic Counseling for Adult Neurogenetic Disease*,
DOI 10.1007/978-1-4899-7482-2_23

NF1 is a congenital condition, though symptoms may not be present at birth. If evaluated by an NF specialist, the vast majority of children born with NF1 meet clinical criteria by the age of 9. Individuals may ultimately be diagnosed with NF1 after being referred to a specialist due to the presence of one or more signs known to be associated with NF1. Clinical criteria are well-established and dictate that an individual has NF1 if they exhibit at least two of the following [3]:

- Six or more cafe-au-lait spots (>5 mm prior to puberty and >15 mm after puberty)
- Two or more neurofibromas, or one plexiform neurofibroma
- Optic pathway glioma
- Typical bony abnormality (i.e., pseudoarthrosis, sphenoid dysplasia)
- Axillary or inguinal freckling
- Two or more Lisch nodules
- First-degree family relative with NF1

Cafe-au-lait spots, Lisch nodules, and skin fold freckling in the axillary and inguinal regions of the body are the most common first symptoms in childhood, and are present for the majority of people who have NF1. During puberty, most individuals begin to develop cutaneous neurofibromas. These lesions are uniformly benign, but can contribute to significant morbidity depending on their location and number. About half of people with NF1 are thought to have at least one plexiform neurofibroma. These tumors begin as benign lesions, but are associated with a lifetime risk of approximately 10–12 % for malignant conversion. Plexiform neurofibromas can also exert significant mass effect and lead to neurologic dysfunction [3]. They are distinguished from cutaneous neurofibromas by both their location (plexiform tumors tend to involve more than the dermal tissue of the body) and their constitution. They are thought to arise *in utero*, but may not initially be apparent.

A small percentage of individuals with NF1 will have pathognomonic bony lesions at birth, such as tibial bowing, pseudoarthrosis, or sphenoid wing dysplasia [2]. Other complications of NF1 typically present later in life, including an increased risk for vascular complications (hypertension, stroke, renal artery stenosis, AV malformations), breast cancer (in women), pheochromocytoma, gastrointestinal malfunction and GIST, and renal malignancies. The median life expectancy is about 8 years shorter than the general population, likely due to malignancy and vasculopathy [2].

NF1 is a progressive condition and symptoms will typically increase in number, size, and/or severity with age. Therefore, the disease burden of NF1 in adults, and the need for more frequent and varied medical appointments, is often higher than in childhood. NF1 can be highly variable both within and between families. Affected individuals can have any combination of associated symptoms, and there are no means by which to prognosticate symptom development or progression, which is often frustrating to affected individuals and their families [2]. This variability is particularly important when working with adults involved in reproductive decision-making, as prenatal testing can indicate whether a baby has inherited an *Nf1* mutation, but does not provide a means to know how the disease course will unfold for this child. This uncertainty is often troubling to potential parents and is the basis for choices to intervene in pregnancies or pursue other reproductive options.

Pain and neurologic disability can become paramount concerns for some adult patients with NF1. As neurofibromas grow within the nerve sheaths of the body, tumors can impact normal nerve function by means of mass effect or nerve compression. Depending upon the location of the tumor(s) within the central and peripheral nervous system, some patients experience difficulty with mobility, bowel and/or bladder function, and sexual function. Though not typical, chronic pain syndromes can occur for some patients [3].

Adults living with NF1 are often isolated and can have difficulty accessing the support and services that they need to best manage their medical and emotional concerns. Stigma from visible lesions is reported frequently and can impact relationships [4]. Communities in which people have a chance to meet others living with NF1, whether virtual or in person, are of great assistance. Care providers should stress the importance of maintaining a good quality of life and receiving appropriate support, as well as providing resources as appropriate.

Adults with NF1 may also face feelings of guilt and shame as they consider starting a family of their own and grapple with the inherited nature of their condition and concomitant 50 % chance of passing NF1 on to each child. Additionally, some women with NF1 report a noticeable increase in their symptoms during pregnancy, particularly in the number and size of cutaneous neurofibromas and cafe-au-lait spots [2]. This can be a significant factor in reproductive decision-making. Women with NF1 who are pregnant are not considered to be at high risk unless they have uncontrolled hypertension or known tumors located within the reproductive system.

23.2 Diagnosis

Most people are diagnosed with NF1 by clinical evaluation. A skin exam completed by a specialist well-acquainted with features of NF1 and a thorough ophthalmologic exam will be sufficient for diagnosis in most cases. Genetic testing can be used to supplement the clinical evaluation for cases in which diagnostic criteria are not entirely met. MRI and other imaging are not routinely conducted for diagnostic purposes, though images that exist for other purposes may be reviewed at the time of evaluation. Segmental or regional NF1 is diagnosed in individuals who have symptoms of NF1 confined to one region of the body and whose parents are unaffected by NF1. Segmental NF1 is caused by somatic, rather than germline, *Nf1* mutations [2].

23.2.1 Distinguishing NF1 from NF2 and Schwannomatosis

Two disorders related to NF1 are neurofibromatosis 2 (NF2) and schwannomatosis. It is important to distinguish between NF1, NF2, and schwannomatosis, as there are different management strategies and counseling issues for each [3].

NF2 is characterized by multiple benign nervous system tumors, primarily schwannomas, meningiomas, and ependymomas, none of which are seen as part of NF1. People with NF2 can also have juvenile cataracts. The hallmark of NF2 is bilateral vestibular schwannomas, which can cause progressive hearing loss and often lead to deafness in the third or fourth decade. Very little overlap exists between NF1 and NF2. Occasionally, people with NF2 can have cafe-au-lait spots or cutaneous neurofibromas, but tend to have many fewer in number than people with NF1 [1]. The average age of onset of symptoms for NF2 is between 18 and 24 years of age, while people with NF1 tend to show symptoms in the first decade of life. The gold standard for diagnosis of NF2 is a high-resolution brain MRI with thin cuts through the internal auditory canals. If this study shows no evidence of vestibular tumors by the age of 30, the person is unlikely to have NF2 [5]. Molecular testing can also be helpful when distinguishing NF1 from NF2.

Schwannomatosis causes growth of multiple benign schwannomas, which are not part of NF1. In fact, there is no known clinical overlap between NF1 and schwannomatosis. As both NF2 and schwannomatosis can present with multiple schwannomas, the distinction between these two diseases is more challenging. The primary difference between schwannomatosis and NF2 is that people with schwannomatosis do not develop vestibular schwannomas. The schwannomatosis phenotype may not yet be fully appreciated because it is a rare disease and only recently described. A clinical exam by an NF expert, MRI review, and pathology reports from any removed lesions are often typically sufficient for accurate diagnosis. Molecular testing can be helpful, but not always conclusive, as the two genes that have been associated with schwannomatosis thus far do not explain all diagnosed cases [5, 6].

23.3 Treatment

Treatment for NF1 remains symptomatic. Surgery is the mainstay for addressing symptomatic tumors, though in many instances surgically-induced nerve damage results in a poor outcome. For this reason, any adult NF1 patient with a symptomatic tumor should be seen by an NF specialist prior to pursuing surgery. Plastic surgery can be pursued to remove cutaneous neurofibromas and minimize the resultant scarring [3]. Medications can address hypertension and pain. Mind-body therapies, such as acupuncture and biofeedback, can assist with pain management, as well. No known compounds or medications can prevent the symptoms of NF1. Clinical trials for adults are focused primarily on treating aggressive tumors that either have undergone malignant conversion or are not amenable to surgery [3]. Access to support groups or other communities of people living with NF1 can assist with feelings of isolation and stigma, thereby potentially reducing risk factors for depression and anxiety.

23.4 Genetics

(*NF video clip Part 2*)

NF1 is caused by mutations in the *Nf1* gene at 17q11.2. Approximately 97 % of people meeting the clinical criteria for NF1 will be found to have a mutation within this gene. It is thought that the remaining individuals might either have a low level of mosaicism for an *Nf1* mutation or may have a mutation in a control region for this gene that is not found at this locus [2]. Alternatively, a number of individuals with cafe-au-lait spots and skin fold freckling have been found to have mutations in a different gene called *SPRED1*. This constellation of features is referred to as Legius syndrome and can appear to mimic NF1 [7]. However, individuals with Legius syndrome do not appear to be at risk for developing neurofibromas or other tumors within the NF1 spectrum, which is important both for individual prognosis and for reproductive decision-making [7]. *SPRED1* testing is often performed as a reflex test following negative genetic testing for NF1.

Over 500 mutations have been described within the *Nf1* gene, including in-frame, frameshift, and truncating mutations, as well as small and large deletions. Mutations in *Nf1* are thought to be 100 % penetrant by adulthood [8]. Only a few genotype/phenotype correlations exist at this time:

1. Whole gene deletions/NF1 microdeletion: Deletion of the whole *Nf1* gene is associated with a large number and early appearance of dermal neurofibromas, somatic overgrowth, and more severe intellectual impairment than usual [9].
2. A 3 base pair in-frame deletion of exon 17 (c.2970-2972 delAAT) results in typical pigment abnormalities but no cutaneous or superficial plexiform neurofibromas [10].
3. NF1 microduplication results in a lack of NF1 features but possible seizures and intellectual disabilities [11].

The variability of NF1 is probably due to a combination of genetic and non-genetic factors, making genotype/phenotype correlation difficult.

23.5 Genetic Counseling Issues

While genetic testing for NF1 can be of assistance in some cases, it lacks consistent clinical utility. Identification of a mutation within the *Nf1* gene can help to confirm a diagnosis of NF1 and provide information to test other family members, but does not impact management or prognostication of symptoms. Additionally, there are no identified interventions at this time that can prevent or decrease the symptoms of NF1. As symptoms of NF1 tend to occur early in life, issues surrounding presymptomatic testing typically do not arise and clinical evaluation is often sufficient for diagnosis [3].

Genetic testing is important for adults who are considering starting a family and might want to pursue either preimplantation genetic diagnosis (PGD) for NF1 or prenatal testing once a pregnancy is achieved. Both of these options require an individual to have a known mutation within the *Nf1* gene. PGD has not been widely used in the NF1 community, and most couples that choose to undergo prenatal testing are doing so in order to be prepared. As NF1 can be widely variable within a family, understanding that a baby has inherited the mutation from a parent does not allow for prediction of clinical course. Thus, prospective parents may not take the risk of invasive prenatal testing.

23.6 Neurofibromatosis 1 Case History

W.Y. is a 32-year-old man who was diagnosed with NF1 in childhood based on multiple cafe-au-lait spots and bilateral axillary freckling. In puberty, he began to develop cutaneous neurofibromas on his chest, back, and arms. He had some difficulty in school, and required support in several of his subjects in junior high and high school. He is not married and has no children. He is a warehouse manager and has recently noticed significant pain in his left leg at work causing him to have difficulty completing various aspects of his job. MRI revealed a large plexiform neurofibroma growing along the sciatic nerve. The neurologist discussed medical and nonmedical pain management options, as well as the potential need to adjust some of his daily activities. W.Y. told the neurologist that he had some questions about NF1 and was referred for genetic counseling. He presents with his mother.

The counseling session begins by asking W.Y. to explain the reason for referral. He indicates that he wants to learn more about NF1 and how it might affect him. He states that as a child, he had never thought much about it, but by adolescence was bothered by the appearance of the cutaneous neurofibromas, especially those that were noticeable to others. He says that he learned to live with that aspect of NF1, but now he is hearing that he might have to reduce or change his work. He wants to know what else might happen to him in the coming years. He becomes noticeably anxious as he says this. His mother adds that she has always wondered why he has NF1, since neither she nor his dad have symptoms, and there is no other family history of this condition. She muses about whether it had to do with her being sick and using antibiotics while she was pregnant with W.Y.

The genetic counselor acknowledges how scary it is to consider losing a meaningful portion of one's life and to hear that symptom progression might cause the future loss of other abilities. She also validates that it is normal for W.Y.'s mother to wonder what caused NF1 in her son and to blame herself. She explains that she would like to ask some family history questions to understand more about the origin of NF in their family.

As they talk, the counselor notes that there are no other people in the family who have symptoms consistent with NF1. She indicates to W.Y. that this is fairly common, as half of the adults with NF1 are the first person in their family to be affected. The counselor then discusses the genetics of NF1 and uses the family history to normalize W.Y.'s situation.

The counselor asks if W.Y. has ever had genetic testing to locate his *Nf1* mutation. He shakes his head no, so she offers to coordinate testing. W.Y. asks whether it would make any difference to his diagnosis or treatment, and the counselor tells him that testing would confirm the diagnosis, but not change treatment. The discovery of a mutation would provide information for W.Y., should he choose to have children of his own in the future and want to pursue preimplantation genetic diagnosis (PGD) or prenatal testing. W.Y.'s mother seems interested and asks if she could have testing as well. The counselor inquires about her motivation. She replies that it would help "clear her mind" by verifying that she did not contribute to her son having NF1. The counselor agrees that it would be desirable to be able to let go of the self-blame, and reviews that there are no known links between behavior, diet, or medications taken during pregnancy and the development of NF. W.Y.'s mother says that she knows this, but still wants to consider testing. W.Y. says that he doesn't care about testing, but will go ahead if his mom wants him to and if it would be beneficial if he ever wants to have kids.

The counselor inquires about whether W.Y. is involved in a relationship and whether his partner has any knowledge of NF1. W.Y. says that he is not seeing anyone, and comments that he sometimes thinks it might be better for him to stay single and not have children. When the counselor invites him to say more about this, he shares that dating has been hard for him because of his appearance and his feeling that women often judge him or aren't attracted to him because of this, and that he isn't sure how or when to talk with potential partners about the genetic nature of NF1. W.Y.'s mother seems suddenly upset, and interjects that his tumors shouldn't matter because they don't change who he is as a person. She also states that the "right" woman will be fine with all of it. W.Y. rolls his eyes. The counselor asks whether this is a subject that they have discussed before. They both say that it is. The counselor then asks what their experiences have been around these conversations. W.Y. talks about how his mother wants everything to be okay and so always responds to these concerns by saying that he will find someone who will love him for who he is and not care about the disease. W.Y. goes on to say that he worries about it, sees people look at him differently, and has lived through hearing derogatory comments. He ends by saying, "She doesn't understand because she doesn't have NF1." W.Y.'s mother appears frustrated and says that, of course, she doesn't know exactly what it is like to live with NF1, but she does know her son's many wonderful attributes, and it hurts her to think that people wouldn't take the time to see these because of bumps on his skin.

The counselor comments that everything they have shared with her is very typical, and that W.Y. and his mother are both expressing valid and important perspectives. She encourages them to listen to each other and try to understand each other's viewpoint. She asks whether he is connected with any other adults with NF1, and if he is aware of the group that gathers monthly at a local restaurant to talk about living with NF1. She also spends a few minutes brainstorming with W.Y. about how and when it might feel right to him to bring up his diagnosis with a potential partner. By the end of the conversation W.Y. seems more confident that he will know when the situation presents itself.

The genetic counselor asks W.Y. if he is ready to go ahead with testing, and he indicates that he is. She gathers the necessary insurance information and proceeds with an informed consent discussion for NF1 genetic testing. Testing is sent and a follow-up appointment is made for return of results.

Discussion Questions

- How does having both the adult client and his mother present impact the counseling session?
- How important is it to spend time in the session addressing the mother's views on why her son has NF1?
- Given that the client's diagnosis is not in question and he is not considering children of his own right now, should the counselor challenge the client to further consider his decision to pursue genetic testing that has no current clinical utility?
- Is the balance between providing information and providing supportive counseling appropriate in this session? Why or why not?

W.Y. does not return to clinic for his scheduled appointment. The genetic counselor had reviewed results in advance of the appointment and is aware that a mutation in the NF1 gene was found. She phones W.Y. to reschedule and leaves a message. She does not hear back for a week, so she tries again and leaves another message. After another week passes with no contact, the counselor becomes concerned and phones the neurologist who had initially referred W.Y. to her. The neurologist indicates that W.Y. had called about 4 weeks ago due to increasing pain in his leg. He ordered a PET scan and a needle biopsy of the plexiform neurofibroma in W.Y.'s left leg, and he was ultimately diagnosed with a malignant peripheral nerve sheath tumor (MPNST). W.Y. was referred to oncology and is about to start a course of radiation therapy followed by surgical resection, though the neurosurgeon feels that an amputation of his leg would be the best hope for a cure. The counselor thanks the neurologist for the update and indicates that she has genetic test results for W.Y. The neurologist asks if the result could impact the treatment recommendations, and the counselor says no. She indicates that she will call W.Y. once more the following week and if she does not reach him, she will mail the neurologist a letter with his test results.

The counselor phones W.Y. the following week and this time reaches him. She indicates that the neurologist has informed her about his laboratory results. The counselor asks how this news is affecting him emotionally, and he says that he is scared of what might happen and doesn't want to lose his leg. The counselor says that she can understand his reactions to this news. She goes on to ask about his mother and how she is doing with the information. W.Y. states that she is really positive and keeps telling him that he will be okay, but that he knows she is upset and scared too. The counselor inquires about his other support. He has shared this information with friends and the guys at his workplace. He says that they are a second family and have been really supportive. They are planning a fundraiser to help cover his out-of-pocket medical expenses. The counselor indicates that, although this is an unexpected complication and the unknown can be scary, W.Y. is doing a good job accessing his social support system, which will likely be valuable to him during his treatment. She also offers to talk to him at any time. He thanks her.

As the conversation is drawing to a close, the counselor states that she has received genetic testing results, and asks W.Y. if he would like to receive them now. He says he's not sure and that maybe he can call her in the upcoming months so that they can talk about it then. The counselor agrees, and they end the call.

Discussion Questions

- How does a genetic counselor determine the urgency of communicating genetic test results to a patient? How would it differ in situations in which the result might impact clinical management?
- How does an unexpected intervening event, such as a cancer diagnosis, impact the process of returning genetic testing results to a patient?
- When and how should a genetic counselor recontact a patient in a situation such as this?

23.7 Resources for Patients

Children's Tumor Foundation: www.ctf.org
NF Network: www.nfnetwork.org

References

1. Borofsky, S., & Levy, L. M. (2013). Neurofibromatosis: Types 1 and 2. *American Journal of Neuroradiology, 13*(4), 1071–1077. http://dx.doi.org/10.3174/ajnr.A3534.
2. Boyd, K. P., Korf, B. R., & Theos, A. (2009). Neurofibromatosis type 1. *Journal of the American Academy of Dermatology, 61*(1), 1–14.

3. Ferner, R. E., Huson, S. M., Thomas, N., Moss, C., Willshaw, H., Evans, D. G., et al. (2006). Guidelines for the diagnosis and management of individuals with neurofibromatosis 1. *Journal of Medical Genetics, 44*(2), 81–88.
4. Vranceanu, A. M., Merker, V. L., Park, E., & Plotkin, S. R. (2013). Quality of life among adult patients with neurofibromatosis 1, neurofibromatosis 2 and schwannomatosis: A systematic review of the literature. *Journal of Neuro-Oncology, 114*, 257–262. doi:10.1007/s11060-013-1195-2.
5. Uhlmann, E. J., & Plotkin, S. R. (2012). Neurofibromatoses. In S. Ahmad (Ed.), *Neurodegenerative diseases* (pp. 266–277). New York, NY: Spring Science Business Media.
6. Piotrowski, A., Xie, J., Liu, Y. F., Poplawski, A. B., Gomes, A. R., Madanecki, P., et al. (2014). Germline loss-of-function mutations in LZTR1 predispose to an inherited disorder of multiple schwannomas. *Nature Genetics, 46*, 182.
7. Brems, H., Pasmant, E., Van Minkelen, R., Wimmer, K., Upadhyaya, M., Legius, E., et al. (2012). Review and update of SPRED1 mutations causing Legius syndrome. *Human Mutation, 33*(11), 1538–1546.
8. Patil, S., & Chamberlain, R. S. (2012). Neoplasms associated with germline and somatic NF1 gene mutations. *The Oncologist, 17*(1), 101–116.
9. Leppig, K. A., Kaplan, P., Viskochil, D., Weaver, M., Ortenberg, J., & Stephens, K. (1997). Familial neurofibromatosis 1 microdeletions: Cosegregation with distinct facial phenotype and early onset of cutaneous neurofibromata. *American Journal of Medical Genetics, 73*(2), 197–204.
10. Pasmant, E., Vidaud, M., Vidaud, D., & Wolkenstein, P. (2012). Neurofibromatosis type 1: From genotype to phenotype. *Journal of Medical Genetics, 49*(8), 483–489.
11. Moles, K. J., Gowans, G. C., Gedela, S., Beversdorf, D., Yu, A., Seaver, A. H., et al. (2012). NF1 microduplications: Identification of seven nonrelated individuals provides further characterization of the phenotype. *Genetics in Medicine, 14*(5), 508–514.

Chapter 24
Tuberous Sclerosis

Amanda Bergner

Tuberous sclerosis complex (TSC) is the second most common primary neurocutaneous syndrome, with an estimated incidence as high as 1/5,800 and approximately 50,000 affected individuals in the USA. TSC is an autosomal dominant genetic condition that is expressed in individuals harboring a mutation in either the *TSC1* or *TSC2* gene, found at 9q34.13 and 16p13.3, respectively [1]. About 15 % of people who meet the clinical criteria for TSC do not have a mutation in either *TSC1* or *TSC2*, indicating further genetic heterogeneity. TSC is thought to be fully penetrant with variable expressivity both within and between families, likely due to modifying genes and microenvironmental factors. Approximately two-thirds of people with TSC have *de novo* mutations, while the remaining one-third have inherited a mutation from a parent [2]. TSC is pan-ethnic and affects men and women equally, though women tend to have milder disease than men [2]. The majority of diagnoses are based on highly specific and sensitive clinical criteria. As the diagnostic criteria have become more specific over the past several decades, and clinicians are better acquainted with TSC features, the incidence estimates have increased due to the detection of many previously undiagnosed individuals with milder features. Genetic testing can assist diagnosis in cases involving individuals who do not yet meet clinical criteria.

Electronic supplementary material Supplementary material is available in the online version of this chapter at 10.1007/978-1-4899-7482-2_24. Videos can also be accessed at http://www.springerimages.com/videos/978-1-4899-7481-5.

A. Bergner (✉)
Department of Neurology, Johns Hopkins University School of Medicine, 600 North Wolfe Street, Phipps 117, Baltimore, MD 21287, USA

McKusick-Nathans Institute of Genetic Medicine, Johns Hopkins University School of Medicine, 600 North Wolfe Street, Phipps 117, Baltimore, MD 21287, USA
e-mail: abergne1@jhmi.edu

J.S. Goldman (ed.), *Genetic Counseling for Adult Neurogenetic Disease*,
DOI 10.1007/978-1-4899-7482-2_24

24.1 Clinical Presentation

TSC is a progressive condition in which symptoms typically worsen with age and affected individuals can have any combination of associated symptoms, making it difficult to predict disease course for an individual. However, *TSC2* mutations typically cause more severe symptoms than *TSC1* mutations [2]. Additionally a higher number of cortical tubers are generally correlated with a higher level of cognitive impairment and a greater seizure burden [3].

The diagnostic features of TSC primarily involve the skin (i.e., ash leaf spots, facial angiofibromas, Shagreen patches, ungual/periungual fibromas), the kidneys (i.e., renal cysts, renal angiomyolipoma), the lungs (i.e., lymphangioleiomyomatosis), the heart (i.e., cardiac rhabdomyoma), and the brain (i.e., cortical tubers, subependymal giant cell astrocytomas, subependymal nodules) [4]. There can also be retinal lesions including hamartomas and achromic patches; though these findings are common for people with TSC, they are typically asymptomatic [4]. Even when symptoms are not present at birth, TSC is considered a congenital condition. In childhood, the two most common presentations of TSC are seizures/infantile spasms and autism with developmental delay [1]. Occasionally, children may be diagnosed because of renal or cardiac dysfunction. Once children come to medical attention and a full evaluation is undertaken, most are found to have hypomelanotic macules and brain lesions consistent with TSC. As children age, they can acquire additional cutaneous manifestations, such as facial angiofibromas and forehead plaques. The facial angiofibromas of TSC are the most disfiguring and can lead to social-emotional concerns, but none of the skin lesions of TSC cause medical complications.

Certain brain lesions can progress over time, causing further medical complications. Seizures can begin at any age and continue throughout life. When individuals are diagnosed prior to the onset of seizures, families may experience a great deal of anxiety as they "wait" for this particular and frequent feature to present. Most individuals require multiple antiepileptic drugs for treatment; seizures associated with TSC are often medically intractable [4]. Status epilepticus is a major cause of premature death.

Some individuals with TSC have cardiac rhabdomyomas, which develop *in utero* and begin to regress after birth. In a minority of cases, these growths can cause arrhythmias or infant sudden cardiac death. Dependent on the size and location of the rhabdomyoma, tumor resection may be considered [1]. Otherwise, these masses are asymptomatic and require no treatment.

Kidney complications continue to progress throughout the lifespan, and kidney failure and hemorrhages are the second most common causes of premature death for people with TSC.

Lung features can become evident in the third and fourth decades of life, and almost exclusively affect women; estrogen has been identified as a possible source of proliferation of particular cells in the lung [5]. Lymphangioleiomyomatosis (LAM) is a progressively degenerative pulmonary disorder that causes reduced lung capacity, thus limiting daily activities. Some people progress to respiratory failure and death, and currently no treatment other than lung transplantation exists [1]. Bronchopneumonia is another major cause of premature death for people with TSC.

Psychiatric manifestations of TSC in childhood are primarily autism and developmental delay; some children exhibit signs of hyperactivity or attention-deficit hyperactivity disorder (ADHD). A significant proportion of these individuals will go on to be diagnosed with mental retardation; very few adults with TSC are cognitively intact [1]. Adults with TSC have a higher rate of depression, aggression, schizophrenia, and bipolar disease than the general population [4].

Most adults with TSC do not function independently. They may live in specialized group homes or require ongoing support from family, and can benefit from employment and vocational rehabilitation services. Incarceration is not uncommon for adults with TSC due to aggressive or violent behaviors that are frequent psychiatric manifestations of their condition. Some adults with TSC have a milder presentation with less cognitive and psychiatric burden [4]. Adults living with TSC are often isolated and can, therefore, have difficulty accessing the support and services that they need to best manage their medical concerns. Virtual or in-person TSC support communities can be beneficial. The medical team should address how to maintain a good quality of life and access appropriate support, and provide resources as needed [4].

Given the frequency of significant medical problems, many adults with TSC do not have children. Those who do may face feelings of guilt, shame, and fear as they grapple with the inherited nature of their condition. Many couples consider preimplantation genetic diagnosis (PGD) and/or prenatal testing, as symptoms of TSC cannot be predicted and are known to vary within a family. Therefore, an affected adult cannot presume that their child will have similar symptoms. In fact, a child who inherits TSC from a parent has a fairly high likelihood to develop at least one significant medical problem, such as seizures or kidney disease. Depending on their symptoms and medication, women with TSC who are pregnant may be managed as high risk, particularly those with seizures. The balance between maintaining seizure control and limiting the risk of birth defects in the unborn child due to the known teratogenicity of multiple antiepileptic medications can be challenging [1].

24.2 Diagnosis

TSC diagnosis is made by clinical evaluation, and the classification of definite, probable, or possible TSC is based on the features detected at the time of evaluation [4]. In most cases, a skin exam completed by a specialist well acquainted with features of TSC, an ophthalmologic exam, and kidney and brain imaging are sufficient for diagnosis. Genetic testing can supplement the clinical evaluation for cases in which diagnostic criteria for definite TSC are not met. Individuals with TSC may not receive a definitive diagnosis for many years; delayed diagnosis can complicate adjustment to the disorder and lead to increased anxiety in individuals and families as they wait for other potential symptoms to develop. Surveillance is continued during this time, and anxiety should be addressed and treated.

24.3 Treatment and Management

Treatment for TSC remains symptomatic. Brain tumors may require surgical resection. Renal ultrasounds are used for surveillance to detect masses or cysts, which, if over a certain diameter, are resected to reduce the risk of hemorrhage and renal failure. Poly-drug anticonvulsant therapy is standard for patients with seizures, and epilepsy surgery may be considered for individuals whose seizures remain resistant to medication [4]. Oopherectomy can be considered for women with LAM to reduce the exposure to estrogen; oxygen supplementation and lung transplantation are other possible treatments [1]. Multiple research protocols using chemotherapies and anti-angiogenesis factors, such as mTOR inhibitors, are currently underway and will hopefully lead to other treatment options for patients.

24.4 Genetics

Two genes have been implicated in TSC: *TSC1* and *TSC2*. Approximately 85 % of people with definite TSC will harbor a mutation in one of these two genes. About 31 % have a mutation in *TSC1* and 69 % have a mutation in *TSC2* [5]. *TSC1* mutations are primarily small deletions, insertions, and nonsense mutations, while *TSC2* mutations include large deletions or rearrangements [4]. Genetic testing should be pursued by first sequencing both genes and, if negative, following up with deletion/duplication analysis of both genes.

Some individuals who receive negative genetic testing results may actually have a low level of mosaicism for a mutation in one of the two genes; empiric data based on multiple studies estimates the frequency of somatic mosaicism to be about 1 % of all people with TSC [2]. Alternatively, individuals with negative testing for the two known genes may have a mutation in a gene that has not yet been described. Some individuals have a deletion that encompasses both the *TSC2* locus and the adjacent *PKD1* locus, which has been implicated in autosomal dominant polycystic kidney disease (ADPKD). Individuals with this molecular finding will have features of both TSC and ADPKD [1].

TSC is thought to be 100 % penetrant by adulthood. Several genotype/phenotype correlations exist at this time. However, the variability of TSC is likely due to a combination of genetic and stochastic factors, making genotype/phenotype correlation difficult. The following correlations are known:

- *TSC2* mutations generally produce a more severe phenotype than *TSC1* mutations, including increased likelihood of renal malignancy, intellectual disability, autistic disorder, and infantile spasms [1].
- Women with mutations in the carboxy terminus of the *TSC2* gene are more likely to develop LAM, or to have more significant symptoms of LAM [6].
- Renal cysts occur more frequently with *TSC1* mutations, small *TSC2* mutations, and large deletions/rearrangements of the contiguous genes *TSC2* and *PKD1*.

24.5 Genetic Counseling Issues

Genetic testing for TSC can provide information for families, but lacks consistent clinical utility. As with most genetic testing, an affected individual is generally tested first in order to have the best opportunity to locate the mutation in that family. Identification of a mutation within the *TSC1* or *TSC2* gene can help to confirm a diagnosis of TSC. However, determining the specific mutation does not impact management choices or prediction of symptoms, other than the likelihood that manifestations of TSC due to mutations in *TSC2* will be more severe. Additionally, no interventions exist at this time to prevent or decrease the symptoms of TSC. As symptoms of TSC tend to have an early onset, issues surrounding presymptomatic testing do not frequently arise and clinical evaluation is often sufficient for diagnosis.

Genetic testing is important for adults who are considering starting a family of their own and might want to pursue either PGD or prenatal testing. Both of these options require knowledge of the individual's specific mutation. As TSC can be variable within a family, understanding that a baby has inherited the mutation from a parent does not allow for prediction of clinical course. Thus, prospective parents may not risk invasive prenatal testing unless they are considering pregnancy termination.

If there is an affected parent, recurrence risk of TSC is 50 %. If a child is diagnosed and thought to be the first person in the family with TSC, both parents should undergo a comprehensive skin exam, retinal exam, kidney imaging, and brain imaging to assess for a mild phenotype that has not yet been diagnosed [4]. If molecular testing in the child reveals a mutation, parents should undergo genetic testing. If neither parent is found to be affected or carry a *TSC1* or *TSC2* mutation, the recurrence risk for a future pregnancy is about 5 %, which represents the estimated rate of germline mosaicism in this population [7].

When coordinating genetic testing for TSC, it is important to understand the relative frequency of mutations in each of the two implicated genes, as well as the most appropriate methods by which to undertake molecular analysis. Additionally when interpreting a negative test result, the possibility of somatic mosaicism should be recognized [4].

24.6 Case History (Fig. 24.1)

K.Y. is a 21-year-old woman who has a family history of TSC. Her older brother was diagnosed as a child and followed by the local neurologist for seizures. K.Y. has recently become engaged and has questions regarding her risk of having a child with TSC, so the local neurologist referred her for genetic counseling. She presents for her genetic counseling appointment with her fiancé.

The genetic counselor opens the appointment by asking K.Y. to describe her reasons for coming. K.Y. indicates that her brother is 25 years old and has had seizures since he was about 8. He takes medication, but sometimes still has seizures. When she was about 15 years old, her mother told her that her brother had TSC. Since her engagement, she has become concerned about transmitting TSC to future children and wants more information.

The counselor asks K.Y. what it was like growing up watching her brother manage the symptoms of TSC. K.Y. recalls that his condition was a big part of her childhood, and it often scared her to see her brother have a seizure. She frequently attended her brother's medical appointments and recalls that she secretly wondered if he was going to die. As he got older, she noticed some growths on his face and wasn't sure if she could "catch" whatever it was that he had. Later when she was told that her brother's symptoms were due to TSC, she went online to learn more, and discovered that TSC is genetic. This information has caused her to worry that she might have a child with TSC. The counselor says that it can be very scary to have a sibling with a chronic medical condition, and that K.Y.'s emotional experience is typical. She also affirms that it is reasonable to wonder about her own risk of having a child with TSC.

The counselor asks K.Y. how her brother is doing now. K.Y. indicates that he had some learning and behavior difficulties in school, so he never finished high school. He still has seizures occasionally, and has recently become more

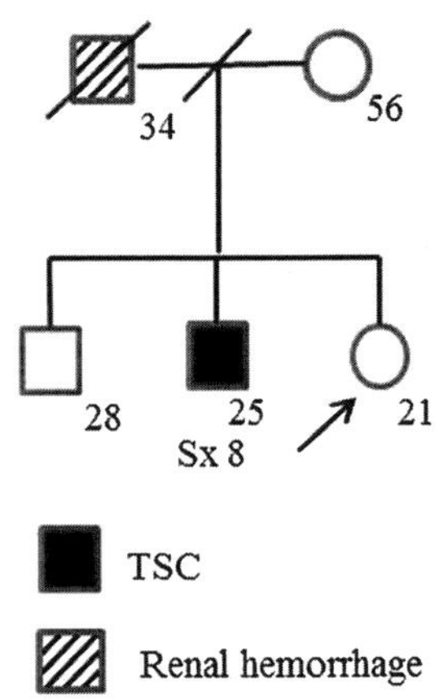

Fig. 24.1 TSC case history pedigree

aggressive. He was living at home until last month when his mother chose to move him into a specialized group home because she could no longer manage his challenging behavior. Though the house is calmer and she feels safer, K.Y. says that she and her mother are both sad and miss him. The counselor listens and reflects back that, although this transition is hard right now, it seems that K.Y. has been able to identify some positive aspects of the change as well.

The counselor suggests that they start by reviewing K.Y.'s family history. K.Y. has another brother who is 28 and in good health. Her mother has hypothyroidism, but no other medical concerns. Her father died when she was a baby, and her mother and stepfather raised her. She has several stepsiblings who are all well. K.Y. indicates that she has had migraines since she was a teenager and was recently diagnosed with asthma, but has no other medical concerns. There is no other family history related to TSC. When asked about the cause of her father's death, K.Y. indicates that she isn't sure, but thinks it had something to do with his stomach. The counselor asks K.Y. if her brother or her family has done any genetic testing for TSC. K.Y. isn't sure, but says she can ask her mother.

The counselor reviews the family history with K.Y., indicating that it is possible that her brother is the first person in her family to have TSC, which is the case for about 2/3 of people who have this diagnosis. She also discusses that, without knowing more about K.Y.'s father and his cause of death, she cannot exclude the possibility that K.Y.'s father also had TSC. She then states that understanding which of these possibilities is most likely will influence the calculation of her recurrence risk. If her father had TSC, K.Y. would be at a 50 % chance of having inherited a gene mutation from him. If he did not have TSC, she would have a 5 % chance. Her lack of seizures, learning problems, or other major medical concerns is a good sign, but she will likely need further evaluations to determine whether she has a mild form of TSC.

The counselor then reviews the genes involved with TSC and the process of genetic testing. She indicates that K.Y.'s brother should be tested first, and then, if a mutation is identified, K.Y. can pursue testing. K.Y. agrees to ask her mother about whether her brother has had genetic testing and about her father's health and the cause of his death. She will also gather any relevant medical records that she can for review. A follow-up appointment is scheduled for the following month.

K.Y. presents 1 month later for follow-up. The counselor summarizes the prior appointment and asks whether K.Y. was able to locate any further information. K.Y. indicates that her mother does not think they have done any genetic testing for her brother. She then presents her father's medical records, including a hospitalization note. The hospital report indicates that her father had multiple renal cysts and lists his cause of death as renal hemorrhage. The counselor says that in light of these records, it is more likely that her father had TSC, and, therefore, a higher chance that K.Y. herself could have inherited a gene mutation from him.

The counselor inquires whether K.Y. thinks that her brother could undergo genetic testing. She says that their local neurologist sees him regularly and perhaps could coordinate this at his next visit. The counselor provides K.Y. with written information for the neurologist about testing and K.Y. agrees to follow up with the counselor again once her brother's genetic testing has been completed.

Discussion Questions

- How can the experience of growing up with a sibling who has a significant chronic disease impact an individual's attitude about the possibility of having a child with the same disease?
- How can a thorough investigation of family history affect coordination of genetic testing and calculation of recurrence risk?

K.Y. returns to clinic 5 months later. In the meantime, her brother has undergone genetic testing for TSC and no mutations were found in either the *TSC1* or *TSC2* gene. The counselor reviews the lab report and confirms that both genes were tested by sequencing and by deletion/duplication analysis at a lab familiar with TSC testing. The counselor reminds K.Y. that about 15 % of people with TSC will have negative genetic testing, but that they still have TSC. The counselor goes on to tell K.Y. that her brother's results mean that K.Y. cannot have genetic testing for TSC. In the absence of any other information, her recurrence risk could be estimated, but not specifically determined. K.Y. asks how she might be able to gather more information to further refine her risk for carrying a TSC mutation. The counselor indicates that she could undergo a series of evaluations, including a skin and eye exam, and brain and kidney imaging to determine whether she has any mild symptoms of TSC. K.Y. elects to pursue this option and the counselor agrees to have their clinic assist in coordinating these evaluations. They agree to meet again once the evaluations are complete.

Over the next several months, K.Y. undergoes the recommended evaluations and her records are forwarded to the counselor. As the counselor prepares to see K.Y. in follow-up, she reviews the results and learns that K.Y. is found to have five hypopigmented macules, a retinal achromic patch, and multiple kidney cysts. The counselor reviews the records with the geneticist with whom she works, who agrees that K.Y. appears to have TSC. The counselor knows that this will be new information for K.Y. and so prepares for the clinic visit by blocking the appointment following K.Y.'s in case they need extra time.

K.Y. returns to clinic to review her results. The counselor indicates that, according to the skin evaluation report, the renal ultrasound report, and the ophthalmology report, K.Y. has a mild case of TSC. K.Y. appears surprised and doesn't say anything for a moment. Then she says, "Are you sure?" The counselor replies that she is sure and has reviewed the records with a knowledgeable physician. They then review the common features of TSC and what is likely to arise for K.Y. in the future. The counselor reminds her that it is difficult to predict specific symptoms given the variability of the condition.

K.Y. then asks about her future children. The counselor indicates that she probably has a 50 % chance of passing a mutation to each child. Because her brother's genetic testing was already completed and no mutation was located in *TSC1* or *TSC2*, PGD and prenatal testing for TSC are not possible. The counselor reviews several findings that can sometimes be seen on prenatal ultrasound, but says that these are not always present and so cannot be considered a reliable form of diagnosis. The counselor reminds her that even if they knew whether the baby had inherited a TSC mutation, they would not be able to predict the course of the disease. K.Y. begins to cry and the counselor comforts her. K.Y. indicates that she is okay, but wants to think about all this for a while, and then come back with her fiancé to discuss their options. The counselor agrees that this sounds reasonable and they set a follow-up appointment for 2 month's time.

Discussion Questions

- What are some of the challenges in disclosing a diagnosis of an inherited condition to a fiancé?
- What responsibility does the genetic counselor have to ensure that the lab tests, radiology scans, and clinical evaluations are complete and reliable, as this is the information upon which the diagnosis and recurrence risk are based?
- How does a lack of mutation identification affect a counseling session, and would you have discussed other reproductive options without the presence of the fiancé?

References

1. Lendvay, T. S., & Marshall, F. F. (2003). The tuberous sclerosis complex and its highly variable manifestations. *The Journal of Urology, 169*(5), 1635–1642.
2. Sancak, O., Nellist, M., Goedbloed, M., Elfferich, P., Wouters, C., Maat-Kievit, A., et al. (2005). Mutational analysis of the TSC1 and TSC2 genes in a diagnostic setting: Genotype–phenotype correlations and comparison of diagnostic DNA techniques in Tuberous Sclerosis Complex. *European Journal of Human Genetics, 13*(6), 731–741.
3. Goodman, M., Lamm, S. H., Engel, A., Shepherd, C. W., Hauser, O. W., & Gomez, M. R. (1997). Cortical tuber count: A biomarker indicating neurologic severity of tuberous sclerosis complex. *Journal of Child Neurology, 12*(2), 85–90.
4. Manohara, D. (2012). Primary care management of tuberous sclerosis complex in children. *Journal of the American Academy of Nurse Practitioners, 24*(7), 391–399.
5. Van Eeghen, A. M., Black, M. E., Pulsifer, M. B., Kwiatkowski, D. J., & Thiele, E. A. (2012). Genotype and cognitive phenotype of patients with tuberous sclerosis complex. *European Journal of Human Genetics, 20*(5), 510–515.
6. Strizheva, G. D., Carsillo, T., Kruger, W. D., Sullivan, E. J., Ryu, J. H., & Henske, E. P. (2001). The spectrum of mutations in TSC1 and TSC2 in women with tuberous sclerosis and lymphangiomyomatosis. *American Journal of Respiratory and Critical Care Medicine, 163*(1), 253–258.
7. Leung, A. K. C., & Robson, W. L. M. (2007). Tuberous sclerosis complex. A review. *Journal of Pediatric Health Care, 21*(2), 108–114.

Part VIII
The Clinical Evaluation

Chapter 25
The Neurological Examination and Testing

Jacinda B. Sampson

Genetic counselors working in neurology should be informed about the neurological examination. They can help explain findings to patients, but also may be called on to collate outside medical records for the clinical team. For the adult patient, this could be decades of records from multiple physicians. When sifting through piles of medical records inches thick, what information is relevant? Which studies or findings will the neurologist or geneticist need, and why were they ordered? An understanding of the general and neurological exam, and commonly ordered tests and studies, can help find the relevant records or, importantly, which ones are missing. This chapter is not meant to be a substitute for medical school, but to orient the genetic counselor to exams and tests encountered in daily practice.

25.1 The General Physical Exam

Suspicious exam findings may direct the doctor from an environmental or acquired cause of disease toward a genetic one, prompting the neurogenetics referral. In the interview portion of the visit, the review of systems queries subjective symptoms related to the major body organs and functions. The physical examination, from top to toe, seeks objective signs of disease. Exam elements are chosen based on the patient's reported symptoms, so they often vary from patient to patient.

Electronic supplementary material Supplementary material is available in the online version of this chapter at 10.1007/978-1-4899-7482-2_25. Videos can also be accessed at http://www.springerimages.com/videos/978-1-4899-7481-5.

J.B. Sampson (✉)
Department of Neurology, Columbia University Medical Center, 630 W. 168th St., Box 16, New York, NY 10032, USA
e-mail: js4171@cumc.columbia.edu

J.S. Goldman (ed.), *Genetic Counseling for Adult Neurogenetic Disease*,
DOI 10.1007/978-1-4899-7482-2_25

25.1.1 Cardiovascular Exam and Studies

The cardiovascular exam begins with the vital signs of heart rate and blood pressure. *Auscultation* of the heart may detect rhythm irregularities and murmurs, or bruits may be heard over the carotid or other arteries. The pressure of a finger can inform about peripheral pulses, the return of color to blanched skin about capillary refill, and residual indentation in the skin about edema.

Complaints of dizziness, fainting, dyspnea upon exertion, chest pain, or palpitations may prompt cardiac referral or further testing. A normal *cardiac catheterization* (coronary artery angiogram) in the setting of congestive heart failure (CHF) may be the "dog that did not bark," alerting the referring physician that a genetic etiology, rather than coronary artery disease, may be responsible.

A 12-lead *electrocardiogram* (ECG) detects the electrical activity of the heart. A *Holter monitor* or event monitor is worn for a longer period of time and is a more sensitive test for episodic rhythm abnormalities. Mention of a pacemaker or pacer/defibrillator suggests that a medically significant arrhythmia was found. Arrhythmia may be genetic in origin (Brugada and long QT syndrome) or an element of a syndrome (Kearn-Sayre syndrome and myotonic dystrophy).

An *echocardiogram* is an ultrasound that shows the muscular function of the heart. A *transthoracic echocardiogram* is a noninvasive test in which the probe is applied to the chest wall. A *transesophageal echocardiogram* is performed by inserting a probe down the esophagus to the level of the heart, which gives a better view of the cardiac valves and aortic root; it can be informative in an obese individual when the transthoracic technique does not adequately visualize the heart. Alternatively, a *cardiac MRI* can detect the early fibrosis of cardiomyopathy. The heart muscle is affected in certain muscular dystrophies, mitochondrial, and storage disorders.

25.1.2 Pulmonary Exam and Studies

Decreased breath sounds at the lung bases, abdominal paradoxical breathing, use of accessory muscles of the neck in breathing, and interruption of speech for breaths may indicate weakness of intercostal muscles and the diaphragm. Lung function is prognostically important in many neuromuscular disorders. An example of a genetic disorder for which respiratory impairment may be the presenting symptom is acid maltase deficiency.

Pulmonary function testing (PFTs) quantifies lung volume and breathing strength, and can distinguish asthma and emphysema (or chronic obstructive pulmonary disease, or COPD) from neuromuscular respiratory weakness.

A home overnight *oximetry* is a screening test for nighttime breathing problems. *Polysomnography* (a sleep study) may reveal hypoventilation or obstructive breathing pattern due to weak bulbar muscles of the neck and throat.

25.1.3 Dermatologic Exam

The skin may be a superficial organ, but can be deeply meaningful in the diagnosis of neurogenetic disorders (e.g., café-au-lait spots in the neurofibromatoses). Other symptoms, such as ash-leaf spots in tuberous sclerosis, may only be visible when illuminated by a Wood's lamp (ultraviolet light). The skin can be a clue to vascular abnormalities (e.g., angiomata in Fabry's disease, arteriovenous malformations in hereditary hemorrhagic telangiectasia, port-wine stains in Sturge-Weber syndrome, and caput medusa veins in end-stage liver failure).

Skin elasticity, the appearance of scars, and even skin texture (velvety skin, or follicular hyperkeratosis) can suggest a connective tissue disorder such as Ehlers-Danlos syndrome, Marfan's syndrome, or Ullrich muscular dystrophy. A history of unexplained poor wound healing or surgical incision dehiscence (pulling apart) would be significant for these disorders.

25.1.4 Orthopedic Exam

Skeletal proportions (Marfan's), stature (tall in Marfan's, short in mitochondrial disorders), and joint mobility can be meaningful. Spine abnormalities such as scoliosis, joint abnormalities, such as the presence and pattern of contractures (e.g., at the elbows for Emery-Dreifuss muscular dystrophy, but also the deep finger flexors for Bethlem myopathy), or hypermobility or history of dislocation can be meaningful in connective tissue and muscular dystrophies.

25.2 Neurologic Examination

The neurologic exam is designed to localize a neurological problem within the "black box" of the brain, spinal cord, peripheral nerves, and muscles [1]. Areas of the brain testable by the neurologic exam are considered "eloquent" (i.e., the exam findings "tell" the examiner localizing information). However, portions of the brain remain ineloquent, and for these areas, ancillary testing can aid localization.

25.2.1 Mental Status and Neuropsychiatric Evaluation

The mini mental status exam (MMSE) and *Montreal Cognitive Assessment* (MoCA) exams are brief screening tools for cognitive function, and can be performed in a routine neurology visit. In contrast, a neuropsychological evaluation may take 6 h or several sessions and is composed of multiple tests assessing different areas of cognitive function, such as language, visuospatial function, construction, motor function, verbal and nonverbal memory, attention, abstract thinking, and executive function [2]. Depending on the test, weaknesses can localize to the frontal, temporal, or parietal lobes, and to cortical or subcortical areas. Neuropsychological testing may help identify developmental and learning disabilities. It can help distinguish memory problems related to depression, dementia, or feigned symptoms. Repeated neuropsychiatric evaluation can document cognitive decline (see Chap. 26 for more detailed explanation of testing).

25.2.2 Cranial Nerves

Cranial nerves (CN) serve the special senses, sensation of the head and other areas, and muscles of the eyes, head, and some of the neck [3].

The olfactory nerve (*CN I*) is not routinely tested (which is why medical records documentation may read "cranial nerves II through XII intact"). Patients may be unaware of loss of smell, or report a loss of taste instead. However, degeneration of the sense of smell can be an early finding in dementias and Parkinson's disease.

Ophthalmologic exam (*cranial nerves II, III, IV, and VI, and more*): The eye is not just a poetic "window to the soul," but also a direct view of the optic nerve (CN II), which is an extension of the brain, as well as of the retinal vessels representing the circulatory system. Using the exam room's direct ophthalmoscope, the eye can be panned from the anterior portion to the back of the orb. Tortuous vessels in the sclera may suggest ataxia telangiectasia. Swirling opacities of the cornea may indicate Fabry's disease. Dislocation of the lens may be a symptom of Marfan's syndrome, and cataracts may suggest a number of diagnoses. The "Christmas tree" cataracts of myotonic dystrophy were a diagnostic sign before genetic testing became available. The optic nerve, if swollen (papilledema), may indicate increased intracranial pressure and an emergency situation. If pale, the optic nerve may attest to a genetic optic atrophy or demyelination, such as in multiple sclerosis. Degeneration of the macula, the portion of the retina that serves central vision, can have a genetic basis, as can the abnormal pigmentation of retinitis pigmentosa. A "cherry red" spot is a red flag for lysosomal storage disorders such as hexosaminidase deficiency. The arteries and veins of the retina can display the changes from systemic disease: hypertension, atherosclerosis, diabetes, vasculitis, and even arterial emboli. So, if the neurologist seems to spend an inordinate amount of time peering in the patient's eyes when the chief complaint is elsewhere, she may be using the ophthalmoscope as a detective's magnifying glass seeking a specific clue. An excellent online reference for eye findings is the Neuro-ophthalmological Virtual Library (http://library.med.utah.edu/NOVEL) [4]. As retinal imaging becomes more routine, printed retinal photos may accompany the medical records. An *electroretinogram* (ERG) tests the responses of retinal ganglion cells, which can be informative in retinal degenerative and mitochondrial disorders.

Eye movements (*CN III, IV, and VI*): Decreased range of motion of the eyes is seen in the mitochondrial disorders, chronic progressive external ophthalmoplegia (CPEO), and Kearns–Sayre syndrome. Some abnormal eye movements, such as nystagmus (rhythmic beats), or abnormal saccades (eye movements from switching gaze directions), as seen in ataxias and some dementias, localize to the motor control upstream of the cranial nerves III, IV, and VI.

The trigeminal (*V*) controls sensation of the face, cranial vessels, and meninges, as well as the muscles of mastication. It is also the nerve that conveys the sensation of headache.

The facial nerve (*VII*) controls facial strength, a tiny muscle controlling tension of the eardrum, and taste. Upper facial strength is tested with eye closure and brow furrowing and lower facial strength by smile or cheek puff. Facial weakness can be a feature of some muscular dystrophies or a central neurological insult, such as stroke.

The acoustic nerve (*VIII*) serves hearing and vestibular function. This can be screened at a visit by testing hearing with the sound of finger rubs or a tuning fork. *Audiometry* can give additional information about symmetry and affected wavelength ranges. Deafness has many genetic causes, and hearing loss can be an element of a syndrome, such as a mitochondrial disorder or facioscapulohumeral muscular dystrophy.

Grouped together, bulbar muscles control speech and swallowing, and are controlled by *CN IX, X, and XII*. The glossopharyngeal nerve (CN IX) delivers sensation from the mouth and taste from the back of the tongue. The glossopharyngeal and vagus (CN X) together control salivation and swallowing muscles. The hypoglossal nerve (XII) controls the tongue. Slurred or nasal speech can be signs of bulbar dysfunction. Tongue fasciculation, from the loss of CN XII input, can be seen in amyotrophic lateral sclerosis (ALS); bulbar weakness can be an initial symptom of ALS, as well as some muscular dystrophies.

The vagus (*X*) *nerve* extends into the chest and abdomen, and is difficult to isolate in direct testing. The vagus nerve controls the vocal cords, and delivers sensation from the throat, and viscera—heart, lungs, and most of the gastrointestinal tract, but its predominant function is autonomic.

The spinal accessory nerve (*XI*) controls the sternocleidomastoids (strap muscles of the neck) and part of the trapezius muscles, which are tested with strength of head turn and shoulder shrug. Examples of disorders that cause weakness of the CN XI muscles include facioscapulohumeral muscular dystrophy and amyotrophic lateral sclerosis.

25.2.3 Autonomic Examination

The autonomic nervous system includes sympathetic and parasympathetic functions, which control many "housekeeping" functions of the body, the examination of which is incorporated into other areas of the general and neurologic exam.

Autonomic fibers extend along the cranial nerves and down a plexus alongside the spinal cord. The cranial nerve exam tests autonomic fibers that travel with those nerves and which control pupil responses, facial sweating, tears, and saliva. Autonomic functions dominate vagal (X) nerve functions, and include heart rate variability, blood pressure regulation, and gut motility. Outside of the cranial nerves, the autonomic system controls skin sweating, the lower gastrointestinal tract, urination, and erectile function.

Tilt table testing examines autonomic control of cardiac function and vascular tone. *EMG* testing of superficial skin responses tests sweat function. *Thermoregulatory sweat testing* with alizarin dye can show regional changes in sweating. Clinical examples of genetic disorders involving the autonomic nervous system are the hereditary sensory autonomic neuropathies (HSAN), and Riley–Day syndrome [5].

25.2.4 The Motor Examination

Motor testing requires the cooperation and effort of the patient when asked to push, pull, grip, lift, and walk. Muscle examination not only includes strength, but also muscle bulk and tone. The examiner looks at muscle bulk for hypotrophy (low muscle bulk from birth), atrophy (loss of muscle bulk), or pseudohypertrophy ("woody" texture due to fibrosis). Testing for tone, or resistance to passive movement, actually tests descending inhibition from the brain or spinal cord; its absence results in increased tone, or spasticity. The pattern of muscle weakness (proximal, distal, symmetry, involvement of facial, speech, or swallowing muscles) gives significant clues for diagnosis of neuromuscular disorders (refer to http://neuromuscular.wustl.edu).

25.2.5 The Sensory Examination

Sensory testing requires the patient to report what can or cannot be felt. The examiner can use cotton balls, safety pins, tuning forks, or the cool metal of the reflex hammer, and move toe or finger joint position to test the modalities of light touch, pain, vibration, temperature, and proprioception. Deficits in all or some of these modalities may localize to nerve fiber size, spinal cord level, or peripheral nerve length. *Electromyography* (EMG) or *nerve biopsy* described later can give additional details about peripheral nerve function.

25.2.6 *Reflex Exam*

Deep tendon reflexes are typically tested at the biceps, triceps, brachioradialis, patellas, and Achilles tendons, and can be thought of as a circuit test of the synapse of the sensory and motor nerves in the spinal cord, "tuned" by inhibition descending from the brain down the spinal cord. Brisk reflexes can indicate loss of that descending inhibition; lost reflexes can indicate a loss of the "circuit" at the peripheral nerve or muscle, such as in peripheral neuropathies and muscular dystrophies.

Spinal reflexes also can indicate an upper motor neuron defect. Hoffman's reflex is elicited by flicking the middle finger, and watching for reflex spread to the thumb; crossed adductors are present if tapping the adductor results in spread of reflex to the opposite side. The Babinski sign is tested by looking for upward movement of the great toe when the sole of the foot is scraped, and is a primitive reflex that is normal in infancy before corticospinal tracts are fully myelinated. However, it is abnormal in adults.

Other primitive reflexes include glabellar (failure to suppress blinking when tapped between the eyebrows), rooting or snout (lip puckering when the cheek is stroked or lips are tapped), and palmomental (chin twitching when the palm is scratched), which are normally present in infancy, but disappear as the brain matures. Their reappearance can signal brain injury or a degenerative process involving the frontal lobes.

25.2.7 *Coordination and Gait*

Coordination testing can include asking the patient to tap their fingers or feet, but also more complex movements such as handwriting. Gait testing includes not only a normal walk, but also walking on a line and on heels and toes. Gait is a complex task requiring cooperation of many brain functions: strength, sensation, tone, coordination, and motor planning.

During the interview, and even during the walk from the waiting room, the physician will observe the patient's movements. Findings of movement disorders can be detected through all portions of the neuro exam: blinking frequency may be decreased in Parkinson's disease, increased in tics, or prolonged in blepharospasm. Eye movements may be abnormal in ataxias and Huntington's disease, to the point where a patient may turn their head, rather than their eyes, to change the object of their gaze. Speech may be soft in Parkinson's, changed in rhythm and volume in ataxia, or interrupted by outbursts in Tourette syndrome. Tremor types may be distinguished by their frequency (speed), or whether they are worse at rest or with action. Dystonia can vary by time of day (Segawa syndrome) or worsen with an action (writer's cramp). The neurologist uses all manner of exam techniques to try to bring out a movement disorder: examining writing, different rhythmic movements, distraction, and stress, asking a patient to take or hold a medication before an exam, or scheduling a visit early or late in the day, to both diagnose and optimize medication management.

25.3 Neuroimaging

Imaging can further define lesions localized to eloquent brain regions or discover lesions in non-eloquent regions. Different imaging modalities are used for brain, spine, and peripheral nerves and plexi; the area and suspected abnormality will determine which imaging modality will be most helpful [6].

25.3.1 Computed Tomography (CT)

Computed tomography (CT) is an X-ray based modality that sensitively detects hemorrhage and calcifications. It is not well suited for imaging the cerebellum, spinal cord, or peripheral nerve, but is excellent at imaging the vertebral column.

An intravenous dye (contrast) can give details about whether a brain lesion enhances on a CT scan. *CT angiograms* give excellent information about brain vessels; *CT perfusion scans* can detect regions of abnormal blood flow to the brain. Allergies to iodine or contrast, and renal function must be assessed before ordering contrast with a CT scan.

For even more detailed information about brain vessels, a conventional *angiogram* (performed via arterial catheterization) may be done, which can give dynamic information about blood flow for familial arteriovenous malformations, or deciding on management of aneurysms.

25.3.2 Magnetic Resonance Imaging (MRI)

Magnetic resonance imaging (MRI) is based on the response of water or paramagnetic elements (such as iron) to magnetic fields. Different protocols (such as T1, T2, proton gradient, and FLAIR) provide different structural information. Some protocols might need to be specifically requested: *gradient recall echo* (GRE) protocols give additional information about iron deposition (such as in neurodegeneration with brain iron accumulation) or iron left behind by microhemorrhages (such as cerebral amyloidosis). Iron is an important element in the enzymes making dopamine, and the iron-rich stripe of the substantia nigra can be seen to fade on MRI GRE in Parkinson's disease as those cells are lost.

Diffusion-weighted imaging protocols detect loss of cellular control of water permeability. This imaging can be abnormal in prion disease (Creutzfeldt-Jakob disease), metabolic disorders (MELAS), or ischemia.

MRI scans can also be done with contrast that is chemically different from CT scan contrast. A lesion that is highlighted by contrast indicates a loss of the blood–brain barrier, and can distinguish active from older multiple sclerosis plaques, and differentiate between brain tumor types, and infectious and inflammatory processes.

25.3.3 Magnetic Resonance Spectroscopy (MRS)

Magnetic resonance spectroscopy (MRS) is able to determine certain biochemical signatures within a selected volume of brain tissue, such as lactate (which can be elevated in mitochondrial disorders) and choline-to-creatine ratio (which are distinctive in tumors and demyelination).

25.3.4 Single-Photon Emission Computed Tomography or SPECT

Single-photon emission computed tomography or SPECT uses a radioisotope to detect blood flow in the brain. It is, therefore, a method of functional imaging. A *DaTscan* is a SPECT that uses a radioactive drug to measure dopamine availability in the brain. This scan can distinguish between dopamine-deficient diseases, such as Parkinson's disease, and those without dopamine deficits.

25.3.5 Positron Emission Tomography (PET)

Positron emission tomography (PET) scan detects isotope decay of radio-labeled compounds and can add functional information to structural information on CT or MRI scans. Fluorodeoxyglucose (FTG) is labeled with 18-fluorine and shows areas of higher metabolic activity or areas of asymmetry. Pittsburgh compound B (or PiB) is an 11-carbon-labeled compound that binds to amyloid, and is useful in imaging dementia.

25.4 Neurophysiology

Neurophysiology testing is based on the innate electric nature of the brain, nerves, and muscles (analogous to electrical wiring, insulation, and circuits). Abnormalities in the function of the central and peripheral nervous systems and muscle can be localized based on their electrical activity or by observing their response to depolarization [7].

25.4.1 Nerve Conduction Studies (NCS) and Electromyography (EMG)

Nerve conduction studies test peripheral nerves by applying small electrical shocks to the proximal part of the nerve, and detecting the speed and amplitude of the nerve's response distally. NCS studies can distinguish between the demyelinating (type 1) and axonal (type 2) forms of Charcot–Marie–Tooth disease. EMG detection of low amplitude, complex discharges is characteristic of myopathy. Irritability upon needle insertion can signal a myositis. Large-amplitude motor units and decreased recruitment can indicate a neuropathic or denervating process. Defining regions of denervation is part of the El Escorial Criteria for amyotrophic lateral sclerosis. Unusual muscle electrical discharges, such as myotonia, can be seen in the myotonic dystrophies and acid maltase deficiency.

25.4.2 Electroencephalography (EEG)

Electroencephalography (EEG) is the detection of cortical electrical discharges by surface electrodes. EEG recordings can be done as an outpatient or inpatient with video recording to capture seizure semiology. Sometimes several EEGs must be done before capturing seizure discharges. EEG is often normal in neurodegenerative disorders. EEGs are also used to detect other abnormal cortical activities, such as periodic lateralized epileptiform discharges (PLED) and slowing, such as seen in encephalopathies.

Evoked potentials use EEG surface electrodes to test sensory pathways. *Somatosensory evoked potentials* (SSEPs) test the integrity of the sensory pathways in the spinal cord. *Visual evoked potentials* (VEPs) use alternating black and white grid patterns to test the visual pathways. Auditory evoked potentials use audible clicks to test hearing, and are the basis of the newborn hearing screening.

25.4.3 Transcranial Magnetic Stimulation (TMS)

Transcranial magnetic stimulation (TMS) uses magnetic stimulation over the skull to activate the motor cortex; the speed and amplitude of the signal are then measured over its course to the limbs. It can be valuable in characterizing upper motor neuron function in hereditary spastic paraparesis and primary lateral sclerosis.

25.5 Cerebrospinal Fluid Studies

Cerebrospinal fluid (CSF) bathes and cushions the brain and spinal cord. Routine studies on CSF obtained by lumbar puncture (commonly termed a "spinal tap") include cell count, glucose, and protein. Oligoclonal bands are an indication of an inflammatory process in the CNS. CSF studies can be useful in excluding non-genetic disorders, such as multiple sclerosis, paraneoplastic disorders, or neoplasm. Another CSF biomarker, protein 14-3-3, can be elevated in prion diseases, but also in other disorders. Neurotransmitter metabolites can be detected in CSF, and are abnormal in dopamine-responsive dystonia. Measurements of amyloid and tau proteins are now useful in distinguishing Alzheimer's disease from other forms of dementia.

25.6 Biopsy

Muscle biopsy can be useful in the diagnosis of muscular dystrophies. Small fibers, central nuclei, and increased intramyofascial connective tissue indicate a dystrophic process. Antibody staining for sarcolemmal proteins, such as dystrophin, dysferlin, merosin, emerin, the sarcoglycans, alpha dystroglycan, and caveolin 3, can be diagnostic for the muscular dystrophies caused by defects in those proteins. Other features found on muscle biopsies, such as cytoplasmic inclusions including central cores, rods, rimmed vacuoles, or ragged red fibers, can be diagnostic or be a diagnostic clue. When mitochondrial disease is suspected, muscle biopsy also allows measurement of muscle respiratory chain enzymes. If fiber-type grouping is found, muscle biopsy can reveal a neurogenic process.

Nerve biopsies are carefully selected to decrease the chance of leaving a region of numbness or weakness served by that nerve. Nerve biopsies can help distinguish a demyelinating from an axonal neuropathy or a multifocal process. They can show if reinnervation or remyelination is occurring. Non-genetic, systemic disorders, such as inflammatory disorders, sarcoid, amyloid, and vasculitis, can also be diagnosed by muscle or nerve biopsy.

25.7 Conclusion

Sifting for clues to a genetic diagnosis in a medical record that spans years of medical reports and tracking down results for important studies not included with the initial referral can be time consuming. However, knowing what to look for, both to exclude and include, can help narrow the differential diagnosis list and avoid redundant and expensive testing. Knowing what was found previously can make the patient's initial visit more productive, closer to definitive diagnosis, and allow more clinical time for other services to the patient and family, such as education, counseling, and plan of care.

References

1. Campbell, W. W. (2005). *DeJong's the neurologic examination* (6th ed.). Philadelphia, PA: Lippincott Williams and Wilkins.
2. Vakil, E. (2012). Neuropsychological assessment: Principles, rationale, and challenges. *Journal of Clinical and Experimental Neuropsychology, 34*(2), 135–150.
3. Wilson-Pauwels, L., Akesson, E. J., & Stewart, P. A. (1998). *Cranial nerves: Anatomy and clinical comments*. Toronto, ON: Decker.
4. Neuro-ophthalmological Virtual Library (http://library.med.utah.edu/NOVEL).
5. Mathias, C. J., & Bannister, R. (1998). *Autonomic failure: A textbook of clinical disorders of the autonomic nervous system* (4th ed.). Oxford: Oxford University Press.
6. Osborn, A. G. (2012). *Osborn's brain: Imaging, pathology, and anatomy*. Philadelphia, PA: Lippincott Williams and Wilkins.
7. Preston, D. C., & Shapiro, B. E. (2012). *Electromyography and neuromuscular disorders: Clinical-electrophysiologic correlations* (3rd ed.). London: Saunders.

Chapter 26
The Neuropsychological Evaluation

Elise Caccappolo

Neurological diseases are often associated with changes in cognition and behavior. The evaluation of an individual's cognitive and emotional function is performed via neuropsychological testing, which uses a battery of standardized measures that possess a high degree of predictive validity. Neuropsychological assessment provides more detailed information than mental status testing, given the breadth of assessment that occurs, and is more sensitive, given the use of standardized administration procedures and normative data for interpretation purposes.

26.1 Purposes of Neuropsychological Testing

26.1.1 Diagnosis

With its high degree of sensitivity, neuropsychological assessment is particularly valuable when a thorough, precise evaluation of cognitive function is required. In this way, neuropsychological assessment often serves as a diagnostic tool. The pattern of scores obtained on tests can help differentiate between various conditions. In cases where standard neuro-diagnostic procedures, such as the neurological exam, mental status testing, EEG, or imaging, are negative, neuropsychological assessment may offer valuable information regarding strengths and weaknesses in cognitive functioning, which often detects or helps to confirm suspected neurological disease. Subtle cognitive changes, identified through neuropsychological testing, often represent the earliest symptoms in patients at risk for neurodegenerative disorders, including Alzheimer's disease (AD), frontotemporal dementia (FTD),

E. Caccappolo (✉)
Department of Neurology, Columbia University Medical Center, 710 West 168th Street, New York, NY USA
e-mail: ec668@cumc.columbia.edu

J.S. Goldman (ed.), *Genetic Counseling for Adult Neurogenetic Disease*,
DOI 10.1007/978-1-4899-7482-2_26

Huntington disease (HD), Parkinson's disease dementia (PDD), dementia with Lewy bodies (DLB), cortical basal degeneration (CBD), vascular dementia (VaD), including CADASIL, as well as other conditions such as multiple sclerosis [1–12].

Like many specialized tests, neuropsychological assessment cannot identify the etiology of impairment in isolation, i.e., solely based on the pattern of test scores, but requires interpretation that is grounded on other information such as clinical symptoms, imaging data, or lab findings. In this context, data obtained from a neuropsychological evaluation can provide information about etiology. In neurodegenerative disorders, the pattern of impairment on testing can assist with differential diagnosis as each disorder leads to circumscribed atrophy in distinct neural networks, which affect cognitive functioning in characteristic ways. Testing can also differentiate between specific conditions such as dementia and depression (previously referred to as "pseudodementia").

26.1.2 Patient Care and Planning

Results from neuropsychological testing are often used to assist in treatment planning and care for patients. Assessments can be made regarding an individual's insight and capacity for self-care, including his or her ability to follow a medication or other therapeutic regimen (e.g., rehabilitation), maintain or return to school or employment, safely operate a motor vehicle, or manage finances. Characterizing an individual's specific cognitive strengths and weaknesses and identifying psychiatric or emotional conditions that may be a factor in one's functional status can contribute to the development of a management plan. Caregivers and patients can then use this information to make informed decisions about the future.

26.1.3 Documenting Change in Cognitive Status Over Time

Neuropsychological evaluations are often repeated at regular intervals to assist in monitoring disease progression. Data from serial testing provides valuable information regarding the status of a neurological condition; that is, comparisons of performance across time, considered in the context of measurement error and practice effects, can help to reveal whether a condition is changing and if so, at what rate and in what ways. Longitudinal clinical testing is particularly useful in cases where there is a memory complaint or a suspicion of dementia, as it can assist in differentiating between normal age-related cognitive decline, mild cognitive impairment (MCI), and dementia. A decline on repeated testing is often used to identify conversion from MCI to dementia. In neuro-oncology patients, neuropsychological scores have been found to be more sensitive to tumor growth than MRI [13].

26.2 The Neuropsychological Evaluation

While predesigned batteries exist, most neuropsychologists select a battery of tests to be used for individual patients based on the referral question. A battery typically consists of paper and pencil tests and may also include questionnaires and computerized tasks. A comprehensive neuropsychological evaluation typically includes assessment of the following areas, which are categorized into cognitive domains and will be described in greater detail below: Intellectual functioning, attention and concentration, memory, language, visuospatial skill/visuoconstruction, and executive functioning.

26.2.1 Screening Tests

Cognitive impairment is often broadly assessed by means of screening batteries, rating scales, and inventories. These measures are beneficial in that they are brief and can provide an overall estimate of the patient's level of general cognitive ability while also alerting the clinician to specific areas of cognitive function that will require more formal assessment [14]. The Mini-Mental Status Examination (MMSE) is likely the most frequently used brief screening instrument in both research and clinical settings, and is particularly useful as a dementia screen. The MMSE uses a 30-point scale to assess orientation, word recall, language abilities, attention and calculation, and visuospatial ability, but has been criticized for its lack of executive function measures and its focus on the domains of orientation and language, which are often preserved in MCI and even dementia [15]. The MMSE is most effective when differentiating dementia patients with moderate or severe deficits from controls, as opposed to differentiating controls and mildly impaired patients [16]. Recently, screening instruments have been developed to more adequately assess for dementia. The cognitive portion of the Cambridge Examination for Mental Disorders (CAMCOG) includes all of the items from the MMSE so as to allow for the calculation of an MMSE total score (subsequently, the two measures correlate strongly), but assesses additional cognitive areas such as perception (recognition of famous faces and objects from unusual angles) and abstract thinking (identifying similarities between objects) as well as functional status [17]. The Montreal Cognitive Assessment (MoCA) was specifically designed to assess for mild cognitive dysfunction and as such includes measures of executive functioning [18]. In this way, it may be a more useful cognitive screening test for neurological diseases that affect younger populations.

26.3 Formal Neuropsychological Evaluation

26.3.1 Intellectual Abilities

General intellectual functioning, or IQ, is assessed to provide, among other items, an estimate of an individual's level of pre-morbid functioning so as to allow for comparison for other test scores. Specific measures, such as word-reading tests that include irregularly spelled words, are resistant to brain damage and can also be used to assess an individual's abilities pre-injury or disease state. Intellectual ability measures such as those on IQ testing allow for comparison between verbal and nonverbal abilities, which, roughly speaking, localize hemispherically, and assess processing speed and working memory. An individual's IQ is typically assessed with the Wechsler Adult Test of Intelligence (WAIS). Nonverbal measures, such as tasks that require conceptual thinking, are less commonly used, but are available for nonverbal patients or for those who do not speak English to assess general intellectual function.

26.3.2 Attention and Concentration

The ability to sustain or divide attention is often affected by brain disorders. A patient with attentional difficulties may present as distractible or complain of having difficulty maintaining concentration. Increased vulnerability to interference may affect an individual's ability to maintain attention. Slowed processing speed, manifesting as slowed reaction time, may underlie an individual's difficulty with dividing attention. Common tests of auditory attention include the Digit Span subtest of the WAIS, in which the patient is required to repeat increasingly longer strings of numbers read aloud by the examiner. Working memory becomes involved when the patient is asked to repeat a string of numbers in reverse. Many elderly patients, and even those with severe brain damage, are able to perform similarly to normal controls on this measure due to its reliance on immediate memory which is, overall, often immune to the effects of aging and frequently remains intact in brain-damaged patients. Other tests that require oral alphanumeric sequencing, such as the Letter-Number Sequencing subtest from the WAIS, provide a more sensitive measure of mental tracking and working memory. Tests that incorporate scanning and visuomotor tracking, such as the Trail Making test, provide measures of divided attention. Computerized vigilance tests, such as the Continuous Performance test, assess reaction time and accuracy.

26.3.3 Memory

Comprehensive memory testing is multi-faceted given that the concept of learning and memory is generally understood from a dual-function point of view, where declarative/explicit memory is differentiated from nondeclarative/implicit memory [19]. Declarative memory can be further divided into semantic (memory for facts) and episodic (autobiographical) memory, while nondeclarative memory is categorized into item-specific and procedural memory subsystems [20, 21]. Neuropsychological assessment of memory is performed via tests of verbal and nonverbal (i.e., visual) learning and retention. Verbal learning and recall can be assessed with tests of prose, where the patient is read aloud a story and asked to recall it following a brief delay as well as following a longer delay period. Rote learning is assessed with word-list tests, where a list of words is repeated numerous times to the patient so that a learning curve can be obtained, as well as a measure of the patient's immediate and delayed retention and recognition. Other word learning tests incorporate cues, such as the Paired Associates subtest of the WMS. Tests of visual memory attempt to assess learning and retention with similar means, i.e., by presenting the patient with stimuli to be learned and freely recalled or recognized following a delay. The assessment of visual memory is often confounded by verbal associations that are not easily removed, even with the use of abstract designs. Many visual memory tests require stimuli to be reproduced or copied by the patient following immediate and longer delay periods.

26.3.4 Language

Neurologic patients may present with deficits in expressive or receptive speech (aphasia). Patients may complain of a decline in the speed and ease of verbal production; tests of expressive speech include measures of confrontation naming which require specific word retrieval ability. Patients with anomia are unable to adequately retrieve words or names, and often make phonemic or semantic paraphasic errors when attempting to name a particular item. Fluency of speech is assessed by asking the patient to generate as many words as possible that belong to a particular group within a short time frame. Phonemic fluency testing requires that the individual produce words that begin with a particular letter. Semantic fluency tests require the generation of words that are included in specific categories, i.e., "tell me as many animals/fruit/types of clothing as possible." Pure writing deficits, i.e., acquired agraphia that occurs separately from a motor cause, are relatively rare. Repetition is assessed with tests of varying syntactic complexity. Problems with receptive language may manifest as comprehension difficulties that can be assessed with a variety of tasks designed to assess verbal comprehension. Acquired alexia, or the inability to read, can be measured with various reading tests that examine speed, word recognition, and comprehension.

26.3.5 Visuospatial Skill/Visuoconstruction

Many aspects of visual perception can be affected by neurological disease. Patients with spatial changes may present with difficulty navigating new or even familiar routes (topographic disorientation) or an increased tendency to forget where an object was placed. Patients with hemispatial neglect are unable to attend to one side of their body, usually the left, and may be unable to "see" objects on the left side of space. In neuropsychological assessment, visuoperceptual tests assess the ability to recognize abstract shapes and designs, familiar and unfamiliar faces, and angular relationships. Perceptual organization is assessed with copying tests or tests that require visual organization of disarranged pieces. Facial processing is tested with tasks requiring facial perception and discrimination ability. Tests of visuoconstruction, where the patient is instructed to copy two- and three-dimensional figures with increasing complexity require perceptual, spatial, and motor abilities. Three-dimensional building tasks such as the Block design subtest of the WAIS involve the spatial component of perception and require motor execution.

26.3.6 Executive Functioning

Executive processes are integral to higher order processing, so that executive dysfunction is reflected as impairment in the ability to strategically plan, self-monitor, formulate goals, regulate (activate and inhibit) responses, and coordinate complex cognition and motor control. Generation and follow-through can be assessed with tests of verbal fluency or design fluency. Impairments in set shifting ability are a notable feature of executive dysfunction and can be assessed with sequencing tasks requiring the individual to alternate between items, either verbally or motorically, in order to complete tasks requiring flexible thinking. Problem solving, abstract thinking, and judgment are evaluated with tests requiring higher order information processing, or the ability to apply generalized information to specific situations, sometimes while integrating feedback. Response inhibition is assessed with tests that require the patient to suppress an automatic action, like responding to a stimulus or naming the color that a word is printed in as opposed to reading the word aloud (Stroop effect). Decreased response inhibition is also tested with tests of motor programming, and can be manifest as stimulus-bound behavior, e.g., compulsive imitation of the examiner's movements or utilization behavior. Executive dysfunction is also associated with emotional dysregulation, which can manifest as chronic depression, anxiety, or hyperemotionality.

26.3.7 Personality/Emotional Functioning

Changes in personality and behavior often accompany neurological diseases, either as a direct effect of a brain disorder or as a secondary reaction to an individual's experiences of loss or frustration. It may be difficult to tease apart the specific causality of emotional distress given the interactions between these processes. Questionnaires are frequently used to assess the patient's subjective mood state or to evaluate for psychiatric (axis I and axis II) disorders.

26.3.8 Effort

Motivation and effort are often assessed as part of a formal neuropsychological evaluation, particularly when clients are seeking financial compensation for injuries, or cognitive complaints are not typical of the associated injury or illness. Forced choice tests or symptom validity tests are used to identify malingering or insufficient effort. Pattern analysis, or the analysis of test performance patterns, is also used [22, 23].

26.4 Interpreting Neuropsychological Test Performance

Test scores are evaluated within an empirical frame of reference. In this way, an individual's performance on neuropsychological tests is interpreted by comparing his or her scores to the mean performance of a large sample of "normal" subjects, i.e., normative data, which is usually organized by age and education and, at times, by gender and race. This process allows an individual's performance to be compared to that of appropriate peers.

Neuropsychological testing is not without its shortcomings. A primary drawback is the length of time required to perform a thorough assessment. A formal neuropsychological evaluation can take anywhere from 2 to 8 h, depending on the ability level of the patient, the nature of the referral question, and the intended purpose of the evaluation results. The neuropsychologist must be attentive to the patient's energy and motivation to be confident that a valid assessment of an individual's true ability is obtained. The effects of cultural differences on test performance represent another major obstacle in providing valid assessments for individuals who were not born and raised in the USA. Neuropsychological tests, while standardized, do not have adequate norms for minority populations. Cultural differences contribute to a high degree of variability in test performance, often leading to lower scores on tests. While the availability of tests in languages other than English has increased over the past two decades, most tests are administered in English and are normed on English-speaking populations, putting nonnative English speakers at a disadvantage given that the effects of biculturalism and bilingualism on test performance are not fully understood.

26.5 Patterns of Test Performance

Traditionally, neuropsychological profiles have been roughly categorized into "cortical" and "frontal-subcortical" profiles. Cortical dementias, which include Alzheimer's, frontotemporal dementia, and the asymmetrical cortical atrophies, typically present with deficits involving the cerebral cortex and may include aphasia with confrontation naming difficulty, impaired memory, deficits in complex visuoprocessing, including poor visuoconstruction ability, and executive dysfunction such as poor insight and judgment. Other dementias, including most forms of VaD and dementia associated with movement disorders such as PDD, CBD, PSP, and DLB, present via a "frontal-subcortical" profile and are characterized by slowed speed of processing and executive dysfunction as well as memory impairment that reflects a pattern of poor encoding and retention as opposed to a retrieval problem. Finally, mood changes including depression, apathy, and amotivation are more common in subcortical than cortical dementias.

Other neurological disorders besides dementia are characterized by specific profiles on testing. Mild cognitive impairment, amnestic subtype, is diagnosed when the patient demonstrates memory impairment but no other areas of deficit; that is, tests within all other domains are performed within normal limits, and there is no significant functional decline. Non-amnestic MCI is diagnosed when subtle impairment is observed across one or more domains other than memory. Cognitive deficits associated with MS can vary and may present as slowed information processing, memory deficits, executive impairment, or even visuospatial difficulties. Depression manifests as slowed processing and psychomotor speed and poor effort throughout testing.

26.6 Summary

Obtaining an understanding of the role of the neuropsychological evaluation in the diagnosis of genetic disorders illustrates its value, not only as a sensitive diagnostic tool, but also as a means of providing recommendations for treatment care to patients with neurologic diseases and their caregivers.

Glossary

Alexia Loss or impairment of the ability to read.

Anomia The inability to name objects or to recognize the written or spoken names of objects.

Agraphia An acquired disorder of writing or spelling.

Aphasia Acquired language impairment resulting from neurologic damage.

Declarative (explicit) memory Events, experiences, or facts that can be consciously recalled, such as episodic or semantic events.

Measurement error The difference between the actual value of a quantity and the value obtained by a test.

Nondeclarative (implicit) memory Memory that is altered without conscious mediation, such as procedural memory, priming, and classical conditioning.

Phonemic paraphasia Substitution of a word that sounds similar to the intended word (kite for mite)

Semantic paraphasia Substitution of a related word for the intended word (wife for husband)

Stimulus-bound behavior Difficulty disengaging or focusing attention or behavior from one stimulus in the perceptual field to another.

Malingering Intentionally feigning or exaggerating symptoms for external gain.

Pseudodementia A psychiatric condition that resembles dementia. Often results from depression but may be associated with other psychiatric disorders.

Utilization behavior The act of grasping or using objects that are within reach or in the field of vision, regardless of whether they are related to the present task. Associated with bilateral frontal lesions, particularly inferior frontal lesions.

Working memory A limited capacity system that stores information temporarily so as to allow for its manipulation, especially with complex tasks such as learning.

References

1. Elias, M. F., Beiser, A., Wolf, P. A., Au, R., White, R. F., & D'Agostino, R. B. (2000). The preclinical phase of Alzheimer disease: A 22-year prospective study of the Framingham Cohort. *Archives of Neurology, 57*(6), 808–813.
2. Weder, N. D., Aziz, R., Wilkins, K., & Tampi, R. R. (2007). Frontotemporal dementias: A review. *Annals of General Psychiatry, 6*, 15.
3. Hahn-Barma, V., Deweer, B., Dürr, A., Dodé, C., Feingold, J., Pillon, B., et al. (1998). Are cognitive changes the first symptoms of Huntington's disease? A study of gene carriers. *Journal of Neurology, Neurosurgery, and Psychiatry, 64*(2), 172–177.
4. Brandt, J., Inscore, A. B., Ward, J., Shpritz, B., Rosenblatt, A., Margolis, R. L., et al. (2008). Neuropsychological deficits in Huntington's disease gene carriers and correlates of early "conversion". *The Journal of Neuropsychiatry and Clinical Neurosciences, 20*(4), 466–472.
5. Williams-Gray, C. H., Evans, J. R., Goris, A., Foltynie, T., Ban, M., Robbins, T. W., et al. (2009). The distinct cognitive syndromes of Parkinson's disease: 5 year follow-up of the CamPaIGN cohort. *Brain, 132*(Pt 11), 2958–2969.

6. McKeith, I. G., Dickson, D. W., Lowe, J., Emre, M., O'Brien, J. T., Feldman, H., et al. (2005). Diagnosis and management of dementia with Lewy bodies: Third report of the DLB Consortium. *Neurology, 65*(12), 1863–1872.
7. Litvan, I., Grimes, D. A., Lang, A. E., Jankovic, J., McKee, A., Verny, M., et al. (1999). Clinical features differentiating patients with postmortem confirmed progressive supranuclear palsy and corticobasal degeneration. *Journal of Neurology, 246*(Suppl 2), II1–II5.
8. Possin, K. L., & Kaufer, D. I. (2010). Parkinsonian dementias. *Continuum (Minneapolis Minnesota), 16*(2 Dementia), 57–79.
9. Chaves, M. L., Ilha, D., Maia, A. L., Motta, E., Lehmen, R., & Oliveira, L. M. (1999). Diagnosing dementia and normal aging: Clinical relevance of brain ratios and cognitive performance in a Brazilian sample. *Brazilian Journal of Medical and Biological Research, 32*(9), 1133–1143.
10. Buffon, F., Porcher, R., Hernandez, K., Kurtz, A., Pointeau, S., Vahedi, K., et al. (2006). Cognitive profile in CADISIL. *Journal of Neurology, Neurosurgery, and Psychiatry, 77*(2), 175–180.
11. Piras, M. R., Magnano, I., Canu, E. D., Paulus, K. S., Satta, W. M., Soddu, A., et al. (2003). Longitudinal study of cognitive dysfunction in multiple sclerosis: Neuropsychological, neuroradiological, and neurophysiological findings. *Journal of Neurology, Neurosurgery, and Psychiatry, 74*(7), 878–885.
12. Glanz, B. I., Healy, B. C., Hviid, L. E., Chitnis, T., & Weiner, H. L. (2012). Cognitive deterioration in patients with early multiple sclerosis: A 5-year study. *Journal of Neurology, Neurosurgery, and Psychiatry, 83*(1), 38–43.
13. Armstrong, C. L., Goldstein, B., Shera, D., Ledakis, G. E., & Tallent, E. M. (2003). The predictive value of longitudinal neuropsychologic assessment in the early detection of brain tumor recurrence. *Cancer, 97*(3), 649–656.
14. Folstein, M. F., Folstein, S. E., & McHugh, P. R. (1975). Mini-Mental State: A practical method for grading the cognitive state of patients for the clinician. *Journal of Psychiatric Research, 12*, 189–198.
15. Jefferson, A. L., Cosentino, S. A., Ball, S., et al. (2002). Errors produced on the Mini-Mental State examination and neuropsychological test performance in Alzheimer's Disease, Ischemic vascular dementia, and Parkinson's disease. *Journal of Neuropsychiatry and Clinical Neurosciences, 14*, 311–320.
16. Galasko, D., Klauber, M. R., Hofstetter, C. R., Salmon, D. P., Lasker, B., & Thal, L. J. (1990). The Mini-Mental State Examination in the early diagnosis of Alzheimer's disease. *Archives of Neurology, 47*, 49–52.
17. Huppert, F. A., Brayne, C., Giill, C., Paykel, E. S., & Beardsall, L. (1995). CAMCOG-A concise neuropsychological test to assist dementia diagnosis: Sociodemographic determinants in an elderly population sample. *British Journal of Clinical Psychology, 34*, 529–541.
18. Nasreddine, Z. S., Phillips, N. A., Bedirian, V., et al. (2005). The Montreal Cognitive Assessment, MoCA: A brief screening tool for mild cognitive impairment. *Journal of the American Geriatrics Society, 53*(4), 695–699.
19. Clark, R. E., Manns, J. R., & Squire, L. R. (2002). Classical conditioning, awareness, and brain systems. *Trends in Cognitive Sciences, 6*(12), 524–531.
20. Baddeley, A., & Wilson, B. A. (2002). Prose recall and amnesia: Implications for the structure of working memory. *Neuropsychologia, 40*(10), 1737–1743.
21. Mayes, A. R., Daum, I., Markowisch, H. J., & Sauter, B. (1997). The relationship between retrograde and anterograde amnesia in patients with typical global amnesia. *Cortex, 33*(2), 197–217.
22. Millis, S. R., Ross, S. R., & Ricker, J. H. (1998). Detection of incomplete effort on the Wechsler Adult Intelligence Scale-Revised: A cross-validation. *Journal of Clinical and Experimental Neuropsychology, 20*(2), 167–173.
23. Mittenberg, W., Rotholc, A., Russell, E., & Heilbronner, R. (1996). Identification of malingered head injury on the Halstead-Reitan battery. *Archives of Clinical Neuropsychology, 11*(4), 271–281.

Index

J.S. Goldman (ed.), *Genetic Counseling for Adult Neurogenetic Disease*,
DOI 10.1007/978-1-4899-7482-2_1